THE [illegible] INTO

NLN PRESS

THE EMERGENCE OF FAMILY INTO THE 21ST CENTURY

Patricia L. Munhall

President, International Institute
of Human Understanding
Psychoanalyst
Columbia, South Carolina

Virginia M. Fitzsimons

Professor,
Department of Nursing
Kean University of New Jersey
Union, New Jersey

JONES AND BARTLETT PUBLISHERS
Sudbury, Massachusetts
BOSTON TORONTO LONDON SINGAPORE

National League *for* Nursing

World Headquarters
Jones and Bartlett Publishers
40 Tall Pine Drive
Sudbury, MA 01776
978-443-5000
www.jbpub.com
info@jbpub.com

Jones and Bartlett Publishers Canada
2406 Nikanna Road
Mississauga, Ontario
CANADA L5C 2W6

Jones and Bartlett Publishers International
Barb House, Barb Mews
London W6 7PA
UK

ISBN: 0-7637-1105-5

Library of Congress Cataloging-in-Publication Data
Munhall, Patricia L.
The emergence of family into the 21st century / Patricia L. Munhall, Virginia M. Fitzsimons.
p. cm.
Includes bibliographical references and index.
ISBN 0-7637-1105-5
1. Family—United States. 2. Family Life—United States. 3. Twenty-first century—Forecasts. I. Fitzsimons, Virginia Macken, 1943–. II. Title.
HQ535 .M86 2000
306.85'0973—dc21 00-36832

Production Credits
Acquisitions Editor: John Danielowich
Production Editor: Rebecca S. Marks
Editorial/Production Assistant: Christine Tridente
Director of Manufacturing and Inventory Control: Therese Bräuer
Marketing Manager: Lynn Protasowicki
Cover Design: AnnMarie Lemoine
Design and Composition: Carlisle Communications, Ltd.
Printing and Binding: Malloy Lithographing
Cover printing: Malloy Lithographing

Printed in the United States of America
03 02 01 00 10 9 8 7 6 5 4 3 2 1

FOREWORD

When Dr. Patricia Munhall began to collect the papers that you will read in this book, she asked me if I wished to participate beyond the kind of prefatory note that I am writing here. I told her that the decision would not be an easy one, that I felt extremely ambivalent toward the family, especially toward the bourgeois American family, and most especially toward my own.

Now, there is a kind of personal journalism that would allow me to talk about my experiences within the context of larger social, cultural, and health concerns. But even that possibility slipped away from me as I began to take notes. The ground simply gave way.

In returning to my origins, I returned to the trauma of World War II, which I did not experience directly, and the Holocaust, which I learned of by innuendo or invective during family discussions and more directly by what I saw on television newsreels. The newsreels were more frightening to me than any of the Hollywood horror pictures that were then the rage. The countless images of emaciated corpses and concentration camp survivors told of a human horror beyond compare. Death was not a unique event but a social catastrophe that served to crush what I held, and still hold, so dear: the idea of an individual self.

As a child, I could not face that fact of political life in the mid-20th century—a fact that seems ever contemporary as we begin the 21st century, since genocide has become a measure of the effectiveness of war. The decades between then and now have done little to erase my pain and the burden of rebellion I place upon myself in the name of preserving the man I believe I am against social and economic pressures and moral compromises of every sort.

My capacity to persevere is as much a result of my family upbringing as my conflicted relationship with that upbringing, and this is, I assume, little more than a sign of the times. That I have done so with variable success—some triumphs, some defeats—is also cause for reflection. That I have written and spoken about the family as a confusion of relationships—some more or less compassionate, some more or less antagonistic—does little to offer a way out or in, depending on your point of view.

Perhaps there is only a certain kind of mediated clarity that I can bring to my own sense of family, knowing all the while that as I do so, I also do less than

I believe I do; that I and the family—my family, the families I know and trust or distrust—exist at arm's length, arms that can as easily embrace as withhold love.

But one thing is very clear to me. Family life, which does not have to mean life with children, is an origin and reflection of the world in which we live. It is a refuge from the world, a wound within the world, a mediation with the world, and a cause of the pleasures and horrors of this world. It is not a "safe" place but a place that we have perhaps more safely tucked away within each of us, or not so safely tucked away, and in which, by which, and through which our fantasies come to life or shatter against life.

I learned from my family what I own and disown; what is mine and not mine; and how in the space between me and another human, rapport can grow or degenerate, flower or die. At the same time, I learned also that the family is just itself, that it offers few solutions and many more questions and is, by its own complexity, incapable of much more. If history is a nightmare from which we cannot awaken, just how deep is the sleep of the family within the visions we grant it, and within which it lives out its life, our lives, my life?

And this, more than anything else, is what prompted me to work with Patricia Munhall toward the completion of the book now before you: an offering of views and contrasts, complicities and vagaries, analyses and recollections. Incomplete by design, it is thus perhaps a more truthful panorama of family life on the verge of entering the 21st century.

Allan Graubard

Preface

Well, here we are on the other side of the 21st century, and we are pleased to introduce the second of three volumes focusing on the phenomenology of women, family, and men as we mark this time in our history. The first volume, *The Emergence of Women into the 21st Century,* was published in 1995; and the third volume, on men, will be published shortly. The change of century, and most believe the start of a new millennium, is an occasion to reflect on the meaning of being human in the socially constructed time and place in which we are alive. Therefore we have attempted to provide a snapshot, a slice-of-life trilogy to assist us in understanding some of the contingencies of our lives. Depending on our individual contexts, we each have varying reasons for such a description and interpretation. Our own subjective perception will alter the understanding gleaned; we may agree with a given author, or disagree entirely. Both responses are equally valid.

These snapshots are guided by a post-modern perspective in which experience is understood through the theoretical concepts of contingency and situated context. The constructs in the discussion of the family that need to be considered as part of each chapter include health, relationships, culture, age, education, social conditions, political contexts, and economic status, among others. So if we ask whether these pieces about the family are representative, the only logical response is "It depends."

The trilogy is phenomenologically based: the reader need not be overly concerned with its generalizability. Each experience is unique to the individual and to that family. However, we do find similarities and commonalties. Through them, and through the differences as well, we can come to a better understanding of the meaning of the family at the entrance to the 21st century.

When we gather contributors for our volumes, we ask our authors to stay close to the experience, to search for material that reflects the experience—in this case, the family experience. We place the theoretical literature at the beginning of these volumes so that readers can have a theoretical foundation against which to read the experiential pieces. The pieces may be read in any order. In phenomenology, the literature review is part of the data collection, so to speak, but the most faithful phenomenology is through the language of individuals who tell their story and attach meaning to the experiences of their lives. We are on sacred ground and would never attempt to influence a narrative.

Some of the contributors are experienced in phenomenological writing, and their pieces may be a composite of different individual experiences. Others, having been asked to tell us their own story, provide us with a first-person narrative and their interpretation of its meaning. We believe that readers will be quite moved by many of these family stories. We learn and come to understand through storytelling—an ancient and yet post-modern way of coming to know. Through phenomenology we learn what science cannot provide for us: the affective, the deeply personal, the subjective, and intersubjective. In other words, we come to meaning.

This volume, like the first, is guided by an overwhelming concern for the human condition. If we are concerned with the human condition, we need to understand the meaning that individuals attach to experiences. Through the narratives and storytelling we are guided to think through ways that take in the interior lives of individuals and that can therefore help us to approach families not just with specific variables or statistics but with an understanding of all the complexities of a human life.

In this volume, voices become the discourse, the platform for understanding. We have attempted to select papers that capture many possibilities of family life that occur simultaneously. Multiplicity, multimind, and interpretation runs the gamut, and you are invited to add your own interpretation. Antithetical ideas and theories become possible and inevitable as a reflection of the nonarguable state of the world: one characterized by flux, disorder, ambiguity, chaos, confusion, and tension. Our daily media actually exploits these characteristics, yet we are aware on our own personal level of the validity of these claims.

This book does not pretend to make sense of this chaos, but it does offer a reading, a hearing, of the voices of family situated in this context. To understand the changes that have occurred, whether over the last hundred or the last thousand years, is to recognize how laws, truths, theories, assumptions, and myth are time-bound and have undergone dramatic change.

We offer these narratives and interpretive pieces to help our readers understand these dramatic changes—and those experiences that may not have changed all that much. We hope to enhance our readers' reflective capacity on the family, and perhaps, as we aspire, to be more fully present to families and those who may need us.

Through understanding the complexities of family, both the good and the bad, the contributors to the larger narrative begin to give us an agenda from which to contribute to programs that encourage life-enhancing, peaceful, loving, free, and liberated families. May you, as we, feel inspired, motivated, and moved enough to add another small effort toward alleviating pain or suffering within families and family organizations. We recognize the incredible importance of all our contributors' efforts—efforts magnified to become a magnificent tapestry.

Lastly, we wish our readers a meaningful family life, in whatever construction it may take, and thus as we enter this new century, we will indeed find meaning in emergence.

Patricia L. *Munhall*
Virginia M. *Fitzsimons*

Introduction

As authors and editors of other works we feel compelled to share with the reader some interesting dynamics that occurred in the compiling, cajoling, and coordinating of this particular volume. Having not experienced such dynamics in other writing ventures and beginning to feel some "familiar" (no pun intended) feelings, we began to reflect on the evolution, partial dissolution, and eventual resolution of a project that took three times longer to complete than any other similar volume. Soon we began to suspect that the processes entailed in this "putting together," or development, forces both positive and otherwise, paralleled the subject of the book, namely, the family.

Of course, there were coincidences, if one perceives the context of what was occurring at the time to be coincidental. (However, a family does not exist without those outside influences either.) The book took about two and a half years to complete. Chapters had to be returned to authors to insure that they were still accurate! Changes had to be made, because the two and a half years *did* make a difference—in some statistics, for example. That was minor, however, compared to the changes in the lives of the first coeditor and seven of the contributors.

Somewhere in the middle of this, we realized that we were experiencing feelings similar to being a parent, a child, a sibling, relating to many individuals and organizations who were also in roles as parent, child, and sibling. The book took on a life of its own. It became a process of family dynamics, with encouragement and cooperation, but also with resistance, acting out, and misunderstandings all the way up to and including the production process. We asked ourselves, does the actual word "family" stir up unconscious feelings and cause us to act out on those feelings? Individuals argued, did not meet deadlines, were uncooperative, and in the end rallied—all "normal" family dynamics.

For example, what prevents a family from actualizing itself? What does that mean anyway? Why is it common to hear that *all* families are dysfunctional in some way? Of course, they could not be otherwise in the context of pop psychology. In this volume, with the exception of about seven contributions, the real pathology that we have witnessed in families was not articulated. So we come to a subject that, for the first time, individuals were reluctant to speak about.

To begin, let us address the first dynamic, that of the contingencies of the editor and first coeditor. In a particular place I will call Oz, Mother had disrupted the worlds of so many of the people involved in this project that we came to see that the effects of having a "sick" mother can never be underestimated. The first coeditor suffered so much undeserved abuse, arbitrarily heaped upon him by this sick mother, that he became as bewildered as any abused child. Thankfully, this was temporary, yet another coeditor had to come on board.

In Oz, family dynamics of jealousy, paranoia, a lust for power, a lack of spirituality, and self-interest all trumped the benefits of a "good" family. The father of Oz (the wizard) became the inconsistent betrayer of his own words, for fear of mother's reprisal and well-known temper. Do we not see this in family life? What was most striking in this first consideration of our own contingencies was the obvious correlation of family dynamics played out in the workplace. This of course is not a new interpretation but does remind us of the importance of analyzing many workplaces and organizations from a family theory perspective. For many of us in this book we were rocking from our *other-than-family* contextual world.

This is to call to our awareness the things that break the spirit, interfere with camaraderie, and impede development. This is to raise to consciousness that the family and the workplace are very similar and in many ways interconnected. "Leave it at the office" is as simplistic as "Just say no to drugs." This interplay caught us all off-guard and could be a volume unto itself. For the moment, though, we need to heighten our awareness of what we bring from the family to the workplace and vice versa.

Also in the situated context was the selling of the National League for Nursing Press. Like a family, we grieved with Allan Graubard, the former editorial director of the press, who had guided us and so many others through the laborious process of "giving birth." Another family metaphor for work! For a period of time, we lived as though we were in a family that was divorcing and we did not know where, or if, we were to find a home. We just had to wait it out. Then the switch to a new family once again paralleled the psychodynamics of resistance tempered with hope.

Why do we share this with the reader? Because the book is phenomenologically grounded and the situated context bears description. There may be as much to contribute to human understanding through the process of writing as through the actual writings. From its inception to its completion (and we do not claim completion of the topic), many contributors and editors were part of a family, experiencing much of what it is like to be a part of a pathological family. Eight of us in this book experienced the family-work connectedness and no longer reside in Oz.

The second notable dynamic in putting this volume together was the absence of individuals who were willing to take on sensitive issues. The papers in Voices Seven and Eight do give "voice" to some very painful family experiences. In "Shadow Families" and in "Through the Distance," Brown, Siccardi, and Evertz articulate the emotional trauma of untreated or unrecognized family problems. "Cancer of Violence" speculates that the recent push to return to the family values of the 1950s invokes the family value of loyalty: what is in the family *remains* in the family. These family secrets wreak havoc under the rubric of loyalty. Is this what occurred for individual contributors? We suspect that there is a great reluctance to reexperience, or even write about in the second person, some of the pain associated with past family experiences. However, those who wrote of these family horrors call upon us to become involved and seek solutions. When we know of family cruelties, we need to know that each of us belongs to a larger family of all humankind and have a social and political responsibility to alleviate pain and suffering in any way we are able.

But maybe we are the ones who are off the mark. Perhaps the family is a wonderful grouping and we are altogether too harsh. After all, at the turn of the 20th century, families did not endure for very different reasons. A much shorter life span resulted in marriages that lasted, on average, 14 years. Unbearable hardships caused and followed the death of members of the family; mothers frequently died in childbirth; and children often died before the age of 5 of diseases that have all but vanished today.

Yet, there are gnawing questions about the family. Does the family reflect the flux of our times? The family of the 21st century emerges in antithetical images. No longer are we confined to one image—and a mythical one at that—but to multiple images of family. Multiple perspectives arising from a polyglot of individuals produce a polyvocal song, and a new freedom to create families and to live through the evolving possibilities of what kind of structure will hold us near, respect our individuality, and provide the love that is needed and the knowledge that an individual is not alone, not alienated. Notable in this volume is the notion of love—the desire of humans to be with other humans in a nurturing and unconditional manner, one that fosters mutual growth and generosity of spirit.

Most academics and observers of the family know very well that the family is undergoing unprecedented change. Considering that the concept of the family in the last century was quite limited, we are optimistic that the new social construction of families might very well offer the goodness of rich family life to evolve in more natural ways than the stereotype construction that had previously limited possibilities. "Through the Eyes of Catherine at 7" is testimony to the enlargement of the concept of family.

Trying to come to closure or envelope to our satisfaction the subject of family as it takes shape in this new century has been quite a challenge. Accepting the limitations of this project, we came to believe, reflected the limitations of what can be openly described by other individuals and ourselves. We had one conversation that spoke to this point. Could we tell our own stories? Not in print, and to those who did, you are braver souls than we.

However, we did believe that writing this introduction with candor could assist the reader in placing this volume in perspective. Perhaps it is just the first volume of family voices: the laying down of the theoretical, followed by experiential—some experiences tragic, others more comfortable. We hope our readers come to enhance their understanding of the meaning of family in this temporal context. Your own story may be here, or that of your friend or neighbor. The writers in this volume give voice to the balance of family experiences and to the tragicomic nature of us all, as human beings, struggling, yet challenged, to make meaning from our desires for healthy and enhancing families in all their complexities.

We thank them for sharing their knowledge and stories to illuminate the emergence of the 21st century family. Yes, as phenomenologists we wonder have we captured the essence of family experience? Beyond the limitations of page limits we know there is more—more variations, more thoughts—as we recognized some notable absences which we have observed in the empirical world but does not appear in the telling of experiences.

Notable absences may represent our subject, yet within the phenomenological approach to research, we need to look beyond the appearance of what is within this volume and look for what may have been inadvertently or accurately included or excluded. For example, reading this book on the family, we note an absence of religion and spirituality as main themes. Is this true for the 21st century family? Does religion play a minor role in the family today? A broader call to readers may or may not substantiate that observation. There are other absences as well. So we recognize a need to engage in dialogue with the reader of this volume. Recognizing that knowledge is perspective in nature, we are motivated to search for additional viewpoints so as to capture more of our heterogeneous family multiple realities. So we invite readers to tell us their unique family experiences for the next volume.

We imagine an enlargement of this album of stories will further our understanding of the dramatic changes of the emergence of the family into the 21st century.

We invite readers to engage in storytelling as research and contribute to an ongoing dialogue towards understanding the traditional, cultural, and changing construction of the family. Since some individuals are not able to write, perhaps someone could tell their story for them, so their voices are not silenced. Otherwise this description of the family is bounded and determined by specific abilities and resources. We need to learn about the missing links in this volume and why they are not spoken aloud. Responses to stories within this volume, with permission to publish, are also welcomed. This is to be a dialogue, where we do engage in exchange of interpretation and experience. This is to be an ongoing search for meaning within family experience.

ACKNOWLEDGEMENTS

EDITORS

Patricia Munhall
President, International Institute of Human Understanding
Psychoanalyst
Columbia, South Carolina

Virginia Fitzsimons
Professor
Department of Nursing
Kean University of New Jersey
Union, New Jersey

CONTRIBUTING AUTHORS

Carolyn Brown
Vice President,
International Institute of Human Understanding
President, TriHealthEd CuberAge
Boca Raton, Florida

Marilyn Burk
Researcher
Randolph, New Jersey

Daniel R. Collins
Author
Barneget Light, New Jersey

Joan Davis
Director, Graduate Nursing
Franciscan University of Steubenville
Steubenville, Ohio

Maureen Duffy
Associate Professor and Chair of the Department of Counseling and Human Resources Development and Administration
School of Education
Barry University
Miami Shores, Florida

Lynne Hektor Dunphy
Associate Professor
College of Nursing
Florida Atlantic University
Boca Raton, Florida

Ellen Goldschmidt Ehrlich
Associate Professor
Faculty Administrator
School of Nursing
University of Medicine and Dentistry of New Jersey
Edison, New Jersey

Julie Evertz
Administrative Vice President
International Institute of Human Understanding
Davie, Florida

Dennis R. Finger
Associate Professor
Department of Psychology
Kean University of New Jersey
Union, New Jersey

Christine Fitzsimons
Graduate Student
Rutgers University
Camden, New Jersey

Susan Folden
Family Nurse Practitioner
Boca Raton, Florida

Edward M. Freeman
Associate Professor
Department of Nursing
Florida International University
Miami, Florida

Sandra E. Gibson
Associate Professor of Nursing
Director, Primary Care School-Based Nursing Center
Miami Shores, Florida

Linda Gonzalez
Family Nurse Practitioner
Miami, Florida

Allan Graubard
Poet, Author, Critic
Washington, District of Columbia

Shelly Green
Associate Professor and Director
Doctoral Program in Family Therapy
Nova Southeastern University
Ft. Lauderdale, Florida

Sherry Hartman
Associate Professor
Community Health and Health Care Administration
College of Nursing
University of Southern Mississippi
Hattiesburg, Mississippi

Catherine Hauri
Elementary School Student
Miami, Florida

Claudia Hauri
Associate Professor
Nurse Practitioner Specialization
Miami, Florida

Shelby Hearon
Novelist
Burlington, Vermont

Sheila Hopkins
Assistant Professor of Nursing
Miami Shores, Florida

Maureen Hreha
Nurse Practitioner
Child Care
Randolph, New Jersey

Sande Garcia Jones
Clinical Nurse Specialist
Mount Sinai Medical Center
Miami Beach, Florida

Sarah Steen Lauterbach
Associate Professor
College of Nursing
University of Southern Mississippi
Hattiesburg, Mississippi

Marilyn Leeds
Family Therapist
Fort Lauderdale, Florida

Judith Mathews
Dean
Muhlenberg Regional Medical Center
Schools of Nursing and Allied Health
Randolph, New Jersey

Patricia R. Messmer
Director of Nursing Research
Mount Sinai Medical Center
Miami Beach, Florida

Evelyn Ortner
Executive Director
Unity House, Inc.
Shelter for Battered Women and Children
Summit, New Jersey

Katherine Parry
Physical Therapist
Hollywood, Florida

Anne Hearon Rambo
Associate Professor of Marriage and Family Therapy
Nova Southeastern University
Fort Lauderdale, Florida

Hilary Rose
Assistant Professor of Human Development
Washington State University
Pullman, Washington

Ganabella Rosetti
Doctoral Candidate
Director and Performing Artist
Department of Theater
City University of New York
New York, New York

Patricia Saccardi
Family Therapist
Boca Raton, Florida

Robert Sitelman
Professor,
Department of Philosophy and Religion
Kean University of New Jersey
Union, New Jersey

POETS

Amanda
Columbia, South Carolina

Carolyn Brown
Boca Raton, Florida

Daniel R. Collins
Barneget Light, New Jersey

kimberly jones
Miami Beach, Florida

JoAnn McKay
Columbia, South Carolina

Patricia Munhall
Columbia, South Carolina

Connie Vance
New Rochelle, New York

Contents

VOICES ONE

Situating the Family in Time

Chapter 1

Families on the Brink, on the Edge

Lynne Hektor Dunphy

I would make the case that each succeeding generation defines the family anew, for itself. Not always an easy birth at that, either. Each generational cohort sets new family "norms," structure tied to function, shaped by societal need. I would argue that function changes first, that structure lags behind. Economic contingencies, in large part, determine function. Homosexuality, for example, has been condemned throughout time as it has always defied function through structure: it did not reproduce. Reproduction, until recent times, was in large part the primary function of the family, its *raison d'être*.

However, even reproduction as function is disconnected from the family today. The postmodern family is situated within the context of *choice*. And with choice comes awesome responsibility—paralyzing at times. Perhaps it is just easier to get pregnant, to have no choice, to be biologically determined. Biology as destiny. Who is really up to the task of defining traditional roles anew? Perhaps adolescent pregnancy is a reflexive gasp, the throes of reproductive determinism, a death struggle. Madonna is a mother, freely chosen, the father a somewhat shadowy, peripheral figure. Their daughter is named Lourdes. Is this truly the dawn of a new matriarchal age? Oprah, however, is thus far childless.

Along with reproductive technologies have come antimicrobials and other life-sustaining technologies. The life span and quality of life in industrialized nations has altered radically in less than a century. All these changes have profound implications for the life cycle of the family and for the function and structure of family life. China reports massive shifts in the population from rural areas to the city—and in that society, family size is legislated. It boggles the mind.

Power structures, meaning who is bigger, travels faster, has more resources to hire "biggers" and keep them armed, has ruled. In a megapolitical view, might makes right. Historically, changes in technology have in turn created shifting and changing power structures on which human relations are based. For example, the development of the small handgun, it can be argued, gave rise to the antislavery movement of the 19th century, as well as the nascent women's movement. It allowed those who were smaller, or fewer in numbers, to overpower the larger and more numerous. Technology continues to free women on a variety of fronts. This has altered, and will continue to drastically alter the function and structure of the family in ways that we can only begin to imagine. Additionally, technology has "freed" man, the worker, the laborer. Job structures and societal roles will be radically altered, and at a more rapid pace than ever before, in the new millennium.

One could speculate that our current epidemic of domestic violence is yet another reflexive, dying gasp of raw male strength, bellowing Samson-like, as its hair, metaphorically, is shorn. Power now resides more clearly than ever in intellect, control in the understanding and operation of technologies not dependent on brute strength, on products whose production is not dependent on the sweat of manual labor. This has profound implications for gender relations the structure and function of the family set free and adrift with reproductive technologies.

Definitions

Webster's *Lexicon of the English Language* (1988) indicates blood bonds in their definition of family: "(1) a group consisting of parents and their children; the children of two parents, (2) a group of people closely related by blood, e.g., children and their parents, cousins, aunts, and uncles, (3) a group consisting of individuals descended from a common ancestry, (4) a household, (5) unit of a crime syndicate usually in a specific geographic location, (6) a group of related genera of animals, plants, languages, etc., and (7) a harmonious group bound together by common interests, i.e., the family of nations." It is noted to be from the Latin *familia*, for household. According to the *Etymological Dictionary of Modern English* (1967), *familia* is from *famulus*, servant. Roget's *Thesaurus of the English Language* (1990) lists "group, household, race, tribe; descent, ancestry, pedigree; parentage, forefathers, offspring, descendants and references, consanguinity, continuity, paternity, and posterity" (p. 180). Taken together, a broad definition could emerge, one not constrained by blood.

The sociologist William Goode (1964) conceptualized the basic purpose of the family as one of "mediation" between the individual and society. In other words, it takes basic societal expectations and obligations and molds and modifies them to some extent to fit the interests and needs of the individual members. Additionally, the family provides new "recruits" for society, preparing children to assume societal roles. Although a number of groups serve a mediating function, the family is conceptualized as of central importance because it is the primary group for the individual. The family, according to Friedman (1992), forms the basic unit of society. This is related to the fact that the family unit, a male and a female, retain replacement or reproductive responsibility. Their role is to procreate and socialize their young for, in part, the larger societal good. The family creates a kinship that helps stabilize society and that may also provide status, incentives, and roles for its members within the larger societal system.

Since the eighteenth century, several elements have been understood as defining the nuclear family: (1) the binding together of a heterosexual couple for purposes of intimacy, including sexual intimacy and (2) the nurture and socialization of children produced from this union. This "marriage" was sanctioned by religious, legal, and social authorities. Additionally, it was supported and recognized by extended kin groups and the community at large. The family's function had changed during this century, from a self-sufficient grouping working together as a social unit for economic reasons to a smaller, nuclear unit, dedicated to satisfying the emotional and relational needs of its members. Hence, the rise of romantic love, with love promulgated as the basis of union and marriage, not the uniting of economic needs and goals.

Although much lip service is paid today to the value of family life, creating such a family, maintaining it, and keeping it intact and viable has become increasingly difficult. This is attested to by an array of statistical data and expert opinion. Community support has declined for a variety of reasons; many family functions have been coopted by the state. The core or center of family life has, in many situations, disconnected; emotional intimacy and sexuality and the raising of children are often compartmentalized. Where will this lead as we enter a new millennium?

In 1996 more than 30 percent of American children were born out of wedlock (it was 5.3 percent in 1960). Today 60 percent of new marriages break up. Conservatives ceaselessly point out that marriage is society's most fundamental institution. Listen to talk radio any day. Naisbitt in *Megatrends* (1984) referred to the 1980s as a "decade of unprecedented diversity" and stated that there is no longer such a thing as a typical family:

> Instead, the diversity in American households of the 1980s has become a Rubik's cube of complexity and, like Rubik's cube, the chances of getting it back to its original state are practically nil. (p. 261)

Increasing bodies of evidence point to the fact that divorce may exact far more of a toll than was previously thought. And the weight is not just borne by the individual family involved but has implications for the very fabric of our society. Each divorce affects family, friends, clergy, neighbors, employers, teachers, and scores of strangers. As novelist Pat Conroy so aptly put it: "Each divorce is the death of a small civilization."

To deal with this shift, broad definitions of family have emerged in the contemporary literature on the subject. Friedman (1992), for example, said, "Family . . . refers to two or more individuals who are joined together by bonds of sharing and emotional closeness and who identify themselves as being part of a family" (p. 9).

A look at the life of the family across the 20th century may prove instructive. For purposes of this discussion, I will limit the analysis to the United States with its own cultural idiosyncracies and unique aberrations. And the story of the 20th-century family is most significant for the changes in the role of the wife and mother.

The Progressive Era

The advent of the 20th century saw the death of Victorian culture and the emergence of the modern age. The rise of modernism correlates with the ascendance of capitalism, molded in a philosophy of materialism, the cult of the individual, technological advancement, honed into the fine mettle of consumerism. For has not *function* essentially come to mean "to consume"? This is nurtured in the more-is-better, growth-oriented belief system. This belief was largely supportable during much of this century when the United States was young and strong and reigned supreme, when optimism flourished and all appeared possible. This characterized the turn-of-the-century Progressive Era, the feminine ideal was epitomized in the Gibson Girl. Though primly dressed in long sleeves and skirts, she nonetheless exuded vitality, she golfed, and she swam.

A darker reality for women, however, underlay the myth. In *Women and Economics*, published in 1898, Charlotte Perkins Gilman analyzed the position of women in marriage and the family in critical terms, without apology. She declared the economic dependence of women on men in marriage as the essential problem confronting women. Personal and intellectual growth in women remained stunted while they cultivated qualities that procured husbands: childlike helplessness and sexual attractiveness. Although Gilman had a small but devoted following, the women's movement remained focused primarily on suffrage. Gilman's argument was perceived as too threatening to the male votes needed to secure the vote for women. The time for Gilman's ideas had also not yet come.

It was around 1912 that women stopped wearing boned corsets. Women were asserting themselves everywhere. By 1900 women constituted 20 percent of the labor force; the average working woman was young and single. Young women left home to work in factories and shops during the rapid growth and consolidation of industrial capitalism. The ideology of "educated motherhood" popularized in the writings of G. Stanley Hall integrated the duties of motherhood with the value of college education for women. Still, it remained difficult for women to combine home and work. Many working women and most college-educated career women remained single. It was still an either-or proposition.

Flappers and Reformers

This elite group of college-educated women such as Jane Addams and Lillian Wald enjoyed a rich support network of women reformists and spearheaded the settlement house movement. But they remained just that—a network of women. Motherhood and family was put aside. Although childless, these women reformers vigorously defended their "womanly" natures and espoused a view of a matriarchal society as more moral and humane. They defended the new ways in "old language." And they were by and large pacifists, opposed to the Great War.

World War I was significant in that more women joined the work force. According to one source, "The girls went to the jobs with gusto." They could not hop on buses and streetcars in long gowns, so skirts were shortened, trenchcoats became modish, and small hats were worn. Near the end of the war, women's long hair came off. There emerged a boyish young woman—slender and short-haired, wearing makeup, smoking and drinking in public: the flapper. These women also breached the double standard. The divorce rate soared. In the 1920s, the United States had the highest divorce rate in the world. These women could not be called lesbians. Sexual fulfillment for women was possible outside of conventional marriage, as was economic independence.

The second wave of "new women" that emerged was far more threatening to existing gender relations. These feminist modernists rejected an older, Victorian female identity tied to sexual purity and sacrifice. Boldly they asserted their right to participate in male discourse, to act as men did—both in and out of bed. Sexual liberation was part of their agenda.

They disowned their rights to female protection in the process, as well as their alliances with the older feminists. This opened the doors for a particularly virulent backlash. By the 1920s, charges of lesbianism had become a common way to discredit women professionals, educators, and reformers. As warnings against lesbianism proliferated, the percentage of women college graduates who married rose between the years of 1910 and 1920, and the percentage of women going on to professional and graduate schools declined. In concert with a retreat from optimism in general wrought by the carnage of World War I, the retreat from professional prominence and economic autonomy for women had begun (Smith-Rosenberg, 1985).

THE "COMPANION-WIFE" AND CONSUMERISM

Fueled by postwar prosperity, an ethic of self-fulfillment and consumerism took hold. Birth control knowledge and usage was on the rise. Families became smaller. The need for more children had been derailed in an urban and industrialized society. Better sanitation and public health measures brought down infant mortality rates. Power relations, long residing in gender issues, were again threatened. Fittingly, male discourse reasserted itself, and a new ideal was promulgated: a view of woman as wife-companion.

At the time, the role of wife-companion seemed a step forward for women. The accomplishments of the Progressive Era, such as suffrage, had not achieved any real structural societal changes for women. The backlash had led to one step forward, two steps backward. University graduate programs remained closed, and the professional job market was reserved for men returning from the war. Women in the 1920s expressed themselves in private and personal terms. Flaunting convention on the dance floor was a good deal more feasible than battling quota systems. If their grandmothers had stormed the saloons, and their mothers had marched for suffrage, they would break tradition in their day by bobbing their hair, smoking, dancing, petting, and raising their skirts.

"Wanted" children were to be an outcome of this romantic love. Birth control à la Margaret Sanger was to be utilized to prevent the drain and drudgery of too many children. Freud was on the horizon as well. Women were cautioned about the dangers of "too much mother love." Behavioral psychologist John Watson traced the disastrous effects in adulthood of "too much coddling in infancy." These effects manifested themselves as invalidism. One pamphlet distributed nationwide by the Children's Bureau in 1928 read "the very love of the mother for her child may be the stumbling block." The "oversolicitous" parent was as disastrous as the stern and forbidding one. And childrearing experts were to be consulted. One's emotions were not to be trusted. The mother was the *least* capable in matters of childrearing, distorted with self-interest and unhealthy emotions. Nursery school was the answer. It would loosen the mother-child bond.

A new-style family emerged, one built on affection, romantic love, and sexuality, as opposed to financial ties and autocratic rule. Once off the farm, so to speak, there was no going back for women. A new approach had to be created to lure women back to conventional marriage and motherhood, "for the good of the family." Of course, keeping the "flame of romance" alive was a burden that fell on the woman.

Clearly, women were in a more untenable position than ever. The world outside the home remained closed off; the world in the home was shrinking. Her dependency on her husband had been recast, but was no less burdensome—if anything, the psychological bonds were more oppressive. Women's sphere of influence had shrunk despite, or perhaps because of, suffrage. The powers of reaction should never be underestimated.

The campus was one of the most important breeding grounds for this new ideology and one of its most powerful popularizers. If women in 1900 learned that poverty could be cured through environmental manipulation and went in droves to the settlement houses, women of the 1930s learned that the crisis in family life could be resolved through a new kind of marital relationship. Sociologists were already stating that the American family was in a state of collapse, having lost its traditional functions and inherited sources of legitimacy. Looking back rather nostalgically to the preindustry family as the center of production and thus solidarity, ruled over by the father-husband patriarch, they conceded defeat. The joint forces of industrialization and democracy had changed the family. The patriarch's control over property had diminished as the family had become a unit of consumption; likewise, his control over the family had diminished because children and wives had been encouraged to fulfill themselves and pursue their own interests. The seeds were sown, even then.

But the answer was still fresh, new. "The distinguishing feature of the modern family," insisted experts, "will be affection." Romantic love and sexuality between husband and wife would be the cohesive force. The decade of the 1920s witnessed the growth of the cosmetic industry and the proliferation of beauty parlors. Charm classes abounded. There was a general disenchantment with reform of all sorts. Postwar disillusionment was rampant.

The 1930s: The Great Depression

The Great Depression in some ways provided temporary relief for women from a constricting scenario. All energies in the 1930s were focused on survival, as unemployment and financial desolation wreaked societal havoc. The slogan "Get the man back to work" was everywhere, keeping women firmly fixed in the home. Nonetheless, 85 million Americans went to the movies every week, many of them as families. The movies were a potent cultural force.

Career women abounded in the movies. The carefree, dance-mad flapper of the 1920s had to go to work. Women who worked were depicted as having intelligence and style. Hair, while still short, became softer. Hems continued to fluctuate. Eyebrows were tweezed, arched, and penciled, often to a fine line. Rarely were women in this decade portrayed as only wives and mothers. Women were detectives and heroines. In part, this was escapist entertainment. But, in part, the strength of women was as important to the family's survival during the Depression as that of men. The family was united in crisis and would remain so through World War II.

Rosie the Riveter: Woman the Worker

World War II led women back again to the workplace. For five long years through the early 1940s women assumed all responsibility on the home and the work front. Skirts shortened; women flew airplanes, served in the military, served as nurses round the world. New talents, energies, capabilities, and self-confidence was released. But then the war ended. The men came home. The United States assumed a role of world leadership, prominence, and prosperity. It was time for women to go home again.

Levittown: The Move to the Suburbs

Postwar times witnessed the resurgence of the cultural apparatus to reinforce the role of wife and mother. Women's magazines abounded, and postwar prosperity again saw an influx of gadgets, appliances, clothes, and luxuries—and all affordable. Mass production destroyed much in individuality of items, but life was homogeneous and comfortable. In the 1950s, the move to the suburbs began. The deprivation of the war years made close family life attractive. Women married younger—even high school marriages became acceptable. The name of the game was security for these children of depression and war.

Both men and women believed that it was women's mission to run a home economically and efficiently. For married women, opportunity meant *not* working. The family was seen as the most important institution in a free and democratic society and, as such, women's caretaking abilities were revered. The vogue for larger families was in full swing. The following is an ode to the American mother published in *Look* magazine in 1956:

> The wondrous creature marries younger than ever, bears more babies, looks and acts more feminine than the "emancipated" girl of the Twenties or Thirties. If she makes an old-fashioned choice and lovingly tends garden and a bumper crop of children, she rates louder Hosannas than ever before.

The percentage of women in American colleges was lower than in any European nation and lower than the prewar figure on U.S. campuses. Nearly two-thirds of matriculating girls dropped out before graduation, while more than half the men stayed. Many coeds left to take menial jobs, supporting male partners. This was called the "Ph.T" (Putting Husbands Through). Marilyn Monroe was this generation's cultural icon of sexuality. In emulating this model, women strove to be sensual, feminine, and unintellectual. Women were childlike, expressing adulthood primarily through their sexuality. This was the era of the "dumb blonde." The Clairol slogan, "If I have but one life, let me live it as a blonde," exemplified the era.

However, clouds already loomed on the horizon of this picturesque scene of family peace and prosperity. Most women already thought that American men did not spend enough time with their children. Most men thought American women were spoiled. The "suburbs" also brought a more isolated lifestyle for some women, accustomed to urban, apartment-dwelling, support with child care, and nearby extended families. Men had to travel farther to work, to "commute." They were home even less. They pursued careers and lifestyles quite different from their wives at home. Between 1950 to 1960 the population in 225 cities rose 8.7 percent; the population in the suburbs of these cities rose 47 percent.

THE WOMEN'S MOVEMENT REAWAKENED

The Feminine Mystique burst on the scene in 1963, rupturing the myth of suburban and marital bliss. Suburban housewives had become prisoners in their own homes. Preoccupied with a routine of endless household chores, they had lost all self-respect. Friedan quoted one marriage counselor who attributed the rise in male-initiated divorces to "the growing aversion and hostility that men have for the feminine millstones hanging around their necks." As a wife-companion, a woman could only find fulfillment through someone else, meaning her husband and children. And personal fulfillment was becoming a valued norm.

Friedan suggested work outside the home as the solution. "The only way for a woman, as for a man, to find herself, to know herself as a person, is by creative work of her own. There is no other way." This did not mean just taking a job. This meant pursuing a career. In 1940, one-quarter of all women worked; by 1974, 46 percent worked. Rapid postwar growth of the service industries provided ample employment opportunities both for men, who rapidly assumed most of the managerial positions, and for women.

The end of the 1960s saw the antiwar movement and the rise of a fresh wave of women's liberation. The birth control pill and other reproductive technologies made their appearance. We were suddenly in an age of sexual revolution. Notions of individuality, rooted in the heart of Western culture, self-fulfillment, and satisfaction predominated. Marriages all over the country split apart, with repercussions that continue today. Abortions became legal in 1973. Women were as free as men to have unbridled and irresponsible sex—and they did, in droves. Sexual freedom again proved a modern delusion, as the sexual revolution evolved into the age of AIDS.

The 1970s and 1980s covered ground that we are all more familiar with. Concerns about the integrity of the family and children, the concerns with the legacy we leave to upcoming generations, dominated cultural discourse.

THE WOMEN'S MOVEMENT RECONSIDERED

The United States, it can be argued, remains rooted in materialism and consumerism. We are successfully selling this "ism" abroad. The family continues to be a manifestation in miniature of this social obsession, the cultural apparatus of a capitalist economy. To keep abreast, both partners *must* work. To work, both partners must have a car, clothes, and assorted professional accoutrements. Again, I would argue that this mode has accelerated and heightened in the United States and will, of necessity, be eclipsed by future developments that remain unclear. Consumerism, however, is in its infancy, a trend just beginning, born amidst the throes of industrial growth in third-world countries around the globe. What are we really "selling"? As Francis Fukuyama theorizes in *The End of History*, certain limits have been reached.

FREEDOM IS TERRIFYING

Camille Paglia asserted, "Happy are those periods when marriage and religion are strong. System and order shelter us against sex and nature. Historians usually do not address the history of a social phenomenon until it is starting to die out as an active social source, until it is losing momentum." John Burnham, a historian himself, likens historians to "vultures" who await social change so that they can "identify and circle the dying social movements of their times" (Burnham, 1996, p. 22). As recently as June 1996, the traditional month for weddings, the "Beliefs" column in *The New York Times* addressed the decline of the two-parent family. The author noted the cultural contrasts that swirled around us as the millennium drew to a close.

The author, Peter Steinfels, cited the June 3rd cover of *The New Yorker* magazine featuring a bride: "Bustling about her are bridesmaids and seamstresses, cheerfully adjusting the billowing white wedding gown to accommodate a very visible pregnancy" (p. 8). He contrasted a concurrent, and very real meeting, being held in Manhattan at the same time, a gathering of scholars, family therapists, religious leaders, and policy people, all mulling over how, in the face of rising divorce and single-parent families, to create a "marriage culture."

Steinfels concluded this short piece with a quote from another source: "Marriage is a deal between a couple and society. . . . If marriage is to work, it cannot be merely a 'lifestyle option.' It must be privileged. That is, it must be understood to be, better on average than other ways of living . . . a general norm, rather than personal taste." The source? An advocate for gay marriage.

THE FAMILY AS DEFENSE AGAINST PRIMORDIAL CHAOS

Reflect on the mediating function of the family in the socialization of children to the society at large. Consider William Golding's *Lord of the Flies*, a lawless band of unobstructed young. Children, without the potentially civilizing effects of intact family structure, may remain monsters of unbridled egoism. The unopposed id is not to be taken lightly! Freud understood this. Psychology, largely sanitized today, has yet to come to grips with the unconscious.

The function of a civilized society is to bring order to chaos. Society is our frail barrier against raw nature. Paglia asserted that freedom is the most overrated modern ideal, originating in the romantic rebellion against bourgeois society. We relived this in the 1960s. But Paglia maintains that only in society can one be an individual. In nature, brute force is the law, survival of the fittest. In society, there is protection for the weak. In her words, "Nature is waiting at society's gate to dissolve us in her chthonian bosom."

Extending this metaphor to the family is very simple. It is society that mediates between nature and the individual, society that attempts to impose a semblance of order on spewing chaos. We *created* social order precisely for this reason. Against this backdrop of demonic nature, our petty rebellions against societal structures are trivialized; perspective is obtained. A civilized society remains our best hope for lives well lived. Likewise, an analogous structure, the family, is our best hope for sanity, for kindness, for nurturance, as originally intended. Conventional marriage, despite certain inequalities, keeps raging sexuality in check. Committed parenthood can, in part, tame the id of the infant, can temper the unbridled selfishness and egoism of the child, can create a person with awareness of the other, can raise responsible children who can nurture themselves and others. Without this basis, all may be lost.

The Family as Regressive, Repressive

However, there are alternate views. The notion of the family as a repressive social force is not new. Florence Nightingale wrote in the classic feminist diatribe *Cassandra* in 1852:

> The family? It is too narrow a field for the development of an immortal spirit, be that spirit male or female. The family uses people *not* for what they are, or are intended to be, but for what it wants for them—for its own uses. . . . This system dooms some minds to incurable infancy, others to silent misery.

The idea of romantic love as the basis of marriage was just developing in the 19th century; the role of the family up to then had not been to provide emotional support for individuals but to preserve and transmit property and to stabilize the working community. Far from being an idyllic unit, it was more easily characterized by the social and economic subjugation of women, numerous cases of infanticide, the selling of wives (and in some cultures, daughters), and repression of individual needs (Calhoun, 1960).

Has anything *really* changed? Are our views of the family past in large part romantic delusions? Are we not as entrapped as ever by conventional notions of order and family structure, particularly women? Women now have lives of "two shifts"—the workday and the home front, care of husband, children, aging parents, home, and hearth. Is there any quality of life or time for a family life of any sorts? Is this where the family of the 21st century takes us?

The Family as New Culture

The family, however, has also long been the most vital context for healthy maturation. It has been demonstrated to have a crucial influence on the development of identity and feelings of self-esteem (Minuchin, 1977). Parents interpret the larger world to offspring and model strategies for dealing with the world at large, some more successfully than others. The family shares a common culture—and each is unique. The rise of multiculturalism amid the theme of diversity implies the same for the culture of the family.

It is best to take the broad view, to recollect, for example, that in the 1930s sociologists had declared the state of the family to be disastrous and were busy "revisioning" the unit. It is important not to forget the longevity of the institution of the family throughout history, its capacity to adapt to new conditions. Mary Ann Glendon, a Harvard law school professor specializing in family law, reminds us:

> However frail and faltering they may currently seem to be, families remain, for most of us, the only theater in which we realize our full capacity for good or evil, joy or suffering. . . . Families expose us to conflict, pain, and loss. They give rise to tension between love and duty, reason and passion, immediate and long-range objectives, egoism, and altruism. But relationships between husbands and wives, parents and children, can also provide the frameworks for resolving such tensions. (quoted in Bellah et al., p. 47)

We must remain optimistic and clearsighted. It is a historical illusion to imagine that there has ever been a single family form. What is important is the quality of the relationships, not the structure in which they exist.

It seems inevitable that we will continue to move beyond gender roles as technology advances. The form the family may take does not rest with the family alone. It is nurtured in a crucible of societal values. A "job" culture, rooted in consumerism, has expanded at the expense of a "family" culture. Only a major shift in the organization of work and in American public policy will enable a measure of balance to be restored. Transformation lies in a conceptual shift from a growth-oriented world to one rooted in values and meaning. Resources do run out. It is nature, reasserting itself. Life is ebb and flow. Historically, this time has come. For us all to survive, an ethic of growth must be replaced by an ethic of sustainability. The family is the testing ground—the redefining of family in harmony with new world views and realities.

References

Bellah, R., Madsen, R., Sullivan, W., Swindler, A., and Tipton, S. (1992). *The Good Society*. New York: Vintage Books.

Burnham, J. (1996). How the concept of profession evolved in the work of historians of medicine. *Bulletin of the History of Medicine*, 70 (Spring): 1–24.

Calhoun, A.W. (1960). *The Social History of the American Family.* New York: Barnes & Noble.

Coontz, S. (1992). *The Way We Never Were: American Families and the Nostalgia Trap.* New York: Basic Books.

Easton, B. (1979). Feminism and the Contemporary family. In N. Cott and E. Pleck, (eds.), A *Heritage of Our Own.* New York: Touchstone Books.

Friedman, M. (1992). *Family Nursing: Theory and Assessment.* Norwalk, Conn.: Appleton & Lange.

Fukuyama, F. (1992). *The End of History.* New York: Avon Books

Gilman, C.P. (As Charlotte Perkins Stetson) (1898/1966). *Women and Economics: A Study of the Economic Relations between Men and Women as a Factor in Social Environment.* New York: Harper & Row.

Goode, W. (ed). (1964). *Readings on the Family and Society.* Englewood Cliffs, N.J.: Prentice-Hall.

Hiestand, W. (1991). Nursing, the family, and the new social history. In A. Whall and J. Fawcett (eds), *Family Theory Development in Nursing.* Philadelphia: FA Davis.

Kalisch, P., and Kalisch, B. (1987). *The Changing Image of the Nurse.* Menlo Park, Calif.: Addison-Wesley.

Lawrence, M. (1936). *The School of Femininity.* Toronto: Thomas Nelson & Sons.

Millet, E. St. Vincent. (1978). First Fig. In N. Sullivan (ed), *Treasury of American Poetry* (p. 476). Garden City, N.Y.: Internat'l Collectors Library.

Minuchin, S. (1974). *Families and Family Therapy.* Cambridge, MA: Harvard University Press.

Naisbitt, A. (1984). *Megatrends.* New York: Random House.

Nightingale, F. (1852/1979). *Casasndra.* Old Westbury, N.Y.: Feminist Press.

Paglia, C. (1992). *Sex, Art, and American Culture.* New York: Vintage Books.

______, (1991). *Sexual Personae.* New York: Vintage Books.

Smith-Rosenberg, C. (1985). The new women as androgyne: Social disorder and gender crisis, 1870–1936. In C. Rosenberg-Smith (ed.), *Disorderly Conduct: Visions of Gender in Victorian America.* New York: Oxford University Press. (pp. 245–296).

Steinfels, P. (1996). Beliefs. *The New York Times,* June 1, p. 8.

Chapter 2

Isolating the Phenomenon of Family

Florence G. Sitelman and Robert Sitelman

Discussions focusing on the shifting role of the family, the extended family, the single-parent family, or the breakup of the family need to be supplemented, if not introduced, by some characterization of what the family is. The *family* consists of individuals who exist in certain kinds of relationships: husband-wife (legal or otherwise), parent-child (natural or assumed), brother-sister (by blood, law, or adoption), outward to grandparents, aunts, uncles, cousins, and so on. The husband-wife dyad may consist of individuals of the same sex, in which case roles may be blurred and the traditional family functions may get variously distributed. Moreover, elements of these interlocking sets of relationships may not be present in any particular family or group of families: there are families that do not have husbands or fathers, wives or mothers, children or parents, brothers or sisters, and so on. Furthermore, roles may mingle: fathers may assume roles traditionally ascribed to mothers; mothers may assume roles normally ascribed to fathers; grandparents, uncles, or aunts may function as parents; at certain points in the family history, children may even function as parents to their parents. Sociologists, psychologists, and cultural historians analyze the changing patterns of the family and the implications of the shifting functions of different individuals in what we might refer to as the "family mix." Be that as it may, whether men assume functions traditionally assigned to women or women adopt the roles traditionally assigned to men, whether such roles are now shared or gender-neutral, or whether grandparents, uncles, aunts, or even neighbors assume the functions traditionally assigned to the natural father or mother, the fundamental nature of the *experience* of the family needs to be explicated.

THE FAMILY: SETTING THE CONTEXT FOR EMERGING CONSCIOUSNESS

The family is, before all else, the primary social unit. It is constituted by a set of relationships that provides a context for defining the most fundamental elements of our lived consciousness, the structured foundations for all mental activity, including all perceptual experience. That means it functions to give specificity and particularity to what would otherwise be vague, abstract, and undefined. This movement toward specificity and particularity occurs on two levels of consciousness: the first with respect to the world that is constituted by the objects of consciousness, including other persons; the second with respect to the consciousness itself that perceives and acts in that world, that is, consciousness insofar as it too becomes an object for consciousness. One of the pitfalls of sophistication is that it forgets its own origins, fails to recognize in the obvious the not-so-obvious. It loses sight of the struggle that helped to forge the obvious. Innocence, once lost, is hard to reconstitute; so it is with some difficulty and, no doubt, with much lost in translation, that we try to resurrect the first gropings of the human consciousness as it seeks to define itself in some kind of organized experience.

In these earliest phases of awareness, when those most basic categories of human thought, prerequisite to the developed consciousness and presupposed in all mature experience, are achieving specificity, the family, as the primary social unit, represents a decisive condition for the evolving articulations that are embodied in mental development. It is within the context of and in alliance with the family, as the primary social unit, that stimuli get converted into initial experience, that response to stimuli is determined, that appropriate reactions are isolated, that behavior is defined and action distinguished, that significance is ascertained, that both individuation and relation get specification. These various activities, which, in fact, constitute the structural progression of mental development, a movement from the most abstract, contentless condition to an enriched particularization that lends meaning to the specific consciousness, proceed within a social context that supports and gives direction to the process. But to the extent that social interaction provides a critical influence on the evolving consciousness and the corresponding maturation of experience, the family, as the primary social unit, plays a decisive role.

THE POWERS THAT BE AND SUBJECT-OBJECT DIFFERENTIATION

In the initial awareness, what is to be eaten is not distinguished from what is not to be eaten; nor is what we desire to eat from what desires to be eaten. This sort of experience, uniting desire with its object, is sometimes expressed by the more sophisticated consciousness in terms that speak of the "desirability" or "undesirability" of things—as if what is desired shares desire with the desirer, that is, "it seeks to be eaten." Consider, too, the ambiguity and double sense of the expression, "it (for example, the fire, the knife, the table edge) hurts."

To put the matter broadly, neither significance nor individuation has been achieved at the early stages of development. A good part of signification is transmitted through imitation, through the bans, prohibitions, allowances, and approvals provided by authorities and powers, by "those in the know." A good part comes through language as it defines functions, chair, table, bed, pencil, writing surface, cup, spoon, food, drink. But these are all developments that are carved out of social interaction. Some powers, of course, such as those discovered by animals—for example, some things are hot or cold or painful or eatable, others not so; some actions hurt, others are pleasant, and so on—may not require social interaction, but these will tend to be limited to certain very basic physical features of our experience. And from such purely physical and very basic features very little significance can be squeezed. Thus, if we remove people from a social context, we incur the prospect of stripping much that we regard as meaning from their lives.

Meaningful Motions

Meaning is conveyed by the idea of "having a point" or moving in a direction and is embedded in the notion of purpose. Meaningless living, or movement that has no significance, is described by people as painful. The real threat of loneliness, retirement, and old age (and the fear of death) is the terror of meaninglessness. To be an outcast or an exile is to live in meaninglessness—unless restoration itself provides some basis for significant behavior. Moreover, insofar as action is movement that has purpose or significance, then an individual stripped of purpose is an individual who can move but has reduced ability to act. Reduced ability to act is an attenuated freedom—the freedom to move is reduced to a freedom to drift: a negative freedom to avoid, to not be constrained or compelled at best, but not a positive freedom girded by a sense of purpose. And, finally, the inability to act, to exercise freedom in a positive way, is a diminution of life inasmuch as being alive is constituted by an ability to act, that is, by an ability to function purposively. A life felt as purposeless is often described as a "living death," as being both dead and alive at the same time, a condition sometimes characterized as worse than death, a living hell.

It is the family, as the primary social unit, that gives initial direction to movement and introduces significance to human awareness struggling to find appropriate responses to its sensory field, responses that give definition to experience. It is the family that initially tells us what to do or not to do with respect to things, and, therefore, what those things are. Conversely, it tells us what things are, and, therefore, what to do or not to do with respect to them.

It is precisely the need to grasp what to do with things that provides the basis for giving things definition. That is, we seek definition so that we may know how to act. With definition comes significance, but definition is acquired within the social unit.

CHARACTER DEVELOPMENT

Failing the social unit, babble replaces speech and drift replaces action. The behavior of individuals lacking an adequately supportive social context will be abrupt, and even violent. Purposive action will not be integrated into or overlain by a coherent arrangement of meanings and purposes to provide a system of checks and balances, a panoply of restraints that will modify purposes and discipline means to ends. To the extent, moreover, that the primary social unit—that is, the family—is in the first instance decisive both in the process of self-particularization, the individualization of the subject, and in the development of the ethical person, if the primary social unit or the primary social group fails, the individual will both lack an adequately individuated subjectivity and will be denied the full articulation of an ethical personhood.

The emerging consciousness individuates itself for itself, that is, it becomes a consciousness of itself, in the context of a significant other that is constituted by other consciousness, that is, in a social context. In this respect, it is unclear how a consciousness would individuate itself as a particular consciousness in a context of mere things. Certainly, it is especially difficult to see how it could emerge as an ethical individual capable of social interaction within a broader community were it to lack the kind of developed self-consciousness initially formed in the context of exchange provided by other consciousnesses. Thus, it is within the context of the initial social experience, for example, the family, that the emerging awareness learns of itself in its most immediate form, and the immediate form in which it individuates itself for itself is in its connection to a social unit of which it is a member. That is, it individuates itself as a member of a family.

The first inklings of awareness must know itself powerless in the presence of living forces and urgings that buffet and condition the initial consciousness. These forces and urgings, moreover, must be highly particular and nonrational, emerging and proceeding from no known laws and revealing no articulated connections. They are without reason and may appear or disappear at any moment. They are, finally, total and life-threatening since they admit no perspectives and are atemporal and all-consuming. The only self-consciousness available to the self at this level must be negative and empty—a not this or that, a passivity detached from the content of its experience and at the mercy of whatever afflicts it, including its own cravings, desires, or movements. The intercession of the family on behalf of the emerging, empty, and helpless consciousness in response to the forces that threaten the very existence of that fragile awareness, executed gratuitously and unnecessarily, in a sustained fashion, and without reason in any practical sense, is love.

It is within the context of the love relationship provided by the family and expressed by a life-sustaining care that the fledgling consciousness individuates itself. It individuates itself in the love relationship that sustains its existence and in connection with the caregivers who represent a source of relief for, and, at the same time, are associated with, its own tensions, desires, and concerns. It is the love relationship that drives a wedge, so to speak, between the subject and its agitations, urges, and cravings, thus providing a liberating function. So defining itself, so separating itself from its urges and cravings, it comes to know itself as a member of a relationship within a social unit in which care is given. This caregiving mingles and is integrated with the care, the desires, and the cravings of the emerging consciousness. One knows oneself in the other and knows the other in oneself, in constituting some part of oneself.

In this situation, what is seen and said of it, how it is treated, is not distinguished from what the emerging awareness knows and, indeed, what it is for itself. Against the supportive and disciplining backdrop of the primary social unit from which it extracts itself only in the most tentative and relative terms, and, indeed, only in relational terms, for example, as son or daughter, or child, primal urgings and agitations will be carved, channeled, and forged into feelings, intentions, and purposes that will later expand into ambitions and aspirations.

Under these circumstances, the evolving consciousness has a twofold basis for self-individuation: it both expresses values and norms and produces behavior relative to those values and norms by which both its actions and its character may be measured. Thus, we will know the subject by what its values are as well as by how it measures up to, is true to, those values. This development of the emerging awareness into a subject is connected with and cannot be disassociated from the emerging articulation of the child's environment as a field of meanings rife with various significations in terms of which personality-forming behavior is given direction, solicited, or checked. The two operations, evolution of self and articulation of environment, are, in fact, all of one piece, the separate articulations of which are only abstractions. To put the matter somewhat differently, subject and object are, in fact, distinguishable from each other only in the abstract and only within a context of other parties, the social unit—and even then only tentatively and in relational terms.

These activities of emerging consciousness will later be augmented by the assignment of the duties and obligations that define the character of the relationships and, at the same time, help to further individuate and particularize the subject.

The Emergent Ethical Person

Taken in its totality, the love relationship of the family unit, marked by care and by a process of self-definition that is realized in relational terms, in which one perceives oneself in others and others in oneself, provides the foundation for an ethical life as well as the basis for successful communal living. If the love relationship is not yet the same as ethical living—which in its most fully realized form entails commitment to principles, duties, and obligation regardless of feelings, and sometimes even contrary to feelings—that initial experience which one undergoes inside the primary social unit is the introduction of the evolving subject to budding notions of mutual caring and regard for others, of concern for the feelings, desires, health, and even happiness and well-being of others, as well as expectations with regard to others as to their behavior with respect to oneself.

As desires, cravings, and needs come into conflict with each other in the context of a social unit in which one is a member, methods of adjudication in instances of clashing interests will be required, techniques for resolution of conflict will be realized, and early, albeit primitive, notions of fairness and justice will be instituted in what one hopes is an integrative, mutually respectful environment. As demands emerge in the form of assertion of rights, and the assertion of rights is a proposal of obligations, a basis for ethical living is actuated, requiring but universalization, that is, articulation as principle, for the realization of a mature ethical life.

It is one thing to crave or demand *x*; it is another thing to assert one's right to *x*. The latter assertion strengthens one's claim and indicates of the demand that it is to be acknowledged and supported by others. To assert a right to *x* is to require of others that they support the demand that is packed into the assertion. Assertion of rights is a particularly valuable instrument for the weak and frail who lack the power to enforce their desires and cravings on others and wish not to remain subject to the passing whims of others. However, consistency will require that the assertion of rights is attendant to the assumption of obligations.

The beginnings of ethical existence, then, may be located, albeit in a highly particularized form, in the evolving love relationship still predicated in its most fundamental terms on feelings, including those of gratitude and dependency. That ethical life will receive full articulation as the individual moves outside the family into the wider community.

THE HUSBAND-WIFE RELATIONSHIP

The relationship in which two individuals—traditionally, man and woman—join together to form a family permits each partner to know him or herself in the other. This self-knowledge is attained not only through the role provided by the relationship, namely, that of husband or wife, and its attendant duties and behavioral forms, but also by the reflection each provides for the other, that is, by the ability of each consciousness to find itself in the other. Insofar as this relationship is characterized by mutual respect, it forms the nub of an ethical relationship, although it is sustained by feelings not yet rationalized into universalized principles; insofar as the relationship is nurtured by feelings, the bond of mutual respect is supported and strengthened by regard and care. This relationship may be, and traditionally has been, expressed, cemented, and further articulated—or particularized—by the joint production of children. In this respect, the child may be seen and understood as an embodiment, realization, and further enhancement of the initial relationship. Here too, and once again, one sees and knows oneself in one's children.

Parents and Children

The parents' love of their children and the children's love of their parents is marked both by the knowledge that the children come from the parents and by the sense of separation and passage each sees in the other—the child to become an independent person with a life of his or her own, the parents to age and die. Separation of the maturing child from the parents is a completion of the parental function and leaves the parents moving toward the close of their lives. Passage and separation are a necessary cost of independence and maturity. Growth, change, passage, and separation inform all aspects of the parent-child relationship even as the child assumes traits in the relationship that will become permanent features of the self. It is a relationship of receiving, holding, and clinging even as it is a relationship of transition and passing away; it is a relationship of separation and passage even as values, aptitudes, and attitudes are passed on. This characteristic of passage, of passing on and passing away, colors and helps to define the love relationship that exists between parent and child. The children must move on out of the house to other relationships, to participation in a wider community, to families of their own making, and perhaps to become parents themselves.

Family Formations

The known aging and passage of the parents, from the point of view of the child, encourages the mature child to reestablish itself as a member of a new family of its own making—as a husband or a wife. Equally important, in establishing a family of its own making, the child consciously elects, with ethical significance, what it first knew as natural and given. In doing so, it both reaffirms the family it takes separation from, resurrecting what it leaves behind, and it assumes the role and attendant functions of someone (a parent) from whom it has taken leave. It is an impulse of a general nature, namely, to be a husband or a wife, to have one's own family, one that may but need not be complemented by physical desire and passion.

In the past, as a general matter, and today, no doubt often enough, the desire to be a husband or wife in a family may be the basis of commitments and relationships not supported by romantic feelings, sexual passion, or love. Sometimes, such a desire may simply be constituted by a need to assume the duties and obligations connected to the role—these latter providing a basis for propriety and respectable social position. In the past, entering into marriage exclusively in order to satisfy such needs was often regarded as particular to women. Sometimes, on the other hand, the relationship may find its basis in passion and physical desire where the concern to find oneself in a marital situation may or may not be a complement to the feeling—a condition that was, whether fairly or unfairly, traditionally assigned to men, who, it was thought, had other bases for establishing respectability and position. Be that as it may, certainly it would not be excessive to suggest that the ideal marriage would be characterized by the presence of both elements, ethical and romantic, in the commitments of both partners. Certainly, the presence of passion for the other—as a particular individual—helps to further articulate the process of finding oneself in one's partner.

Family and Community

The family must finally know itself in and against the backdrop of the larger community that both supports and is supported by the families that help to constitute the community. The family must sustain itself by containing within itself two polar sets of activities, one aimed inward at household functions, as husband, wife, son, daughter, and so on, the other aimed outward at the community, incorporating pursuits, duties, and obligations associated, among other things, with vocation and citizenship, which provide both a new basis for self-realization and a series of norms and values to be brought back into the family.

Here a dialogue must occur between family values, habits, and norms and the rules, laws, and conventions confronted outside the family arrangement. Each then gets modified by the other, by the demands, needs, and purposes each would impose on and reflect in the other.

The dialogue can be smooth or violent; if violent, it can be violent against the family or against the community or against both. If sufficiently violent it can tear apart the individual consciousness that tries to incorporate and integrate the contradictions it must sustain in order to articulate its own inner unity—each individual personality being precisely that, a relatively stable unity of opposing demands and impulses. Whichever way the matter turns, character, one's personhood, will be defined by the actions taken and the roles assumed.

The individual consciousness identifies itself by assuming and taking into itself the roles and connected values associated with those roles, and then by more or less living up to the norms implicit in those roles. That individual consciousness may find itself more fully realized by exercising itself in the life of the larger community. It may perceive family activities as secondary and but necessary adjuncts to the greater role it plays in society or it may feel itself most completely realized within the relative privacy and detail of the family unit while regarding activities within the larger community as a necessity to be endured in order to meet family and community needs.

Traditionally, these diverse family activities—one aimed inward, the other outward toward the encompassing community—were assigned to different family members on the basis of gender—young women to find themselves as wives and mothers, as preservers and conveyors of domestic values, young men to realize themselves as bearers of broader social responsibilities, their careers to be played out in the larger public arena. Needless to say, these assignments were often depicted as natural or divinely ordained, and were often highly romanticized and sentimentalized, imposing unwanted requirements of personality and attitude, generating stereotypes of what constitutes the feminine as opposed to the masculine, determining education and career, often masking much suppression and personal tragedy for both men and women. The contemporary assault both on the traditional separation of familial functions and on their sharp division along gender lines, driven to a great measure by economic forces and fueled by ideas of equality and liberation, has, of course, multiple implications for the way human beings will get to know themselves and for what they will think of themselves, for the manner that consciousness will individuate and particularize itself, for what personality development in the future will become, and for how we will live.

While deferring to others in this present discussion on the implications for human development entailed by the changes that are rapidly reconfiguring the contemporary family, we will note that in time men and women will be more likely to enter into and remain in family arrangements out of personal, voluntary commitment and very particularized feelings of love rather than out of a more general need to know oneself in the relatively abstract relationship of husband, wife, or parent. That is, for both men and women, opportunities for self-realization outside the family will make the decision to engage in family life an expression of personal, highly particularized feelings. This may make families more volatile as they become ever more contingent on feelings unsupported by overriding ideals of duty and selfhood realized through marriage and family. However, insofar as family is predicated neither on fleeting passions nor merely on abstract ideals, but becomes instead ever more a function of a very specific, abiding care in which individuals determine and know themselves in and through another consciousness equally reflecting itself in them, then opportunity for self-realization in the most particularized, articulated form is achieved. For some, family then becomes a more enriching, personalizing arrangement than it generally was in the past. For others, family may become more abstract than ever. In the latter case, the implications for the personality development of children must, by the very nature of things, be highly significant.

CHAPTER 3

Which Story Shall We Tell?

Maureen Duffy and Marilyn Leeds

Stories

People, as individuals and as members of families, groups, and wider cultures, share the history of their experiences in narrative accounts called *stories*. Through stories, they also share their hopes and dreams for their own future and for the futures of those they care about. Such stories are always colored and enriched by the values and outlooks of the storytellers, individuals, or cultures. No situation, no description of another, no point of view can be described in language without both including and revealing the perspective of the describer. According to Schafer (1992):

> Narrative is not an alternative to truth or reality; rather, it is the mode in which, inevitably, truth and reality are presented. We have only versions of the true and the real. Narratively unmediated, definitive access to truth and reality cannot be demonstrated. In this respect, therefore, there can be no absolute foundation on which any observer or thinker stands; each must choose his or her narrative or version. (p. xiv–xv)

Prince (1987) points out that narrative has been present in every human society known to history and anthropology. Bruner (1990) goes even further and suggests that narrative structure is built into the nature of social interaction, even before such interaction reaches a linguistic stage.

A variety of narratives about who families are, what they should look like, and how they should act compete for top billing in our culture today. These narratives reflect the politics and points of view of the groups from which they emerge. Each family story has passionate disciples and vocal adversaries.

In a society in which many competing narratives coexist, adherence to preferred versions of reality takes on a religious quality. Believers are anointed and saved. Nonbelievers become the heretics and the unwashed. Our images of what families should be and our expectations for how they should conduct themselves are embedded in the family narrative we propagate.

"For families to be healthy, members must have daily interactions in which their emotional worlds come into meaningful contact: times when minds meet, when closeness is shared" (Larson & Richards, 1994). This is the vision of family as intimate others for its members. It trades primarily in the currency of emotions. Life is hard, pressures are immense, the family should serve as a place of refuge and self-esteem building—this is a relatively recent contender in the family story sweepstakes that provides us with the more and more familiar snapshot of the family member who is laden with commitments.

It is a sunny Saturday morning and he finishes breakfast in high spirits. It is a rare day in which he is free to do as he pleases. With relish he contemplates his options. The back door needs fixing, which calls for a trip to the hardware store. This would allow for a much-needed haircut, and while he's in town, he could get a birthday card for his brother, leave off his shoes for repair, and pick up shirts at the cleaners. But, he ponders, he really should get some exercise. Is there time for jogging in the afternoon?

That reminds him of a championship game he wanted to see at the same time. To be taken more seriously was his ex-wife's repeated request for a luncheon talk. And shouldn't he also settle his vacation plans before all the best locations are taken? Slowly his optimism gives way to a sense of defeat. The free day has become a chaos of competing opportunities and necessities.

Which Story?

This is the self of continuously multiplying and expanding relationships and opportunities, the self of no fixed point, spiraling out to encompass the multiple others who people its world.

In family life, this "saturated self" (Gergen, 1991) interacts with the other saturated selves in the family, embodying the values, preferences, and perspectives of the countless others who are reflected in the identities of each family member. When the members of this family once in a while sit down to eat dinner together, they come as representatives of the special interests of the multiple relationships in which they are involved.

Words, Stories, and Culture

These narratives of control, refuge, and multiplicity represent the "big stories" about who we are as families in our culture today. In some of these versions of family it is much easier to get typecast than in others. It would be an error to think that we select the version of family that most reflects our goals and values. These stories choose us, and inscribe us as characters in them, just as much as we choose them. Stories derive this power through the language in which they are told.

Words, language, meanings, the individual, and the culture are influenced by and mutually influence each other. White and Epston (1990) remind us that the individual is rarely, if ever, creative and original enough to unilaterally invent the stories he or she performs in life. The culture extends its shaping hands at every turn.

Words

Culture reveals itself in words. The themes and values of our culture are announced in the words we use to describe ourselves and the world in which we live, through the literature that chronicles our times, in our political and religious institutions, and through the stories that are told in our families and schools about what is significant. Meanings and values are embedded in the very language we construct to make sense of and describe our world.

Words and descriptions of ourselves and our ways of living bear the imprint of our culture's history of interactions with itself and its environment. Lopez (1986) comments on the relationship between people, their environment, and the production of language.

A long-lived inquiry produces a discriminating language. The very order of the language, the ecology of its sounds and thoughts, derives from the mind's intercourse with the landscape. To learn this indigenous language, then, is to know what the speakers of the language have made about the land.

The "talk of the town" really is the talk of the town. Language takes into itself the ways that the town feels, thinks, hopes, and dreams and, in turn, discloses those hopes and dreams in words. Language, then, does not represent the world as it is, but rather the world as we have come to know it. Language provides us with maps of the world that we call *Stories*. It is through these story-maps that we know who we are and how we are to live.

Which Story?

"Big stories" about families in our culture might lead us to reflect not only on what these stories are telling us about our cultural view of family, but also on what these stories are not telling us. Interesting questions then arise. As we balance on the beginning of a new millennium, can our families survive the stories we are promulgating about them? Is the repertoire of family stories from which our culture has drawn nearly exhausted? Finally, if we were to construct new stories about families, what might they be like?

The Family as Mainstream Culture Cop

One dominant story suggests that responsibility for molding and shaping the behavior of its members rests squarely on the shoulders of the family. The family is seen as the primary agent of socialization and social control. In this narrative, substance abuse, academic failure, relationship difficulties, and juvenile delinquency reflect the family's failure to adequately socialize its members.

In this narrative, the metaphors of *molding, controlling, and reforming* are dominant. The behavior of family members is required to conform to a larger cultural script. When it doesn't, the mechanisms of discipline, punishment, and treatment are set in motion and applied. Mental health care itself gets ensnared in this narrative of control and management. Fabrega (1989: p. 590) states, "That psychiatry came to be identified with problems involving the control and regulation of the deviant and marginal clearly set it apart from other medical disciplines, and this association is part of its social tradition."

In the narrative of family as social control agent, broader institutions of culture, like medicine, mental health care, and education, are conscripted, alongside the family, into the service of regulation of behavior.

As every teacher knows, children who are troublesome in class are routinely referred to therapy for "treatment." That this treatment is largely in the interests of social control almost never gets mentioned. The therapists, guidance counselors, school administrators, teachers, parents, and physicians involved—all the characters in the script—perform their parts reflexively. In this narrative of control, family members have many more prohibitions about what they cannot be or do than they have prescriptions for what they can be or do.

A Common Story

In popular culture, one of the most vivid representations of the social control narrative and the family can be found in Pat Conroy's (1976) book and subsequent movie, *The Great Santini*. But Meecham, the unforgettable, tough-talking Marine colonel, ran his household as if it were boot camp at Paris Island. Conroy vividly describes the lens through which Meecham measured his children's development: "He analyzed his son's posture with slouch-hating, dust-loathing eyes. When he held inspections, the colonel's business was posture and cleanliness" (p. 90). No infraction was too small to go unnoticed. No opportunity to berate and humiliate was lost. Bull Meecham, like the Marine Corps motto, *Semper Fi*, was faithful to his vision of himself as the responsible party in the work of perfecting the world, especially the world of his wife, children, and home. Yet, when all was said and done, Meecham was every bit as captive to his version of the world as his children were to him.

Comfort and Safe Harbor

Another dominant narrative regards the family as the source and center of interpersonal life and fulfillment (Larson & Richards, 1994; Skolnick, 1991). In this narrative, providing a context and support for relational closeness, intimacy, and the sharing of emotional life are the central functions of contemporary families. Poor communication and lack of mutual support are the signs of failure. The family is viewed as a refuge, a safe harbor from the demands and pressures of the world. Family members are expected to provide comfort and solace for one another in the face of escalating threats from the outside world. This view of the family is founded on romantic notions of the person.

From *Romeo and Juliet* to the spy thrillers of Robert Ludlum, the reification of love as a thing, as a good, has made its indelible mark on our cultural sensibility. People seek love as an object. Young people search for the "right person," for their soul mates. Teenagers commit suicide when a relationship ends because they can't live without the object of their love. Even after leading lives of adventure and danger, the heros and heroines of contemporary fiction fade into anonymity together by setting up house in quiet, tree-lined locations, quite apart from the traffic of ordinary life.

Something Special

These powerful organizing conceptions of romantic love require that personal fulfillment and family happiness be found outside of and apart from the multiplicity of activities and relationships that people are involved in on a daily basis. Work is important and even critical, not because of the goods and services provided through it, but because it is an essential ingredient of a positive self-image, a hallmark of a person of depth. In the romantic tradition, for a person's life to have meaning, it must have depth.

The work activities of the day are necessary, but the core of the day, its heart, can only be found in personal relationships and in family. These are found at home, away from the hurly burly of daily life. In this narrative, the well-functioning family bolsters its members and prepares them emotionally to go back into the fray, the worlds of school and work.

There is also an element of simulation in this narrative of family life. While we could speak of families imitating movies and television, the simulation we are intrigued by is the simulation of therapy. The therapeutic relationship has become the model for proper family relationships. Parents are exhorted to listen to their children, to paraphrase and reflect back to them the feelings and concerns they are expressing. Failure on the part of parents to do so can result in a rupture of the parent-child bond and, worse, damage to the developing psyche of the child.

Couples are taught how to communicate with each other based on much the same principles. Use of "I" messages, acceptance of one's partner's feelings, and avoidance of put-downs and other forms of criticism are extolled as guidelines for fostering intimacy and good communication. The ideals of the nonjudgmental, empathetic, and accepting Rogerian therapist have become the standards for good parenting and relational intimacy.

Cut-and-Paste Versions of the Family

Another "big story" about family is emerging from the lived experience of individuals and families as we enter the twenty-first century. This narrative is the postmodern version of the family.

The postmodern story of the family emphasizes the rapid and unremitting change that swirls at the eye wall of family life. Family members, while still yearning for connectedness with others, may find that such connectedness is found not necessarily in the womb of the home but rather at the intersection of the multiple roles and relationships populating everyday life.

Technology projects and extends the domain of discursive and interpersonal relationships at a dizzying pace, a pace that was unimaginable for most people only a few years ago. No single, unitary view of the world provides stability and direction. The moral compasses of the social control and interpersonal closeness narratives of the family shatter in a thousand directions. The family is subjected to such a proliferation of influences from every quarter that it no longer has the capacity to filter out as in the past.

Which Story?

The "family" has lost control and is no longer steering its own ship, and maybe that's not such a bad thing. Family members can't identify with what they think of as the organizing experiences and principles of their own generation. And they can't identify with those of any other generation either.

Narratives of marginalized groups such as women, gays and lesbians, and people of color each jostle for voice and for validation. People who have been victims of oppression talk back, sometimes very loudly, and push to find openings and space for their stories. Identity and stability are found in rapid change and multiple social relationships, not in predictability and continuity.

A clinical case example is illustrative here. The Goldberg family, consisting of Father and five children ranging in ages from 2 to 16, sought therapy. Little did the family know that as Mom developed her computer skills, their lives were about to change forever.

The 16-year-old son was initially referred for therapy by his high school guidance counselor. His presenting problems were inability to concentrate in class and overwhelming sadness because of his mother's apparently sudden decision to move out of the family home. The day after Christmas his mother had packed and moved to Sioux City, Iowa, to live with a man whom she had met six weeks earlier in a chat room on the Internet. Dad and the five children participated in therapy.

A year later, the son, now 17, is again doing well in school. He has openly engaged his mother in conversations about the ethics of her behavior. He is not as sure now as he was a year ago that his mother's choices represent rejection of him and his siblings. Dad, who was crushed and bewildered by his wife's decision, gives her his frequent-flyer miles so she can see the children more often, even though their divorce was final 10 months ago.

The family has changed religions and finds a lot of support from people in their new church. The small children get teary-eyed for a few minutes when their mother leaves after a visit. In between visits, they occasionally save souvenirs from their daily activities to show their mother when she comes.

Sometimes when she calls them from Sioux City the children are eager to talk to her. Other times they don't come to the phone because they're busy playing with friends or are engrossed in a video game.

Story as Reality

Individual stories and family stories are subtexts of larger cultural stories. They are variations on a cultural theme. Which cultural theme or which combination of cultural themes specific family stories reflect is a function of how particular families are situated in relation to the pool of available cultural stories and which associations and allegiances have attracted them. Foucault (1973, 1979, 1980) has provided an extensive analysis of why some cultural stories are readily available and other stories, what he calls "subjugated knowledges," are not.

Bruner (1986) points out that stories, repeated frequently enough, become realities. The people who live the stories, the characters, may find that the parts assigned to them are rigid and overly defined.

Bull Meecham in *The Great Santini* was hardened into a role that he never commented upon from a position outside of the role. That occasionally he could yield and be flexible never occurred to him. That his son, Ben, was literally dying for more visible signs of Bull's affirmation and love also never occurred to him. Over the course of his life he faithfully enacted an assigned cultural script.

Proliferation of Stories in an Ideologically Interactive World

As the 21st century begins, there is no reason to believe that the number of stories about individuals and families will do anything but proliferate. Access to different perspectives about the world through communications technology involves a geometrically increasing number of people. The new world, the world of the 21st century, will be an ideologically interactive one.

In an ideologically interactive world, no single story about how families should live and about what values families should represent can contain the range of meanings and experiences of the interacting participants. Totalizing stories, while they might maintain some level of popularity, can no longer show the way. And they can't show the way simply because they are disrespectful. They do not acknowledge the presence of others and the implications of such a validation of others.

Totalizing stories specify and describe the other and leave no room for the other to describe himself or herself differently—therein lies their ethical fallowness. The claim for themselves authority over the other and specify the conditions by which the other should live. Such stories make these claims to authority by appealing to "truth" and "objectivity."

Von Foerster (1991) suggests that the foundation for ethics is absent when the other is not fully embraced in dialogue. He states:

> The notions of Truth and Objectivity guarantee the popularity of this position [believing in truth and objectivity], the former promoting authority. . . . "It is as I tell it" . . . the latter removing responsibility. . . . "I tell it as it *is*". . . . When I ask myself, "Am I a part of the universe?" and answer "Yes, I am," I decide here and now that, whenever I act, not only I change, but the universe changes as well. . . . I have adopted the position of being part of the universe because it ties me with my actions inseparably to all others, and thus establishes a prerequisite for a foundation for ethics. (p. 65–66)

In Von Foerster's (1984, 1991) view, there can be no ethics where there is no choice. When the universe is described *as it is*, as if description is independent of describer or storyteller and the character's scripts are preordained and prescribed, there can be no ethics because there can be no choice.

Making Room for Difference

The dominant stories in our culture about families—the family as social control agent, the family as safe harbor, and the emerging postmodern story of the family—will all be challenged in the ideologically interactive new world of the 21st century. Yet, because it does not have a rigid plot line and because it incorporates the possibility of continuously adding and subtracting themes, characters, voices, and points of view, the nod must be given to the postmodern story of the family as we enter the new millennium.

More than the other stories, the postmodern story of the family accommodates choice, the presence of others, and the juxtaposition of differing perspectives. While it may provide a less solid platform upon which to fashion a life than the other contemporary stories of the family, it also provides the exhilarating combination of more freedom and more responsibility for oneself, for others, and for the world.

The postmodern story of the family incorporates, rather than bemoans, the changed circumstances and meanings within which people today must make sense of their lives and identities. Bateson (1990) underscores these changes:

> Today, the materials and skills from which a life [or family] is composed are no longer clear. It is no longer possible to follow the paths of previous generations. . . . Many of the most basic concepts we use to construct a sense of self or the design of a life have changed their meanings: Work. Home. Love. Commitment. (p. 2)

From the postmodern perspective, not only have meanings changed but contradictory meanings may be assigned to the same set of facts by the same describer who resolves the contradiction, as Watzlawick (1984) suggests, by oscillating back and forth between the two views.

Same Beginnings, Different Endings

The families captured by the romantic version of family life and the importance of living out the values of good therapy in their own relationships could begin to develop an appreciation for therapy as a caricature of intimacy. Such an appreciation could open the doors to humor and play as the partners in the relationship consciously attend, for example, to the fact that they are held to a higher standard than the therapist, they are expected to use "I" messages and good communication skills every time they speak to each other while the therapist only has to do so for 50 minutes at a time!

If Lillian, Bull Meecham's wife, were to tell the story of the Santini family from her perspective, the narrative of control and regulation would be subtext to the more important theme of attenuating Bull's harshness and insensitivity in the interests of keeping the relationships in the family alive.

In families governed by the narrative of social control, listening to the voices of the subdued and silenced family members exposes both the strengths and vulnerabilities of all the members. Listening for many voices dissipates the dominance of a single voice.

It is the celebration of the many over the one, the juggler over the pedant, the marginalized over the privileged, that will usher the postmodern story of the family into the 21st century. And in that moment of celebration, the juggler will become the instructor, the one story will be that there are many stories, and those at the margin will find their way to the center of the page.

References

Bateson, M. C. (1989). *Composing a Life*. New York: Plume Books.

Bruner, J. (1986). *Actual Minds, Possible Worlds*. Cambridge, Mass.: Harvard University Press.

———. *Acts of Meaning*. Cambridge, Mass.: Harvard University Press.

Fabrega, Jr., H. (1989). An ethnomedical perspective of Anglo-American psychiatry. *American Journal of Psychiatry*, 146:588–596.

Foucault, M. (1973). *The Birth of the Clinic: An Archeology of Medical Perception*. London: Tavistock.

———. (1979). *Discipline and Punish: The Birth of the Prison*. Middlesex: Peregrine Books.

———. (1980). *Power/Knowledge: Selected Interviews and Other Writings*. New York: Pantheon Books.

Conroy, P. (1976). *The Great Santini*. Boston: Houghton Mifflin.

Gergen, K. J. (1991). *The Saturated Self: Dilemmas of Identity in Contemporary Life*. New York: Basic Books.

Larson, R., and Richards, M. H. (1994). *Divergent Realities: The Emotional Lives of Mothers, Fathers, and Adolescents*. New York: Basic Books.

Lopez, B. (1986). *Arctic Dreams*. New York: Bantam Books.

Schafer, R. (1992). *Retelling a Life*. New York: Basic Books.

Skolnick, A. (1991). *Embattled Paradise: The American Family in an Age of Uncertainty*. New York: Basic Books.

Von Foerster, H. (1984). On constructing a reality. In P. Watzlawick (ed.), *The Invented Reality* (pp. 41–61). New York: Norton.

———. (1991). Through the eyes of the other. In F. Steier (ed.), *Research and Reflexivity* (pp. 63–75). London: Sage.

Watzlawick, P. (1984). The imperfect perfection. In *An Invented Reality* (pp. 169–173). New York: Norton.

VOICES TWO

UNDERSTANDING FAMILIES

This poem attempts to give voice to one of the deepest of all connections.

Mother's Day

Mother's day, ah, so happy, in honor
we acknowledge your selflessness,
your smotherhood, your porridge
burnt just around the edges.

And in honor, we salute you
and your wanton ways
whether real or imagined.
And your vulnerability found in nakedness.

We acknowledge every day your sacrifices,
Made in the name of motherlove
mirroring in intent the crucifixion, yet expecting
little in return, just short of, blind submission.

To all the mothers whose inspirations
and recipes have passed down thru generations,
Creating mother-daughters
who keep the couches occupied,

You are the best mother in the world,
Because we never bled, at least
not to death, and for that
we follow the commandment to love and honor thou.

And on this day and every day
We praise you, we say we love you,
we disobey you, we follow in your path
inhaling the reality that we are you.

—Patricia Munhall

CHAPTER 4

HOW FAMILY SCIENTISTS STUDY FAMILIES: EIGHT THEORETICAL STUDY FRAMEWORKS

Hilary A. Rose

DEFINING FAMILY

It was the first class of the summer quarter. My goal for the class period was to encourage my undergraduate students to define family, and then to introduce the concept of diversity. I described some groups of people and then asked the students to raise their hands if they considered these groups to be a family.

I started with baby Robbie, his mother Sue, and Sue's unmarried partner Sam, all of whom share a home. "Are they a family?" I asked. About a third of these undergraduates agreed that they were. "OK.," I said, "Sam brings home a paycheck to help support Sue and the baby and takes turns feeding Robbie and getting him ready for bed. Is this a family?" Approximately half the hands in the room went up. I told the students that lately Sam, who really loves Robbie, has been thinking of adopting him. By now, most of the hands in the class were up, indicating that Sam, Sue, and Robbie are a family. "Sam's full name is Samantha," I said. "Is this a family?"

Whoosh! Hands descended quickly as students' faces registered a mixture of disgust, shock, and confusion. (Roughly a quarter of the students kept their hands up.) Clearly, the majority of the undergraduates in this class were unwilling to call a same-sex couple with a child a family.

As we enter the 21st century, policy makers and lay people alike are struggling with how family is to be defined. Consider, for example, the recent debate among politicians, religious leaders, and gay activists over the Defense of Marriage Act, a law banning federal recognition of same-sex marriages. In effect, such a law also denies that Sue, Sam, and Robbie are a family.

I would like to thank Charles Halverson, Gary Peterson, Sharon Price, and Jennie Wakefield for their helpful comments on an early draft of this chapter. I would also like to thank Valerie Havill for originally sharing with me the classroom exercise about Sam's family.

Family scientists are also struggling to define family (Popenoe, 1993; Stacey, 1993). Ernest Burgess, one of the earliest family scientists, described the family as "a unity of interacting personalities" and wrote, "The actual unity of family life has its existence not in any legal conception, nor in any formal contract, but in the interaction of its members" (1926:5). Burgess's definition of family is surprisingly contemporary, especially in light of how most Americans define the traditional nuclear family: "legal, lifelong, sexually exclusive, heterosexual . . . with the female as full-time housewife and the male as primary provider" (Popenoe, 1991:50).

The way in which we define family has implications for both how we study the family and how we develop policy affecting families. For example, just over 20 years ago, a married couple was threatened with federal arrest for giving false information on a census form: the couple reported that the wife, not the husband, was the head of the household (Brandwein et al., 1974). And until 1974 in Texas, it was legal for a husband to kill his wife if he found her in bed with another man (Buss, 1995). Similarly, how family scientists view families and theorize about them has implications for how families are studied. The purpose of this chapter is to review different theoretical frameworks used by family scientists.

Wesley Burr (1995), one of the foremost theorists of family science, has written "Families are so complex that it is impossible for any one theory to explain everything" (p. 74). According to Burr, different theories allow family scientists to study different aspects of family life. It is impossible to know and work with all the theories in depth, but it is possible for family scientists to be familiar with several of them, and then use a specific theory when appropriate. Working from Burr's (1995) contention that different theories allow family scientists to explore different aspects of family life, I will survey eight theories of family science (see Table 4–1). For each theory (or theoretical framework), I will present key concepts and a critique and include a research application of one aspect of family life in the United States. First, though, I will address the question of why we use theories at all.

The Value of Theory

Why use theory in the first place? A theory is like a good map, because it tells you what to look for in exploring a concept. But not all maps are alike. Some maps are so general, they give too few details to be useful. Some maps only show landforms without reference to political jurisdictions. Some maps are so detailed, they do not show the big picture. Maps differ because they have different purposes. Your purpose as the map reader will determine which map you choose to view. At the same time, the map you look at will influence how you view the world. A political map, for example, will show a very different world than a topographical map. Theories work the same way.

As a family scientist, you may choose a certain theory because you have a certain research question or because of your training. What theory you choose,

TABLE 4–1 EIGHT THEORIES OF FAMILY SCIENCE AND THEIR RESEARCH APPLICATIONS

Theoretical Frameworks	*Research Applications*
Biosocial perspective theory	Dating and mating
Structural functionalism	Transition to parenthood
Social learning theory	Parent-child relations
Exchange theory	Divorce
Family development theory	Aging families
Symbolic interaction theory	Lesbian families
Family systems theory	Remarriage
Ecological systems theory	Minority families

however, will determine which research questions you ask. Exchange theory focuses on the costs and benefits of choosing between alternatives (for example, the choice of staying in a bad marriage or asking for a divorce). Thus, a researcher who uses exchange theory will ask, "What are the costs of getting divorced?" (Price & McKenry, 1988). A family developmentalist, on the other hand, will be interested in the transition from one stage to another, asking, "What precipitates the transition from being single to being married?" (Rodders & White, 1993).

Thus, theories guide family scientists to what is important, but they can also act as blinders, preventing researchers from seeing, or even considering, anything outside the domain of that particular theory. LaRossa and Reitzes (1993), for example, point out that symbolic interactionism ignores the biological nature of humans. A theory that ignores biology will not guide researchers to ask about hormonal fluctuations or brain structure. Although symbolic interactionism does not guide researchers to ask about the biology of sexual drives, it will guide researchers to ask about the meaning of sexual drives (LaRossa, 1979).

There are many theories used by family scientists. This great variety exists because family science is an interdisciplinary field. Psychologists, such as Gerald Patterson (1975, 1980, 1986), study families using psychological theories, for example, social learning theory. Sociologists, such as Sharon Price (Price & McKenry, 1988), study families using sociological theories like exchange theory.

Some family scientists use no theory at all, and others use more than one (Burr, 1995). Still others use grounded theory, theory developed out of a particular set of data (Glaser & Strauss, 1967). A researcher's choice of theory depends on his or her training and assumptions about how the world operates.

Some aspects of family life can be studied using more than one theory. The transition to parenthood can be studied from a biosocial perspective (for example, differential parental investment), but it can also be studied from an exchange perspective (for example, the costs and benefits of parental leave), or a developmental perspective (for example, the factors that precipitate parenthood). This transition can also be examined from a symbolic interaction perspective (for example, the meaning of parenting), a systems perspective (for example, the introduction of a new member into the family system), or a structural-functional perspective (for example, parenting roles). Even within this one topic, different theories allow researchers to focus on different aspects of the transition to parenthood. A range of family theories follow.

Biosocial Perspective Theory

The biosocial perspective has its roots in Charles Darwin's (1859) ideas about natural selection and survival of the fittest. Principles of Darwin's evolutionary theory contributed to social Darwinism and early 20th-century social reform movements like eugenics or selective breeding, used to justify sexism (Shields, 1975) and racism (Troost & Filsinger, 1993). Early sociologists like Lester Ward attacked social Darwinism, effectively eliminating biological and evolutionary thinking from the social sciences for the first half of the 20th century. Evolutionary thinking continued to blossom in the biological sciences, especially among ethologists (Bowlby, 1969; Lorenz, 1977) and sociobiologists (Wilson, 1975). Alice Rossi (1977), in her controversial presidential address to the American Sociological Association, introduced evolutionary thinking into her discussion of parenting. Since then, family science has "moved out of sociology . . . and has moved to study a wide variety of biological variables in parent-child relationships and human development" (Troost & Filsinger, 1993:682).

Adaptation

According to the biosocial perspective, the family is an evolutionary adaptation to the problem of the survival of human infants and children. "Neoteny together with altricial rearing (the prolonged helpless state of the human infant) imply that in the environment of our arising, family members were there as care givers" (Troost & Filsinger, 1993:685–686). Some of the assumptions of a biosocial perspective on the family are:

1. Biosocial factors are both biological and social in nature.
2. Biosocial factors do not determine human behavior, but they do constrain it.
3. Adaptations in behavior and physiology vary depending on the environment.

Application

In addition to parent-child relations, the biosocial perspective is often used to study dating and mating practices. "Because reproductive competition is central to evolutionary theory, evolutionary theorists are particularly interested in the average differences between men and women in . . . mating behaviors" (Kenrick & Trost, 1993:150). Women, on average, are less aggressive, less promiscuous, and more interested in older, wealthy men. Men, on the other hand, are more aggressive, more promiscuous, and more interested in younger, attractive women (Buss, 1989; Kenrick & Trost, 1993). Differences in mate preferences "reflect sex differences in the adaptive problems that ancestral men and women faced when selecting a mate" (Buss, 1995:18).

Critique

The biosocial perspective has been strongly criticized on a number of grounds. Social Darwinism, and sociobiology in particular, have been criticized for being both sexist and racist (see Bleier, 1984; Shields, 1975; Troost & Filsinger, 1993). Sociobiology has also been criticized as being reductionistic and deterministic (Lewontin et al., 1984). Even some proponents of an evolutionary perspective (Buss, 1995; Troost & Filsinger, 1993) shy away from the extremist views of sociobiologists who believe that "humans possess mechanisms with the goal of maximizing their inclusive fitness, that is, maximizing their gene representation in subsequent generations" (Buss, 1995:9–10).

Structural Functionalism

In their review of structural functionalism, Kingsbury and Scanzoni (1993) wrote that the framework has become "virtually obsolete" (p. 195). They pointed out, however, that its assumptions continue to remain central to family science. For this reason, structural functionalism is included in this review.

Talcott Parsons (1951) believed that humans are moral beings who conform to society's expectations and norms. Such expectations and norms are necessary in order for society to function optimally. The family is seen as "an example of a subsystem that functions, or operates, for the survival and maintenance of society" (Kingsbury & Scanzoni, 1993:196).

Equilibrium

One of the goals of a subsystem like the family is equilibrium, or homeostasis. "Gender role specialization maintained family equilibrium while enabling the family to perform its prime functions of reproduction and socialization" (Kingsbury & Scanzoni, 1993:197).

Based on Freud, Parsons, and Bales (1955) argued that the sexes have different "tasks," or roles, they are expected to perform within the family. Men's tasks are instrumental in that they protect the family and provide for it; women's tasks are expressive in that they nurture children and provide men with a haven from the outside world. Deviance from these gender roles leads to family disorganization such as juvenile delinquency and divorce. Parson's traditional ideas about family structure and function clashed with the social changes of the 1960s and 1970s, especially women's increased participation in the labor force (Winton, 1995).

Neofunctionalists (Alexander, 1985; Boss, 1986) have rejected the Parsonian focus on the status quo and incorporated a dialectic approach with its focus on struggle and change (Kingsbury & Scanzoni, 1993). Nevertheless, "struggle and change include the potential for complete cessation of partners' interactions. That potential returns us to the century-long fear that divorce and its consequences will result in social disorganization" (Kingsbury & Scanzoni, 1993:212).

Application

One application of structural functionalism is the study of the transition to parenthood. In fact, reproduction and the socialization of children are important family functions according to structural functionalism. Feingold (1994) recently conducted a meta analysis of gender differences in personality. Men were consistently found to be more assertive than women, and women were found to be more nurturant than men. This finding lent support to Parson's instrumental-expressive dichotomy. Researchers have also found that new parents typically assume traditional gender roles, as structural functionalism would predict (LaRossa & LaRossa, 1981; Thompson & Walker, 1989).

Critique

Ferree (1991) has argued that feminist researchers reject the traditional Parsonian view of gender roles as fixed and internalized traits of the individual. For example, when it comes to child care, women perform more instrumental tasks (for example, changing babies), whereas men perform more expressive tasks (for example, playing with babies) (Losh-Hesselbart, 1987). Feminist researchers also reject the "separation of spheres," referring to the separate worlds of men (work) and women (home) (Ferree, 1991). Finally, the Parsonian goal of equilibrium has become increasingly difficult to defend in the light of social change (Winton, 1995).

Social Learning Theory

Learning theories have their roots in the Greek philosophy of hedonism, based on the idea that humans seek pleasure and avoid pain. Hedonism, which dates back to Epicurus (Burr, 1995), was echoed by the English philosopher John Locke (1690). Locke (1693) also believed that the human infant is a tabula rasa, a "blank slate" that is written on by the environment.

Based on the ideas of Locke, learning theory (or behaviorism) was articulated by Watson (1919) and Skinner (1974). Social learning theory was developed in response to radical behaviorism (Bandura, 1977). Learning theory explains learned behavior in terms of rewards.

Children are rewarded for certain behaviors, which they then repeat (R. M. Thomas, 1985). Children avoid other behaviors that are punished. Social learning theory, on the other hand, explains learned behavior in terms of modeling.

Children model or imitate the behavior of others. If 4-year-old Maria sees Tanisha being praised for sitting in her seat, Maria will model her behavior after Tanisha's. Behaviors can be learned inadvertently, as when, for example, parents unwittingly "reward" aversive behavior (G. R. Patterson, 1980). A popular use of learning theory is behavior modification (G. R. Patterson, 1975; R. M. Thomas, 1985). "Such conditioning has been employed by parents for socializing their children, by teachers seeking to control pupils' classroom behavior, and by therapists attempting to alter clients' undesirable habits" (R. M. Thomas, 1985:392).

A well-known behavior modification technique is Time Out, the removal of a disruptive child from the reinforcing situation (G. R. Patterson, 1975). Time Out is a mild form of punishment, which if used properly, discourages the child from behaving the same way in the future.

Application

An obvious application of social learning theory is the study of parent-child relations. G. R. Patterson (1980) discussed how distressed parents and children use coercion, or aversive behavior, to reinforce and punish the other's behavior. According to Patterson, "most deviant behaviors . . . are caused by an inept performance of child-management skills" (p. 1). Parents' failure to curb "garden variety, coercive behaviors sets into motion interaction sequences that are the basis for training in aggression . . . the exchanges are such that both members train each other to become increasingly aversive" (G. R. Patterson, 1986:436).

Critique

As with other hedonist theories, social learning theory can be criticized on the grounds that people are motivated to maximize their rewards and minimize their punishments (Burr, 1995). The image generated is one of a calculating, self-seeking individual devoid of compassion, charity, and altruism.

R. M. Thomas (1985) has also criticized behavior modification: "practices are manipulative, violate human rights, and often harm those who are the objects of the conditioning" (p. 392). Nevertheless, social learning theory is evaluated more positively than its predecessor, behaviorism, which devalues "mentalistic" constructs such as cognition and emotions.

EXCHANGE THEORY

Like social learning theory, exchange theory has its roots in the Greek philosophy of hedonism. In the 20th century, exchange theory has been applied to "personal and interpersonal factors that mediate the formation, maintenance, and dissolution of a relationship" (Sabatelli & Shehan, 1993:386). In other words, people are assumed to make cost-benefit analyses of their close relationships.

George Homans (1958) believed that people seek relationships that will be rewarding (for example, because of the status or the attractiveness of the potential partner). The costs of having such a partner, however, must also be calculated in order to determine the likelihood that such a partner will be pursued. Thibaut and Kelley (1959) argued that the attractiveness of a relationship is determined by a comparison between what one puts into a relationship and what one expects to get from it. Peter Blau (1964) assumed that people choose between alternatives, selecting the one with the lowest costs and the most profits.

Relationship stability is a function of attractions (factors that keep people in relationships), barriers (factors that keep people from leaving relationships), and alternatives (factors that draw people away from relationships) (Levinger, 1965). For example, an internal barrier to leaving a relationship would be a sense of obligation to the partner, a promise "until death do us part." External barriers would be legal or financial sanctions that have historically kept people in unhappy marriages: "The higher the social class, the lower the divorce rates. There are high costs involved in the divorce of upper-class people. . . . Each loses a considerable amount" (Winton, 1995:127).

Application

The study of why people divorce is an obvious application of exchange theory. Price and McKenry (1988) have outlined a number of attractions to marriage, barriers to divorce, and alternatives to marriage.

Attractions include factors such as companionship, sexual gratification, and financial security. Barriers include the presence of children, religious beliefs, and economic pressures. Alternatives include economic independence, employment opportunities, and relationship potential. Barriers to divorce have lessened while alternatives to marriage, especially for women (for example, economic independence), have increased, making divorce more attractive.

Critique

Exchange theory is based on the assumption that human beings make rational decisions about important events in their lives (Sabatelli & Shehan, 1993). Exchange theory ignores the nonrational, or emotional, aspect of human decision making. Feminist critics (for example, Hartsock, 1983) argue that exchange theory focuses on the interpersonal, ignoring the larger context that legitimizes male power and status in relationships. Further, "women's experiences . . . bearing and rearing children emphasize human relatedness rather than isolated individuals bargaining out of their own self-interests" (Osmond & Thorne, 1993:602).

Family Development Theory

The earliest developmental position was articulated by the French writer Jean-Jacques Rousseau (1762), who believed that children develop through four distinct stages and that their education should be appropriate to their developmental stage.

Contemporary stage theories of individual development include Freudian, Piagetian, and Eriksonian theories (R. M. Thomas, 1985). During the 1940s, family scientists Evelyn Duvall and Reuben Hill began developing a stage theory of family development based on the family life cycle and developmental tasks (Burr, 1995).

Duvall's (1957; Duvall & Miller, 1985) eight-stage family life cycle pairs each stage with specific developmental tasks. The concept of developmental tasks is borrowed from Havighurst (1953), who wrote: "A developmental task . . . arises at or about a certain period in the life of an individual, successful achievement of which leads to his [sic] happiness and to success with later tasks" (p. 2). Thus, for a family in the childbearing stage of the family life cycle, having and socializing children is a key developmental task. For a family in the launching stage, sending young adults out into the world of work, higher education, or marriage is a key developmental task (Duvall & Miller, 1985).

Recent contributions to family development theory include recognition of the diversity that exists in contemporary families (Carter & McGoldrick, 1989; Mattessich & Hill, 1987). Instead of a linear model, which depicts all families as going through the same stages in the same order, a multilinear model allows for diversity: "People within any society do not follow the same path in their lives: some marry, others don't; some have children, others don't" (Winton, 1995:42).

For example, a multilinear model allows for "boomerang children" (adult children who move back home with their retired parents because of divorce or financial setbacks) or "skip-generation families" (families in which grandparents parent their grandchildren).

Application

An obvious application of family development theory is the study of families in later life. The study of such families is all the more timely because of the aging population (Bengtson & Allen, 1993).

The first members of the baby-boom generation will become senior citizens in the year 2011. Issues for aging families include adjusting to retirement, rebuilding the marriage relationship, and facing the death of a spouse (Winton, 1995). Retirement is of interest as increased life expectancy means people will be retired for longer periods of time. Although studies of retirement typically focus on men's retirement or on wives' adjustment to husbands' retirement, C. A. Price (1996) examined career women's transitions to retirement.

Critique

Critics of family development theory have commented on "the inadequacy of family development theory to incorporate ethnic, racial, and gender differences, as well as its failure to embody the full variability of family forms" (Rodgers & White, 1993:230).

Family development theory has also been described as overly simplistic (Winton, 1995) and deterministic (Rodgers & White, 1993). Thus, the recent reformulation of Rodgers and White offers a more stochastic or probabilistic model. The result is a model of family development that is less able to predict future development but also less prescriptive and value-laden.

Symbolic Interactionism

Symbolic interactionism is a constructionist theoretical framework that developed out of the philosophical work of Charles Cooley, William Thomas, and George Mead in the early part of the 20th century (Burr et al., 1979). These writers rejected the positivistic tradition, claiming that truth is relative, there is no one way of knowing, and there is no objective reality independent of the individual.

The very concept of the social construction of reality (Berger & Luckmann, 1966) owes much to W. I. Thomas's (1928) definition of the situation: how an individual defines a situation will determine how the individual responds to the situation.

Other concepts associated with symbolic interactionism highlight Mead's (1934) concept of role and include role strain, role conflict, role reversal, role distancing, and role transition.

Roles enable role occupants to interact with others by anticipating their behavior (LaRossa & Reitzes, 1993). For example, daughters might well anticipate that fathers will be angry when school-night curfews are ignored.

According to symbolic interactionists, roles are at the heart of one's identity, and changes in roles, or role transitions, can be difficult, especially if they are unanticipated (Stryker & Statham, 1985).

Symbolic interactionism's emphasis on the self is reflected in Cooley's (1902) concept of the looking-glass self, the idea that people develop their sense of self in interaction with other people such as parents and peers. Thus, other people, especially significant others (Mead, 1934), reflect back to the individual a sense of self. If a mother perceives her son's behavior as "bad," she will treat him as though he is "bad," and eventually he will come to believe that he is "bad." Thus, "roles are learned through altercations by which others cast the person into a role and provide the symbolic cues which elicit appropriate behavior" (Stryker & Statham, 1985, p. 313).

Application

One application of constructionism is the study of the current "lesbian baby boom." Kitzinger and Wilkinson (1995) have used a social constructionist approach to study women's transitions from heterosexuality to lesbianism.

These authors described "the ways in which women in transition construct and interpret their changing identities" (p. 102). Lesbian families likewise struggle to create positive identities in a society that renders them invisible (C. J. Patterson, 1995). Lesbians are often denied custody of their own children and refused access to artificial insemination (Tasker & Golombok, 1995), despite a lack of evidence that children of lesbians have developmental difficulties (C. J. Patterson, 1992).

Critique

In their review of symbolic interactionism, LaRossa and Reitzes (1993) mentioned a number of criticisms of the theory. One of these limitations is that symbolic interactionism, like other constructionist theories, overestimates the degree to which individuals and families can create their own reality. This assumption ignores the extent to which humans live in an objective world not of their own making. Another limitation is that symbolic interactionism has overlooked the affective (for example, emotional), biological, and unconscious nature of humans.

Family Systems Theory

Family systems theory has its roots in Ludwig von Bertalanffy's general systems theory, or GST (Whitchurch & Constantine, 1993). Von Bertalanffy (1975) argued that contradictions in the biological sciences can be explained with reference to systems, or sets of "elements standing in interrelation among themselves and with the environment" (p. 159).

One of the key assumptions of GST is holism: the whole is greater than the sum of its parts. For example, "to make a cake, you add butter, sugar, flour, eggs . . . bake the cake, it changes into something that is more than the individual characteristics of the ingredients" (Infante et al., 1990:81).

During the 1950s, researchers and psychiatrists began to observe and apply systemic principles to the growing field of family therapy. Bateson et al., (1956) hypothesized that the origins of schizophrenia were to be found in the double bind, a communication pattern in which verbal and nonverbal channels contradict each other. For example, a mother insists that her daughter give her a hug, and yet the mother's nonverbal signals make it clear that a hug is not welcome.

By the 1960s, a new journal, *Family Process*, appeared featuring research based on systems theory (Broderick & Schrader, 1981).

In addition to holism, key concepts of family systems theory include interdependence and boundaries. Interdependence means that "in families . . . each family member's behavior affects every other member" (Whitchurch & Constantine, 1993:332). Furthermore, each member of the system is equally responsible for what goes on in the system; no one individual in the system is responsible for what occurs. If one member of the system is alcoholic, other members of the system enable the alcoholism.

Systems, by their very definition, involve boundaries that separate one system from another. Boundaries indicate who is in the system and who is not. Confusion over family system boundaries is known as ambiguity (Boss, 1988).

Application

Researchers have applied family systems theory to the study of remarriage and stepfamilies. Establishing family boundaries is an important task for newly formed stepfamilies; not knowing who is in the stepfamily can add to the ambiguity of stepfamily life (Pasley, 1987). A lack of recognized names for stepfamily members (for example, what should you call the adult children of your father's common-law partner?) also contributes to this ambiguity (Ganong et al., 1995).

Conflict is often the result of a lack of shared rules and rituals. If one side of the family insists on a Thanksgiving buffet in front of a televised football game, while the other side wants a formal dinner in the dining room, conflict is inevitable.

Critique

Feminist critics and therapists have voiced a number of concerns about family systems theory. In particular, they have focused on "the failure of Systems Theory to view families in their sociocultural and historical contexts" (Osmond & Thorne, 1993:603). Thus, family therapists often ignore the androcentric bias inherent in our culture. Power relations are also ignored by family therapists who assume that women and men are equally responsible for maintaining dysfunctional behavior. "Even in situations in which women are abused . . . equality is evoked in terms of the 'disguised power' of helplessness" (Osmond & Thorne, 1993:604).

Ecological Systems Theory

Ecological systems theory refers to Urie Bronfenbrenner's (1979, 1992) model of development within a series of contexts. Bronfenbrenner has described the environment as "a set of nested structures, each inside the next, like a set of Russian dolls" (1979:3). Ecological systems theory has its roots in Lewin's (1935) field theory. Lewin argued that behavior is a function of the person and the environment (B = f[PE]); Bronfenbrenner adapted the formula to read that development is a function of the person and the environment (D = f[PE]).

Bronfenbrenner (1979) described four levels of context in which development occurs. The *microsystem* refers to the setting containing the individual and including such factors as time, place, and other individuals. A child's family or day care are examples of the microsystem. The *mesosystem* refers to the interrelations between two or more microsystems (for example, the linkages between home and school). The *exosystem* refers to the linkages between two or more microsystems, one of which does not include the individual, but which has implications for the individual. An example of this type of microsystem would be the child's parents' workplaces. The *macrosystem* refers to the culture or subculture in which the other systems are nested (for example, the social, cultural, or economic climate).

The implications for researchers are clear: research designs must involve the study of the individual in one or more of these systems. As Bronfenbrenner (1977) put it, "If you wish to understand the relation between the developing person and some aspect of his or her environment, try to budge one, and see what happens to the other" (p. 518).

Application

In the late 1960s, Andrew Billingsley introduced a systems approach to the study of Black families. Billingsley (1968) urged that Black families be viewed as "social system(s), embedded within a network of both smaller and larger subsystems located both within the Negro community and in the wider society" (p. 32).

Billingsley's series of nested systems—the Black family within the Black community within the wider society—is a good example of ecological systems. As Billingsley pointed out, "Whatever ails the Negro family is a reflection of ailments in the society at large. The cure for those ills, therefore, is not likely to be found in any single and simple solution" (p. 32).

Critique

Recently, Bronfenbrenner (1992) has recognized a limitation of research in the ecological tradition: researchers have to put the individual (or the family) back into the contexts they are studying.

Important aspects of the individual that need to be taken into account include personality factors and cognitive abilities. At the family level, family values or coping strategies need to be considered (Boss, 1988). Not all individuals or families experience the same environment in the same way. An environment that puts one family at risk, for example, may give another family a developmental advantage.

CONCLUSION

Family scientists use many theories to explain various aspects of family life, predict future development and behavior, and intervene in order to change dysfunctional behavior.

Theories guide family scientists to look at what is important, but they can also blind scientists to aspects of family life that are outside the domain of certain theories. Some theories are better suited to examine certain aspects of family life than others. No one theory can explain all aspects of family life, however; at the same time, no theory is free from criticism. Knowledge of different theories helps family scientists understand family life as we know it.

REFERENCES

Alexander, J. C. (1985). Introduction. In J. C. Alexander (ed.), *Neo-Functionalism* (pp. 7–18). Newbury Park, Calif.: Sage.

Bandura, A. (1977). *Social Learning Theory*. Englewood Cliffs, N.J.: Prentice-Hall.

Bateson, G., Jackson, D. D., Haley, J., and Weakland, J. (1956). Toward a theory of schizophrenia. *Behavioral Science*. 251–264.

Berger, P. L., and Luckmann, T. (1966). *The Social Construction of Reality: A Treatise in the Sociology of Knowledge*. New York: Doubleday.

Bengeson, V. L., and Allen, K. R. (1993). The life course perspective applied to families over time. In P. G. Boss, W. J. Doherty, R. LaRossa, W. R. Schuum, and S. K. Steinmetz (eds.), *Sourcebook of Family Theories and Methods: A Contextual Approach* (pp. 469–499). New York: Plenum.

Bertalanffy, L., von (1975). *Perspective on General System Theory: Scientific-Philosophical Studies*. New York: Braziller.

Billingsley, A. (1968). *Black Families in White America*. Englewood Cliffs, N.J.: Prentice-Hall.

Blau, P. M. (1964). *Exchange and Power in Social Life*. New York: Wiley.

Bleier, R. (1984). *Science and Gender: A Critique of Biology and Its Theories on Women*. New York: Pergamon Press.

Boss, P. (1986). Psychological absence in the family: A systems approach to a study of fathering. In M. B. Sussman (ed.), *The Charybdis Complex* (pp. 11–32). New York: Haworth.

———. (1988). *Family Stress Management*. Newbury Park, Calif.: Sage.

Bowlby, J. (1969). *Attachment and Loss. Vol. 1: Attachment*. New York: Basic Books.

Brandwein, R. A., Brown, C. A., and Fox, E. M. (1974). Women and children last: The social situation of divorced mothers and their families. *Journal of Marriage and the Family*, 36:498–514.

Broderick, C. B., and Schrader, S. S. (1981). The history of professional marriage and family therapy. In A. S. Gurman and D. P. Kniskern (eds.), *Handbook of Family Therapy* (pp. 5–35). New York: Brunner/Mazel.

Bronfenbrenner, U. (1977). Toward an experimental ecology of human development. *American Psychologist*, 32:513–531.

———. (1979). *The Ecology of Human Development*. Cambridge, Mass.: Harvard University Press.

———. (1992). Ecological systems theory. In R. Vasta (ed.), *Six Theories of Child Development* (pp. 187–249). Philadelphia: Jessica Kingsley.

Burgess, E. (1926). The family as a unity of interacting personalities. *The Family*, 7:3–9.

Burr, W. R. (1995). Using theories in family science. In R. Gilbert, B. H. Settles, W. R. Burr (eds.), *Research and Theory in Family Science* (pp. 73–90). Pacific Grove, Calif.: Brooks/Cole.

———, Leigh, G. K., Day, R. D., and Constantine, C. (1979). Symbolic interaction and the family. In W. R. Burr, R. Hill, F. I. Nye, and I. L. Reiss (eds.), *Contemporary Theories about the Family* (Vol. 2, pp. 42–111). New York: Free Press.

Buss, D. M. (1989). Sex differences in human mate preferences: Evolutionary hypotheses tested in 37 cultures. *Behavioral and Brain Sciences*, 12:1–49.

———. (1995). Evolutionary psychology: A new paradigm for psychological science. *Psychological Inquiry*, 6:1–30.

Carter, E. A., and McGoldrick, M. (eds.) (1989). *The Changing Family Cycle: A Framework for Family Therapy* (2d ed.). New York: Gardner.

Cooley, C. H. (1902/1956). *Human Nature and Social Order.* Glencoe, Ill.: Free Press.

Darwin, C. (1859). *On the Origin of the Species by Means of Natural Selection, or, Preservation of Favoured Races in the Struggle for Life.* London: Murray.

Duvall, E. M. (1957). *Family Development.* Philadelphia: Lippincott.

———, and Miller, B. C. (1985). *Marriage and Family Development* (6th ed.). New York: Harper & Row.

Feingold, A. (1994). Gender differences in personality: A meta analysis. *Psychological Bulletin*, 116:429–456.

Ferree, M. M. (1990). Beyond separate spheres: Feminism and family research. *Journal of Marriage and the Family*, 52:866–884.

Ganong, L., Coleman, M., and Fine, M. (1995). Remarriage and stepfamilies. In R. D. Day, K. R. Gilbert, B. H. Settles, W. R. Burr (eds.), *Research and Theory in Family Science* (pp. 287–303). Pacific Grove, Calif.: Brooks/Cole.

Glaser, B. G., and Strauss, A. L. (1967). *The Discovery of Grounded Theory.* Chicago: Aldine.

Hartsock, N. C. (1983). *Money, Sex, and Power: Toward a Feminist Historical Materialism.* New York: Longman.

Havighurst, R. J. (1953). *Human Development and Education.* New York: Longman.

Homans, G. C. (1958). Social behavior as exchange. *American Journal of Sociology*, 63:597–606.

Infante, D. A., Rancer, A. S., and Womack, D. F. (1990). *Building Communication Theory.* Prospects Heights, Ill.: Waveland.

Kenrick, D. T., and Trost, M. R. (1993). The evolutionary perspective. In A. E. Beall and R. J. Sternberg (eds.), *The Psychology of Gender* (pp. 148–172). New York: Guilford.

W. J. Doherty, R. LaRossa, W. R. Schuum, and S. K. Steinmetz (eds.), (1993) *Sourcebook of Family Theories and Methods: A Contextual Approach.* (pp. 195–217). New York: Plenum.

Kitzinger, C., and Wilkinson, S. (1995). Transitions from heterosexuality to lesbianism: The discursive production of lesbian identities. *Developmental Psychology*, 31:95–104.

LaRossa, R. (1979). Sex during pregnancy: A symbolic interactionist analysis. *Journal of Sex Research*, 15:119–128.

———, and LaRossa, M. M. (1981). *Transition to Parenthood: How Infants Change Families.* Beverly Hills, Calif.: Sage.

———, and Reitzes, D. C. (1993). Symbolic interactionism and family studies. In P. G. Boss, W. J. Doherty, R. LaRossa, W. R. Schuum, and S. K. Steinmetz (eds.),

Sourcebook of Family Theories and Methods: A Contextual Approach (pp. 135–163). New York: Plenum.

Levinger, G. (1965). Marital cohesiveness and dissolution: An integrative review. *Journal of Marriage and the Family*, 27:19–28.

Lewin, K. (1935). A *Dynamic Theory of Personality*. New York: McGraw-Hill.

Lewontin, R. C., Rose, S., and Kamin, L. J. (1984). *Not in Our Genes: Biology, Ideology, and Human Nature*. New York: Pantheon.

Locke, J. (1690/1961). *Essay Concerning Human Understanding* (Vol. 1), London: Dent.

———. (1693/1964). Some thoughts concerning education. In P. Gay (ed.), *John Locke on Education*. New York: Columbia University Press.

Lorenz, K. Z. (1977). *Behind the Mirror: A Search for a Natural History of Human Knowledge*. New York: Harcourt Brace Jovanovich.

Losh-Hesselbart, S. (1987). Development of tender roles. In M. B. Sussman and S. K. Steinmetz (eds.), *Handbook of Marriage and the Family* (pp. 535–563). New York: Plenum.

Mattessich, P., and Hill, R. (1987). Life cycle and family development. In M. B. Sussman and S. K. Steinmetz (eds.), *Handbook of Marriage and the Family* (pp. 437–469). New York: Plenum.

Mead, G. H. (1934/1956). *On Social Psychology: Selected Papers*. Chicago: University of Chicago Press.

Osmond, M. W., and Thorne, B. (1993). Feminist theories: The social construction of gender in families and society. In P. G. Boss, W. J. Doherty, R. LaRossa, W. R. Schuum, and S. K. Steinmetz (eds.), *Sourcebook of Family Theories and Methods: A Contextual Approach* (pp. 591–623). New York: Plenum.

Parsons, T. (1951). *The Social System*. New York: Free Press.

———, and Bales, R. (1955). *Family Socialization and Interaction Process*. New York: Free Press.

Pasley, K. (1987). Family boundary ambiguity: Perceptions of adult remarried family members. In K. Pasley and M. Ihinger Tallman (eds.), *Remarriage and Step-parenting: Current Research and Theory* (pp. 206–224). New York: Guilford.

Patterson, C. J. (1992). Children of lesbian and gay parents. *Child Development*, 63:1025–1042.

———. (1995). Sexual orientation and human development: An overview. *Developmental psychology*, 31:3–11.

Patterson, G. R. (1975). *Families: Applications of Social Learning to Family Life*. Champaign, Ill: Research Press.

———. (1980). Mothers: The unacknowledged victims. *Monographs of the Society for Research in Child Development*, 45 (5, Serial No. 186).

———. (1986). Performance models for antisocial boys. *American Psychologist*, 41:432–444.

Popenoe, D. (May 1991). Breakup of the family: Can we reverse the trend? USA *Today Magazine*, pp. 50–53.

———. (1993). American family decline, 1960–1990: A review and appraisal. *Journal of Marriage and the Family*, 55:527–555.

Price, C. A. (1996). Women and Retirement: The Unexplored Transition. Unpublished doctoral dissertation, University of Georgia.

Price, S. J., and McKenry, P. C. (1988). *Divorce*. Newbury Park, Calif.: Sage.

Rodders, R. H., and White, J. M. (1993). Family development theory. In P. G. Boss, W. J. Doherty, R. LaRossa, W. R. Schuum, and S. K. Steinmetz (eds.), *Sourcebook of Family Theories and Methods: A Contextual Approach* (pp. 225–254). New York: Plenum.

Rossi, A. (1977). A biosocial perspective on parenting. *Daedalus*, 106:1–30.

Rousseau, J. J. (1762/1948). *Emile, or Education* (B. Foxley, trans.). London: Dent.

Sabatelli, R. M., and Shehan, C. L. (1993). Exchange and resource theories. In P. G. Boss, W. J. Doherty, R. LaRossa, W. R. Schuum, and S. K. Steinmetz (eds.), *Sourcebook of Family Theories and Methods: A Contextual Approach* (pp. 385–411). New York: Plenum.

Shields, S. A. (1975). Functionalism, Darwinism, and the psychology of women. *American Psychologist*, 30:739–945.

Skinner, B. F. (1974). *About Behaviorism*. New York: Knopf.

Stacey, J. (1993). Good riddance to "the family": A response to David Popenoe. *Journal of Marriage and the Family*, 55:545–547.

Stryker, S., and Statham, A. (1985). Symbolic interaction and role theory. In G. Linzey and E. Aronson (eds.), *The Handbook of Social Psychology* (pp. 311–378). New York: Random House.

Tasker, F., and Golombok, S. (1995). Growing up in a lesbian family: effects on child development. *American Journal of Orthopsychiatry*, 65:203–215.

Thibaut, J. W., and Kelley, H. H. (1959). *The Social Psychology of Groups*. New York: Wiley.

Thomas, R. M. (1985). *Comparing Theories of Child Development* (2d ed.) Belmont, Calif.: Wadsworth.

Thomas, W. I., and Thomas, D. S. (1974). The child in America: *Behavior Problems and Programs*. (3rd ed.) New York: Knopf.

Thompson, L., and Walker, A. (1989). Gender in families: Women and men in marriage, work, and parenthood. *Journal of Marriage and the Family*, 51:845–871.

Troost, K. M., and Filsinger, E. (1993). Emerging biosocial perspectives on the family. In P. G. Boss, W. J. Doherty, R. LaRossa, W. R. Schuum, and S. K. Steinmetz (eds.), *Sourcebook of Family Theories and Methods: A Contextual Approach*. (pp. 677–710). New York: Plenum.

Watson, J. B. (1919). *Psychology from the Standpoint of a Behaviorist*. Philadelphia: Lippincott.

Wilson, E. O. (1975). *Sociobiology: The New Synthesis*. Cambridge, Mass.: Harvard University Press.

Winton, C. A. (1995). *Frameworks for Studying Families*. Guilford, Conn.: Dushkin.

Whitchurch, G. G., and Constantine, L. L. (1993). Systems theory. In P. G. Boss, W. J. Doherty, R. LaRossa, W. R. Schuum, and S. K. Steinmetz (eds.), *Sourcebook of Family Theories and Methods: A Contextual Approach* (pp. 325–352). New York: Plenum.

CHAPTER

5

A PSYCHOLOGIST REFLECTS ON THE FAMILY

Dennis R. Finger

FAMILY DEFINED

What is a family? Today there are so many different kinds of family structures other than the traditional nuclear family of two parents and children. There are mother-led, single-parent households and, increasingly, father-led, single-parent households. Some families are headed by one or two grandparents or another relative such as an aunt or uncle. There are many extended families, which may have a parent, other relatives such as an uncle or grandparent, and children. Traditional two-parent households are no longer in the majority. Children growing up with divorced or separated parents are becoming quite common.

Is it better to have two parents? You might think two is better than one. And it may be. Two parents can share the very challenging tasks and work of being a "good-enough" parent (Winnicott, 1986) and juggling the various parental demands of relating to the child's school, medical needs, emotional and social needs, spiritual and religious aspects, fears and concerns. However, a one-parent family may provide a better, more positive environment for the child. There may be a great deal of conflict and friction in the two-parent environment, creating constant stress for the child. Alternatively, one parent may be absent, neglectful, or emotionally or physically abusive. Of course, children do not choose their parents. It is strictly a matter of chance whether children find themselves in a family situation that is growth-enhancing, growth-inhibiting, or a combination of the two.

MY FAMILY

Let us go from the abstract to the concrete. I was born in Brooklyn, New York, in 1949 to two new parents, Irv and June. Being the firstborn, I was my parents "practice child." Three sisters came after, each about five years apart. The family theory is that each time one of us started school, about age 5 or 6, our mother wanted another child so that she would be able to stay at home and be a mother. June returned to work in her forties; she became a nursing home recreation therapist and administrator.

My father was a bright, hardworking man who became a postal clerk after returning from service in World War II. He stayed in a position far below his capability, although the position provided a reliable, safe living. What was our family like? Each of the four children lived a somewhat different experience. I had a stay-at-home mother and an absent, but hardworking father. My father worked two or three jobs with long hours and few days off. He dedicated his energy, time, and effort to providing for his family. It was rare for him to be at home sick or for personal business. He walked on a straight path, providing food, shelter, and clothing for us.

Early on, we (my mother, my father, and I) lived in a two-family house that we owned. We lived there until I was 7 years old. The upstairs was rented and my parents also rented a room in our own apartment to a mother and her teenage son. I have no memory of the upstairs family or our own renters. This lack of memory bothers me, and I often wonder why I cannot remember any of these people, although I was quite young. I remember staying with my mother, especially curled up next to her as she lay on the couch watching television and eating slices of salami and potato chips and drinking Coca-Cola. Curled up next to her was one of the safest places for me as a young child. I felt warm, protected, snug. When else in my life have I felt such a cocoon-like, warmly wrapped experience? It is hard to duplicate.

Uncle Sidney

For the first five years of my life I lived as an "only" child. My great uncle Sidney built a wonderful, large, blue toy chest for me. Tears come to my eyes as I write about the love shown by my uncle, who died about 10 years ago. Sidney was considered by my parents and other relatives to be a "character," someone who had his own unique, odd eccentricities. Unmarried, Sidney was a sensitive, creative, skinny pharmacist and violinist. He visited our house and played his violin with the air of a seasoned maestro. His visits were a welcome break from our usual daily routine.

Sidney told me he loved a girl when he was in his twenties, but his parents forbade him to marry her because he was too "weak." Parents, of course, can have tremendous power and influence over a child's life, literally changing the life destiny of the child. As we know, in some cultures marriages are arranged by the parents; they choose the child's life mate. I do not know of research on marital satisfaction of prearranged versus nonarranged marriages.

My imagination guided me to different scenarios: cowboys and Indians; cops and robbers; armies and enemies. Also, I had a wonderful train set, which my father and I set up in our basement. The trains became the center of a train world filled with travelers, workers, advertisements, and all sorts of happenings. Oh, how I loved those trains! Some of my happiest childhood moments occurred in my train world. I also liked biking, roller-skating, and playing on the street. The street was the center of my activity. It was a bustling, alive place where neighborhood children gathered to skip rope, play ball and other group games, and just let off steam and run around forever. Whenever my mother called me in to have dinner, I never wanted to leave my friends and the street. The street was so exciting and connected to our family life. As an only child I learned to seek social satisfaction outside the house or use my imagination.

The Dethroner

When I was about 5 my sister was born, and about the same time I started school. I was not prepared for the attention my mother and my relatives gave my sister. Who was this little invader? All of a sudden I was transformed from a 5-year-old kid to someone's older brother with responsibilities for watching my younger sister.

I felt threatened, rejected, and on the periphery of things. I turned to school and became very involved in my elementary school, serving later as a hall monitor, crossing guard (rising to lieutenant rank), and flag bearer (I carried the New York flag but never the United States flag, which was carried by Richard, a big, tall student).

As a psychologist, I have worked with many children and families. The "dethroning" of the firstborn may be a very tough struggle, a major disappointment and an ego-deflating experience for the child: from family center to the sidelines, from the center of attention to sharing the focus. There are also gains for the firstborn, although they may not be readily apparent. These gains may include having a very special relationship with a sibling; getting a less lethal dose of the parental psychopathology; having a family member to share life with after the parents' death; learning to share with others, which is so important in the world outside the family; and other advantages. A sibling may be someone to love and to hate, to cooperate with and compete against, someone who protects and hurts, someone with whom to share experiences.

I remember my sister and I playing gymnastic games and putting on family plays. My sister had a talent for art that was recognized when she was very young. She was awarded an art scholarship to study at the Brooklyn Museum. She carved out a special place for herself in the family. I had no art talent and I was happy if I could draw a straight line.

Each Child a Person

It seems that each child born to a family carves out, or seeks to sculpt, a unique niche in the family. I think this is vital for each child's self-esteem, confidence, and feeling of individuality. You have seen this in numerous families—one child is good at sports, another at dance or theater, a third at academics, and so forth. It is the job of the parents and teachers to help children discover their strengths, talents, abilities, and aspirations.

I remember seeing a videotape about a social worker who worked with women considering abortion. In a personal interview, the social worker talked about her own family and her grandmother in particular. Through her tears, the social worker reflected how her grandmother would hold her granddaughter's hands and say, "What will these hands do? Will they help people who are sick? What good things will these hands do?"

Teachers and parents can help children with their self-in-development, assisting children to see possible future selves. We show children possible future paths in their education, occupation, family life, and school life. We recognize where children are now on the life continuum and where they could be. What do you want to be when you grow up? I remember as a child I wanted at different times to be a cowboy, a doctor, an engineer, or a teacher.

Children can see themselves through their parents' eyes. Hopefully, families are experimental incubators, creating facilitating environments for children's growth (Winnicott, 1965). Unfortunately, our society does a poor job of training adults to become parents. Most parents learn how to parent from their own mothers and fathers. Teachers in classrooms, counselors in therapeutic settings, and others in the child's life may encourage children to develop their best selves. Parents, teachers, and helping professionals need to create a supportive team to raise our children.

Doing Parenting

Having a working, loving family is one of the greatest successes in anyone's life. It takes tremendous sacrifice for parents, especially grueling when the parent is exhausted, stressed, or ill. Sometimes the greatest sacrifices occur when we absolutely cannot give anymore, but somehow find the energy and reserve to give once more.

I remember times when I was able to provide nurturance for my child and other moments when I could not. Many times I review the situation in my head and think of how I could have improved my parenting. I try to allow myself to be open to learning from my own son.

I remember when my son was around 2 years old and he was stacking blocks in uneven, shaky columns. I was concerned that the blocks would fall and I started to straighten and consolidate the columns. I realized that I was intruding on my son's play and relating to him in terms of my own needs for balance, symmetry, and order. Another time, during the summer, I filled a small wading pool for my son. He sat next to the pool and began smacking the water. He was thrilled with the water play. I beckoned him to enter the pool and he rightly resisted my directions. He was having a wonderful time just sitting on the ground, and hitting the water and watching the water jump out of the pool. I finally was able to join him in his water play and delight in his exhilarating experience.

We know that play is a powerful therapeutic tool (Landreth, 1996). In addition, playing together is so important for healthy family relations. Also, I was finally able to empathize with my son, see the world through my son's eyes, attempt to experience his experience as if I stood in his shoes.

Personal Parenting Skills

Empathy is a key to human relations and is vital for families. When we endeavor to empathize, we try to obtain a deeper understanding of another's perspective, of the other's felt world. And yet, how difficult it is to empathize when a parent is in the midst of utter frustration and tested patience. Maintaining empathic parenting is a goal to work toward.

Along with empathy, limit setting is crucial. Children need to feel protected and safe even from their own impulses and misbehaviors. Limits do not hurt children; on the contrary, they help children feel secure. But limits need to be used judiciously. If a child is not hurting herself, others, or property, then limits may not be needed. Loving with limits seems to be a good mix for family success.

And let us include family fun. How did our family have fun? We had family shows. Sunday night was often showtime, with all of us gathered together in the living room of our house in East Flatbush where we lived from when I was 7 through high school. We often laughed hysterically.

In my present-day family, my son has presented magic shows, with me as the magician's assistant and my wife as the audience. We have also performed plays and dance routines for each other. Sometimes my son and I take "walkabouts." These are local adventure walks where we open ourselves up to new experiences. We have discovered "new" parks, met interesting people, encountered local animal life, scanned the skies, found streams and lakes, appreciated the varied architecture, and come to know our town in fresh ways.

I remember the time we walked to the park and ended up playing a spontaneous tennis game with borrowed rackets and tennis balls. Another time we wound up inside a house that was being redone because of a fire and we were given a tour by the owner. These were bonding experiences for us. Family fun is crucial. It is a foundation and continuing resource for cohesiveness, relaxation, and family togetherness. As I live in this moment, family fun seems like a good place to end this reflection on the family.

REFERENCES

Landreth, G., Homeyer, L., Glover, G., and Sweeney, D. (1996). *Play Therapy Interventions with Children's Problems*. Northvale, N.J.: Jason Aronson Publishers.

Winnicott, D. W. (1965). *The Maturational Processes and the Facilitating Environment*. Madison, Conn.: International Universities Press.

———. (1986). *Home Is Where We Start From*. New York: Norton.

CHAPTER 6

The Politics of the Family

Susan L. Folden

As far back as knowledge takes us, human beings have lived in families (Mead & Heyman, 1965:77). Families were created for political reasons. The need to establish lineage for inheritance created the need to clearly differentiate biological families. The traditional biological family was hierarchical and, in most cultures, patriarchal. The political climate of the traditional family simulated inheritance and lineage patterns. The male head of the family retained the majority of the power and influence within the family (Hite, 1995).

Politics

Politics encompasses power and influence. Politics has often been defined as the skillful art of negotiation or the power of persuasion. Political processes essentially act to maintain equilibrium within a system. Political systems outside of the family impact on families and family functioning. Politics within families affects political and social systems in the community.

Families who are socially and politically active have a significant impact on political decision making in communities. This power is often evident when a community board makes decisions about the location of schools, parks, or congregate living facilities. However, families who spend the majority of their resources meeting basic human needs, such as shelter and food, have little time and energy to devote to community politics. These families have little political power (Paolucci, et al., 1997).

The Function of Families

Families have several political functions within society. Families are responsible for the rearing of children and must learn to a coordinate conflicting interests within the family unit. Families are links to society and teach us how to relate to other people (Satir, 1988). Families maintain responsibility for the protection of their members and for maintaining internal and external order.

What is often echoed today is that the government has taken over many family tasks since families no longer assume responsibility for their political functions. Many critics of the modern family attribute this to the increasing number of nontraditional families, especially single-parent families (Winch, 1971). As Americans, we are still debating what role the government should assume in the internal politics of family life. Such issues as child care, elder care, and divorce are family issues being addressed by government today (Mintz & Kellog, 1988).

Politics within the family describes the ability of one family member to influence or control the behavior of other family members. Power is the ability to promote or resist change. Power is often situation-specific. An individual family member may possess power in one sphere of family functioning, such as childrearing, but have little power over the economics of the family (Scanzoni & Szinovacz, 1980). Coercive power is the ability to make others do what you want them to, whether or not they wish to do it.

PERSPECTIVES ON FAMILY

Families remain the basic unit of society today. The idealized family unit in industrialized countries remains the traditional nuclear family living independently in a single housing unit. Marriage signifies the origination of a traditional family in most cultures (Mead & Heyman, 1965). The structure of the family, tradition, and culture influence the politics within the family.

Today, over half of all Americans will live in a nontraditional family at one point in their lives. The emergence of diverse family forms and structures has resulted in various societal changes. Many reasons account for this variance. Immigration has introduced much cultural diversity into our society. Increasing divorce rates and the remarriage of divorced partners has created secondary, blended nuclear families. Many women now choose to remain single and rear children. Many couples choose to cohabit without marriage. Homosexual couples choose to live as families.

Economic realities have forced many young adults back into the homes of their middle-aged parents. Over 20 percent of children today live in poverty and most of these children live in nontraditional families. More than 25 percent of all households consist of a single member because younger adults are marrying later in life and older adults choosing to live alone (Coontz, 1992; Hite, 1995; Mintz & Kellog, 1988).

There is an increasing awareness and acceptance of nontraditional family structures in society today. However, this acceptance of alternative forms of family is not universal. Critics of nontraditional family structures have voiced concerns that the family is in trouble and that families don't work. In answer to these critics, Coontz (1992) questions whether the families of the 1950s were ideal. If they were, why are so many Americans choosing *not* to emulate their families of origin? Nontraditional family forms call upon individuals to restructure the political climate of the family. Traditional families are questioning male dominance and hierarchical versus egalitarian family governance and decision making. Each type of family has its inherent strengths, problems, and possibilities. Patterns lived out in traditional families may not fit into the content of the new family.

Political Power

Political power within the family reflects the personal political power of its members. An individual possessing power in the community is perceived as possessing great personal power in other realms of living. It is very unlikely that any individual with decision-making power in business, institutions, or the community would have little power within his or her family.

Power within the family derives from several sources, and many different types of power operate within each family. Power may be real or perceived; however, the perception that power is centered in an individual is just as effective as the actual possession of power. Power within the family is the ability to influence decision making within the family, control resources, and alter the behavior of other family members.

Power derives from tangible and intangible sources. Tangible sources include commodities such as money and physical strength. Intangible sources include knowledge, self-esteem, and good judgment. Power within the family includes personal, social, parental, and conjugal power (Lamanna & Riedmann, 1988; Raven et al., 1975).

Social power is the power to influence others or inflict one's will on others. It is often derived from one's social and political roles. Social power is a function of occupation and education, knowledge, social position, and prestige. Social power often translates into personal power (Lamanna & Riedmann, 1988). However, a greater force is that of the social power of tradition. Culture influences the lifestyle of families and views of personal autonomy, significance, and responsibility, group structure, and family interaction. The influence of ethnic differences is most evident in immigrant families and is often muted as the family assimilates into the dominant culture. Family roles and tasks are influenced more by social class than by ethnicity (Paolucci, et al., 1997).

Social power within the family can take many forms. *Coercive power* is the ability to punish another person. Family members who believe that they will be punished if they do not obey another family member are relinquishing personal power to coercive power. *The power to reward* others with valued resources is a major source of power in families. In some families, parents reward children with economic resources for good behavior. A great source of power over a spouse is the ability to give or withhold money based on the other spouse's behavior. If a family member can provide valuable resources to other members, he or she has the power of rewarding others.

If a family member is believed to have *expert knowledge or information*, he or she will be given decision-making power over some aspects of family functioning. Power is also found in those with expertise, such as technical skill, knowledge, or information. Many families relegate the decision making about spending and saving money to the person with knowledge of finances.

As a function of fulfilling one's role, such as that of parent, one has *legitimate power*. *Referent power* derives from close association with another family member who has power in a particular realm of family functioning. An individual family member may closely align himself with another family member and emulate the other's beliefs, feelings, and behavior in order to gain personal power in the family. A child who is perceived by other siblings as being "Dad's favorite" possesses power over his siblings (Raven et al., 1975).

Personal power is the power each member possesses. Personal power derives from personal resources such as education, energy, occupation, physical strength, caring and nurturing, and money. Personal power influences the amount of power that an individual possesses in the conjugal relationship. Personal power leaves the door open for domination of one partner over the other.

RESOURCES

Resources defining personal power are not evenly distributed among cultures or between the sexes. Men most often bring the greatest occupational, educational, and financial resources into conjugal relationships even today. If resources are equal in new marriages, childbearing and childrearing can still place the woman in a dependent position (Lamanna & Riedmann, 1988).

Personal power is often centered in gender and traditionally and culturally defined. The head of the household is almost always designated as the male in the home, even in families where women may possess more social, political, and economic power. This societal norm translates into the roles women and men play within the family.

Tradition has defined sex roles within families, and in some families, spheres of influence are understood implicitly to rest within one sex. Women may choose to leave careers for childbearing. Women who work outside of the home have more power in the family's decision making (Lamanna & Riedmann, 1988). Even if a mother continues to work outside of the home, she may not have the time and energy needed to support or promote her political power within or outside of the family. The role of fathers in childrearing has increased over the past decades but has not reached that level assigned to women. The need of many women to maintain the marital bond for the security of the family unit to raise children places many women in a dependent role in the conjugal relationship.

Sources of Power

The source of power in any relationship derives from the need for love or acceptance by its members. A partner who depends on the other for his or her self-worth or emotional stability relegates great power to his or her partner. If children hold any power within the family, love and affection are the major resources from which they derive power. The intense love most parents have for their children gives children immense power in the family. Families choose where they will live based on the educational and safety needs of their children. Most families with children coordinate their leisure time and vacations around their children's school and activity schedules. Rituals and family traditions reach greater significance once children enter the family (Lamanna & Riedmann, 1988).

One function that has been almost entirely ascribed to women in the family is that of nurturing and caring. This function, although claimed as essential for family and community stability, has not always translated to increased power in conjugal relationships or family structures, except in limited areas of family functioning. Most often, this resource is perceived as a weakness within a power structure, making the member feel vulnerable to others.

Parental power is that power exerted by parents over their children. Within the United States, this power is almost absolute. Parents retain the legal, economic, and social right to control their children's lives (Hite, 1995). This unequal power is not questioned in the perspective of the social and political functions of the family to raise children and maintain order within society. Parents have the responsibility to provide for their dependent children and to control their social behavior. Satir (1988) proposed that this power should be used to guide children, not to control them.

Parental power has often been translated as complete power over children. Children with little personal, economic, or social resources have little power for negotiation. The increase in child abuse and neglect revolves around parents' violation of their parental, social, and personal power within families. Children, as well as fragile older adults, are often the victims of an adult's need to seize some kind of power in a world in which they feel otherwise powerless.

Another source of power in families is physical power. Men have greater strength than women and parents have more physical power than young children. Physical power may translate into physical abuse. Physical abuse in the family is facilitated by greater physical power; however, it reflects power inequalities in almost all resources. Women with personal, social, and economic power are less likely to stay in abusive relationships than women without such resources.

Resistance to Power

Unequal power within families caused by unequal distribution of resources challenges the decision-making ability of families and family cohesiveness. When there is unequal power within the conjugal relationship, suspicion and mistrust prevent intimacy in these relationships. Persons without power may submit to the authority or power of another family member, freely accept their lack of power in all realms of family functioning, or acknowledge the lack of power in specific situations. However, if a family member abuses his or her power, or if those without power resent their lack of power, behavior may develop to undermine another member's power. Most of this behavior is not articulated in the family's politics. Unable to challenge rules, family functioning, or policies with negotiation, members who perceive themselves as having little power may choose to use micromanipulation to achieve some level of control. If any resources are held by the least powerful they are rationed or denied in order to manipulate the individual in power. Even if a wife has few economic resources, she may possess enough influence by love and affection, which if withheld from a powerful spouse, becomes a powerful source of manipulation.

Rules are often developed by those possessing power to prevent the unequal members from challenging authority and power. Survival for members often involves only appearing to obey the rules. This type of behavior is often labeled as passive-aggressive behavior. Children who witness this behavior learn quickly how to deceive parents into believing that they are submitting to parents' rules and control.

Another reaction to perceived or real power imbalances within families is the formation of coalitions to seize more power. Children may band together to seek an advantage over the decision-making power of parents. A coalition of one parent with a child or children may be formed to counteract the perceived power of the other parent. This type of coalition severely threatens a strong conjugal relationship. A unified and stable parental coalition has long been cited as the strongest factor in successful parenting (Minuchin, 1982).

Personal Reflections: The Past

Our birth family or our family of origin is the first family to which we belong. It has considerable influence in determining how we construct family politics in those families that we form as adults. Children in most societies have little, if any, political or social power. In most societies they are considered the property of their parents, who assume total responsibility for their growth and development. Although this view of children is changing, most adults were raised in this political climate.

My Story

I grew up in an ethnic neighborhood composed of nuclear families. My parents married at a young age and had five children in seven years and one child seven years later. My father worked two jobs and we saw him at dinner each evening at 5:00 P.M. and on Sunday afternoons, when we went for a family drive. My mother did not work outside of the home. "Children should be seen and not heard" was the rule in our family. My father was the disciplinarian. I remember my father as having all the power and decision-making ability in the family at that time in my childhood. My mother reported our misbehavior and carried out any punishments he dictated.

Our family was not unlike most traditional patriarchal families. Decisions as to where our family would live, vacation, and spend money rested with my father. My mother maintained control of the household. Traditional families were typically antidemocratic and stress obedience, especially obedience to males (Hite, 1995). On the surface, we appeared like most families in our neighborhood. However, our lives changed dramatically the day we found out from a neighbor that my mother was divorcing my father.

My teenage years were spent living in a single-parent household. My mother's parental power and influence over our behavior was continually and often successfully challenged. During our later teenage years, we watched both of our parents remarry. We unwillingly became parts of two different blended families with stepbrothers and stepsisters. Some came to live with our mother, some with our father, others attempted to escape by marrying before completing high school. Neither of my parents' second marriages lasted more than two years. Those of us remaining at home became part of a single-parent family again.

We learned early about the politics of family life. We witnessed power shifts and learned how to form coalitions and how to align ourselves for survival. What we failed to learn in our family of origin was how to negotiate rather than seize power, how to influence with love and respect rather than with fear, and how to be an egalitarian type of family with power spread over the generations.

These patterns influence the operations of the family and the rules by which they function. Family patterns are often idiosyncratic and buried in years of explicit and implicit family negotiations. Most family patterns are supported to maintain the stability of the system, and any massive change is perceived as a threat and is challenged (Laing, 1971). Many families live behind a wall of secrecy. "Family life is something like an iceberg: most people are aware of only about one-tenth of what is going on—the tenth that they can see and hear" (Satir, 1988).

Change

The family has undergone significant changes over the past 40 years. Fewer modern families resemble a traditional family, with a husband, wife, and biological or adopted children living under one roof (Mintz & Kellog, 1988).

Dramatic changes in family structure and power have occurred since the turn of the century. More women work outside of the home; couples are marrying later and having fewer, if any, children. There is less emphasis today on obedience in childrearing. Fewer women are forced to remain in marriages for economic and security reasons (Goldscheider & Waite, 1991).

Families are becoming more egalitarian. Power is distributed more equally among family members. The burden of financial responsibility for the family is now often shared by the adult partners. Childrearing, household purchases, and lifestyle decisions are often shared by both partners. Children today are included in some of the decisions affecting family lifestyle.

These changes have been partially encouraged by women who believe they are effective managers, not only of their own lives but of their family's welfare. Women are receiving increased political power outside of the home, in the political arena, in the workplace, and in social institutions. The employment of women is increasingly influencing how families live their lives. Women are beginning to pursue personal goals independent of the goals they have for their families. Women are entering relationships today expecting an egalitarian decision-making process. When these expectations are not met, some women choose to leave the relationship. Today, individuals are less likely to stay in a family out of a sense of duty, loneliness, or hopelessness than they were two decades ago. Some men have welcomed these changes and gladly relinquished the need to assume total responsibility for the financial security of their families. Many men have assumed some responsibility for the emotional stability of their families.

Despite these advances, most individuals from two-parent families still perceive women (their mothers) as receiving second-class treatment from their fathers (Hite, 1995). Society has traditionally concentrated power in the hands of those with the most economic influence. As family structure reflects societal changes, so does the power structure of the family. Society places value in economic success and prowess. Women, although making strides, are not the economic peers of their male partners in most families. The model of equality for women is in the hearts of many but not always translated to actions (Satir, 1988).

My Family

As I have created my present family with my husband and son, I have struggled with many of the issues facing most women today. In the beginning years of my marriage, I was content to let my husband make the major decisions as to where we would live, how we would raise our children, and how we would spend our leisure time. Later, questioning his authority created conflict. Renegotiating these earlier patterns of being a family has not always been successful. But new and more rewarding patterns are emerging.

The Future

Most of us have been members of different families and family types. Our roles and expectations about family dynamics change as we grow and mature. We are beginning to witness a change in how children are perceived within families, and their power and influence on family lifestyles are increasing. Once merely the property of parents, children are increasingly seen as having individual rights. Despite the slow change, children remain at the mercy of their parents for their physical and emotional growth and survival. Children are witnesses to the politics of their birth family.

More and More

The acceptance of the power of women is slowly becoming a reality. As a society, we are beginning to define and label physical and emotional abuse in the family. We are now beginning to denounce this abuse. We are redefining family, love, and friendship. Family democracy is replacing old hierarchical models of family functioning. Family structure is being redefined—from a rigid, hierarchical, heterosexual, reproductive framework to an ethical, egalitarian, democratized structure. A family framework that provides rights, responsibilities, and power to all of its members is becoming a reality in many modern families (Hite, 1995).

A structure in which all members have power and influence over the family will be realized when all members become equal partners in family decision making. Children must be progressively guided to make decisions about their own activities within a defined arena. As children grow, they should assume a political role within the family. They become part of the decision making about family rules and policies. Through this they learn to bargain, negotiate, and compromise. These skills create strong individuals and strong families.

A strong and united family learns to cope with crises rather than putting all of its energy into preventing crises. Strong, secure individuals contribute to strong families. Children and adults who feel powerful within their family will become powerful influences within their communities.

Families are places to develop people who learn to treat themselves and others with dignity. Families teach us how to connect, survive, and develop intimacy. Families are our first teachers of the rules of politics.

References

Coontz, S. (1992). *The Way We Never Were*. New York: Basic Books.

Goldscheider, F. K., and Waite, L. J. (1991). *New Families: No Families*. Berkley, Calif.: University of California Press.

Hite, S. (1995). *The Hite Report on the Family*. New York: Grove Press.

Laing, R. D. (1971). *The Politics of the Family*. New York: Pantheon Books.

Lamanna, M. A., and Riedmann, A. (1988). *Marriage and Making Family Choices*. Belmont, Calif.: Wadsworth.

Mead, M., and Heyman, K. (1965). *Family*. New York: Macmillan.

Mintz S., and Kellog, (1988). *American Family Life*. New York: Free Press.

Minuchin, S. (1982). *Families and Family Therapy*. Cambridge, Mass.: Harvard University Press.

Paolucci, B., and Hall, 0. A. (1997). *Family Decision-Making Ecosystem Approach*. New York: John Wiley & Sons.

Raven, B. H., Center, R., and Rodrigues, A. (1975). The basis of conjugal power. In R. Cromwell and D. H. Olson (eds.), *Power in Families*. New York: Sage Publications.

Satir, V. (1988). *The New People Making*. Mountainview, Calif.: Science & Behavior Books.

Scanzoni, J., and Szinovacz, M. (1980). *Family Decision Making: Developmental Sex-Role Model*. Beverly Hills, Calif.: Sage Publications.

Winch, R. F. (1971). *The Modern Family* (3d ed.). New York: Holt, Rinehart & Winston.

CHAPTER 7

PREPARING MODERN PRACTITIONERS FOR POSTMODERN FAMILIES

Sherry Hartman

POSTMODERNISM DEFINED

Recent discussions about the family in the literature have included changing family patterns with expanded, more inclusive, and less traditional definitions of family. These family changes have emerged concurrently with society's departure from the modern world of the industrial age into what is now frequently called the postmodern age.

The term *postmodernism* has been of interest in a variety of fields partly because it brings focus to major transformations taking place in contemporary culture. Some scholarship has included postmodernism in relation to families, but in other areas it has been neglected or paid only slight attention. If postmodern insights occur with frequency across the human and social sciences, their relevance to families in general is important as well.

Practice with families and understanding of families may be moving into the future with outdated assumptions about "reality" and the realities of families in particular. This may be the case especially for those attempting to practice in more inclusive, holistic ways. The potential for dialogue in rectifying this absence is imminent.

POSTMODERNISM AND FAMILIES

To begin understanding postmodernism in relevant contexts, it is useful to summarize some recent descriptions of postmodern family life and follow with an account of developments in postmodern thought related to family therapy.

Adapted from S. Hartman, Preparing modern nurses for postmodern families, *Journal of Holistic Nursing*, 9 (4):110–118, 1995.

The balance of this chapter provides descriptions, in a postmodern vein, of vital roles that can be taken in understanding and working with families.

Everyday Life in the Postmodern Family

The days are past when family members could be assumed to share highly congruent outlooks, values, and beliefs about themselves and the rest of the world. The postmodern family can be depicted by a metaphor of the individual and family trying to stay afloat in an increasingly elaborate "cultural soup." The ingredients for this postmodern soup consist of pluralism, democracy, religious freedom, consumerism, mobility, and increasing access to news and entertainment. As technology has shrunk the physical world, it has expanded and made complex the individual experience of the cultural and social worlds.

Individuals are personally connected to significantly more people and varied ways of life, stretching over wider geographical space. Embedded in an unprecedented multiplicity of relationships, one is offered an exciting but daunting mélange of worldviews, beliefs, and realities. To turn on the radio, view a movie, open the newspaper, receive a fax, correspond by e-mail, or look at the late-night news is to become immersed in the other.

We come to understand the opinions, values, fears, doubts, needs, aspirations, and personalities of movie stars, concentration camp survivors, champion athletes, strippers, African famine victims, Nobel Prize winners, AIDS activists, feminist authors, Chinese students. We listen, empathize, and absorb. We gain the potential for understanding the opinions, appreciating the possibilities, and experiencing the feelings of thousands of peoples whose very existence our grandparents, or even our parents, could scarcely have imagined. In effect, we become copulated by others and acquire an infinity of fragmentary and often competing selves.

The new context in which we find ourselves can be contrasted with what we left behind. Gone are the clear directions offered by premodern times, in which people saw themselves mirrored in the details of their world. The psyche was anchored in the myths of the cosmos and each person had a clear role and reason for being. There were few struggles about identity and belief. Gone, as well, is the relative simplicity of modern life in which the individual lost connection to a greater cosmos as the rational self became the bearer of value.

The project of the Western modern era was truth, freedom, and autonomy gained through control and rational order. The self could have many parts, but identity had to be integrated and ordered.

The New Worldview

In contrast to what has gone before, a society enters postmodernism when it is forced to see that there are many beliefs, multiple realities, and a profusion of worldviews. Faith in absolute truth is weakened. Adaptive members become multiply epistemological, able to find validation, relevance, and meaning in various ways. Some seem to enjoy the new freedom, while some try to escape it. Some feel weakened by the ambiguity, seeing fragmentation, disintegration, meaninglessness, vagueness, and social chaos generating deep uncertainty about what, if anything, is real.

There seems less likelihood of drawing objective conclusions about anything. For each person, ethnic group, community, political group, and economic class, little if anything counts as truth outside its own idiosyncratic, partial views. These changes raise the possibility that the emerging character of family life will be described as an increasing vulnerability to what is called the *saturated family*.

Four characteristics of such families can be identified: chaos and discontinuity, ambiguous boundaries, blurred ideals, and a weakened capacity to solve conflict. Saturated families are populated by individuals who no longer believe in themselves as singular, autonomous individuals. So many pieces have been assembled to construct the self that the pieces no longer fit well together and may even contradict each other.

Moving from one relationship and worldview to another produces a self in continuous alteration. Available technology gives members the opportunity to be in various states of mind and motion at will. Everyday household life becomes an intersection of multiple lives, arousing a sense of fragmentation, as if the members of the family were being scattered by the centrifugal force of postmodern life.

In addition to this pervasive, contemporary, and almost unremarkable chaos, many family members belong to what can be labeled as a floating family, a formless array of familial relationships in a continuous state of flux. Boundaries become porous as family-like relationships develop with work colleagues, the child's day-care worker and baby-sitter, a friend across the continent who counsels by e-mail, club members, covolunteers on service projects, and classmates.

Ties are developed that extend and change the web of significant others. Feelings of closeness come and go with changing circumstances. While a designated family is physically together, any number of them may feel not quite present, alienated, emotionally absorbed by other attachments and wishing they were with people who really knew them. The structural fragility of family relationships is due to dependence on voluntary commitments, which can be modified, broken, or abandoned as interests change.

Of Family Life Values

The variety of viable pictures of family life have challenged any exclusive rights to exemplify a correct image of the traditional family. With this loss of a sense of the proper family has come a blurring of ideals. The virtues of the traditional are becoming less easy to see, especially in the images portrayed by the media as they explore the marginalized and parody the mainstream. In a continual quest for variety, the media also tarnish the image of the traditional family and values associated with it through sheer repetition.

In the family so described, there is more vulnerability to conflict. Relating to others slowly transforms our identities; the more others there are, the more we are transformed and the further away from home geographically, emotionally, and intellectually we find our relationships, the greater the potential for quarrels in our family of birth.

Mutual standards for solving conflict vanish with the decline of shared realities and of agreed-upon values and moral ideals to guide judgments. The former refuge of accord and shared perceptions becomes instead a place of collision and contested meanings. Members are divided by gender, choice of lover, education, family of birth, political beliefs, spiritual beliefs, work settings, and childhood community. Standoffs are made more difficult to solve.

Power

Power defined modern and premodern families, with parents (usually fathers) as the traditional decision makers. But postmodern family members have been exposed to the conflicts, doubts, weaknesses, and uncertainties of adults and other authorities. Television especially has seen to it that children lose trust and confidence in authority as they are exposed to the myths of adult wisdom and competence.

It is easy to see why a return to the traditional family has been a strong rallying cry for many of today's political candidates. But short of moving to a deserted island, the majority must learn to live in the postmodern family and world.

It can be pointed out that postmodernism itself is a repudiation of the belief that the contemporary experience is just a temporary phase of disorganization that will be reordered and then rationally progress toward some resolution.

Rather, the mélange of contradictions that indicate a postmodern family seem likely to remain with us indefinitely, perhaps even grow. Communication and media experts tell us daily that our present capabilities for relating electronically and expanding our connections to others are only the beginning. Nostalgia for former modern and premodern families is probably overly sentimental.

Health-care professionals are well aware of the multiple problems that have existed in the authoritarian, oppressive, inflexible, sexist, and intellectually stultifying modern family. What has been lost are the ideals associated with it: safety, security, dependability, a sense of rootedness, and the availability of an unquestioned source of truth and values.

Modernism and Family Therapy

Merely describing the social situations out of which postmodern families emerge is not sufficient for preparing the modern person to work with these families. It further requires providing at least a rudimentary familiarity with how postmodern approaches in the social sciences have influenced the exploration and explanation of those very families.

For those who think more easily along modern lines, it requires turning around one's thought processes. A usual place to start in this undertaking is with the modern tradition from which postmodernism emerged and against which it reacts.

Modernism was itself a critique of the moral certainty of metaphysics (a reality beyond day-to-day experience) and religious truth of the Victorian era. But the critique did not divest modern thought of the notion of true and universal knowledge, as sought though science.

Family theory, especially theories of family systems, is a product of the mid-twentieth-century modernist social science culture. Early family theories focused on the microenvironment of family interactions and processes. Cybernetics provided a sophisticated model for intricately analyzing these processes. The focus was on minute instances of actual family interactions while particularities of race, culture, ethnicity, and gender were ignored.

This approach fulfilled the desire for purity, order, and clarity inherent in the modernist value placed on the ability to reduce (by reason and logic) a complex phenomena to manageable elements. Analytic abstraction was valued in the embrace of reason and logic as a universal human mode of thinking.

The search for universals continued in the form of structuralism sustained by the belief that there was a basic form to all families regardless of context waiting to be charted. Structuralists believed that all healthy families exhibited objective organizational patterns, like clear boundaries between parental and child subsystems, unambiguous divisions of functions within the family, system differentiation, hierarchies, and boundaries, through which children were socialized and achieved adult identity.

Structural family therapists emphasized the system over the individual. The idea of a universal organizational pattern in families presupposed something "out there" separate from the direct experience of individuals. By positing something beyond personal experience the metaphysics rejected by modernism was continued but not acknowledged.

In the modernist view, the one who held the knowledge and ability to delineate and relate these parts of the family also held the responsibility and power for establishing goals and direction for families in need. In family theory such beliefs also find expression in the constructivist movement, which argues that objective descriptions of both microlevel family processes and underlying family structures are illusory.

Family reality for constructivists is a social construction with no facts that exist independent of human perception and invention. Constructivism in family therapy has led therapists to be more interested in narrative and the stories that families tell about themselves than in underlying family structures. Stories can be reconstructed and coconstructed with others.

Postmodernism Themes

Themes that can be found in postmodernism include diversity and multiplicity; relativity; a focus on the language of discourses; suspicion and skepticism about claims to certainty, knowledge, and all encompassing worldviews;

questions regarding modern claims to progress and superiority over all; and a move away from the obvious to focus on what has escaped attention such as the marginal, ignored, decentered, and powerless.

Development in family therapy related to postmodern themes has signaled an end to purely, reductionist systems thinking and a recognition of the larger family context; a trend toward eclecticism in interventions; greater interest in the meaning, narrative, and history of stories told by families; a rethinking of the role of the therapist as a neutral, authoritative expert; and a reflection on the purposes and consequences of therapy.

The Postmodern Model

Postmodernism is particularly suspicious of grand or all-encompassing claims of modern thought referred to as *metanarratives*, or *metavocabularies*. These are vocabularies that seek to "rise above the plurality of appearances in the hope that, seen from the heights, an unexpected unity will become evident; a unity which is a sign that something real has been glimpsed, something which stands behind the appearances and produces them." (Rorty, p. 12)

Postmodern critiques reveal how useless those final vocabularies are, which indulge in patterns of ideas that seek to express, convey, grasp, or define something ultimate or total. Modern discourse makes claims about the scientific mind. By means of order, progress, objective knowledge, and the human capacity for reason, observation, prediction, and control we can have certainty and intellectual authority. The voice of objective truth will prevail.

It is this discourse that has been a target of postmodern critique. This critique aims not at an alternative set of assumptions, but rather at registering the impossibility of establishing any such underpinning for knowledge.

The postmodern condition of uncertainty arrives as the modern discourse deconstructs. Similarly, modern discourses of the family deconstruct and leave the family as largely a product of its culture's habits of thinking in certain linguistic patterns about relationships.

Postmodernism and Family Therapy

Connections between the postmodern approach and holistic practice with families are more than possible—they are desirable. As noted above, the postmodern critique of modernism was a response to reductionist, mechanistic beliefs and the theories following from those beliefs. Interest in holistic approaches grew out of a recognition that particularistic approaches were not adequate or desirable for understanding many human phenomena.

In health care, holistic thinking regarding health and healing was a reaction to the reduction of human systems to disease and deficit categories in medical science models. Placing practice with families in a postmodern context is placing it safely within the purview of holism.

The following draws inspiration from the work of Guba and Lincoln (1987), who delineated the roles of the "fourth-generation evaluator." Those roles were based on evaluation models sharing a belief in value pluralism. Practice roles with families that are congruent with postmodernism share many similarities to those Guba and Lincoln attributed to fourth-generation evaluators.

ROLE PERSPECTIVES

The following roles are believed to be most relevant when the family is the unit of care, that is, when a family system focus is adopted. They will also be useful in those family applications in which either the family or the individual is the focus of care with the other becoming the context for the focus.

Technical Roles

The practitioner retains the technical functions often associated with the helping process, but these are carried out in new ways. Traditionally, practitioners have been viewed as knowledgeable about the relevant foci for assessing dimensions of family health and health processes. They are also considered to be familiar with, and proficient in, the use of the various techniques and instruments for observing, collecting, and analyzing valid and reliable data about the family, as well as in devising intervention plans that meet the professional standards of colleagues. But when practitioners are caring for postmodern families, the focus of activity becomes the claims, concerns, and issues raised by multiple and competing family members, and these are far from predictable.

Practitioners must see themselves as the most accessible and valuable form of instrumentation. If the situation is made complex by diversity and multiple claims, then practitioners must rely on their abilities to collect, organize, prioritize, and analyze by continuously processing data. They must see themselves as capable of reacting rapidly and flexibly to competing issues and situations.

Description Roles

Practitioners play a major role in meeting families' needs to have situations clarified and information shared. Adopting a postmodern approach alters this activity from an objective scientific mode to one closer to an illuminative and historical mode. In this approach, skills are employed not in telling but rather in suggesting and cocreating. These are skills not for fixing images, providing insights, clarifying boundaries, or prescribing tasks but for illuminating scenes, for helping families to appreciate new meanings and to rectify problems.

For example, in helping a family cope with chronic disease a practitioner may become a literary consultant who "uses new language forms, letters and questions to stimulate the family's imagination and liberate it from stale plot lines." (Doherty, 1991) The practitioner's descriptions can instill expectations and counter negative impressions, allowing the family to view itself not as a flawed and disabled group of people but as a healthy unit struggling against a difficult outside problem.

Decision-Making Roles

Ideally, the stance that practitioners have always taken with families eschews the role of judge in favor of a collaborative role, with the families making decisions, especially those involving values.

The practitioner's role enlarges when engaged with postmodern families because of the pluralism and complexity. The role for many becomes more like a mediator of the judgment process. Action can often be taken only after some compromise or consensus is reached. A skilled practitioner is in a position to be an orchestrator because of his or her interactions with all family members and, presumably, because of having gained the family's trust.

Teacher-Learner Roles

Teacher-learner roles are interrelated, with the practitioner moving back and forth between them. Early on, the practitioner has little knowledge regarding any family members, what constructions and values they hold, or what claims, concerns, and issues may be operative in the family.

The learner role is one of having an open posture and of soliciting information. Predictions are impossible and questions only exploratory. As insights, understandings, and initial constructions of one's own are gained, the role becomes one of teacher, postmodern-style, as these tentative constructions are shared not only with family members from whom they came but also with other members. Thus the practitioner teaches family members about themselves, about each other, as well as about herself. The difference these roles take when working with the postmodern family is both in the content and methods. Out of multiple interests and contacts family members bring their own expertise based on their different sources. Unique areas of expertise and dispersed knowledge make learning more egalitarian. A broader, increasingly varied understanding of their world and context is gained and in a more participative way.

Reality-Sharer Roles

While constructions and stories from members initially reflect only their perceptions and values, the practitioner, in teaching and sharing them with other family members, will reshape and modify them. Thus the practitioner and family members actually produce family health outcomes through their interrelationship. Outcomes are better conceived and more comprehensive when informed by the perspective of all participants.

Mediator and Change-Maker Roles

Change in a modernist, developmental sense implies a movement to some preferable state, in other words, movement toward a goal. Traditionally, models conceptualize such goals as consensual units representing the best interests of all members. In contrast, the situation in which postmodern families most often find themselves is one of goal conflict and multiple views of reality. Their potential for agreeing on the true and the good is slight.

Family practice literature addresses the need to consider conflicts between practitioner and family values when family consensus is not in question; but little is said about negotiating goals with family members whose values may remain in conflict. The practitioner as change agent can present his situational knowledge of each family member's interests as though it were a case study that includes an agenda for negotiation. "Findings" (constructions; value positions; and data relevant to stated claims, concerns, and issues) provide the avenue to consensus on needed change and goals.

Political-Activist Roles

Postmodern thinkers are sometimes criticized for relativizing all values, leaving caregivers without justification for the causes they think worth advocating. Practitioners often have goals they strongly prefer and pursue, for example, the improvement of their profession. They also have preferences about fulfilling their roles as citizens. It is possible, in relation to families, for postmodern approaches to ignore or deny the relevance of material reality, history, and power.

Constructivist approaches, related in some ways to postmodernism, can be difficult to apply in situations involving the use of power. If the reality created by family members and carrying its own meaning is viewed as only an interpretive description, then are attributions of meaning by each family member of equal value?

Consider an example from family life with an abuser. It seems difficult not to believe that the abused wife or child's story is more likely to reflect an accurate account than the limited story of the abuser. Is relativity in postmodernism so pervasive as not to allow practitioners such preferences? Morals and values do not escape conditions of contingency. However, according to Fish (1993), "The value of narrative/conversational techniques would not be diminished by situating their use within theories which also addressed material context, history, and the use and abuse of power."

The role of political activism recognizes that family members do not make their stories and narratives just as they please, but are constrained by the larger discourses. These discourses are often thought to be oppressive and harmful. Practitioners must begin to recognize discourses that are harmful to the family, to individuals in families, or to practitioners' work with families, and work politically to eliminate them.

Self-Reflexivity Role

A core requisite for the postmodern stance, self-reflexivity may more rightly be called an attitude rather than a role. It requires practitioners to acknowledge their own influence and authority in creating narratives related to families and health. To be unaware and thus refrain from speaking is in itself taking a stance.

Like therapists, when practitioners are "unaware of the embeddedness of their views and how they participate in discursive practices, they are unlikely to be open to alternatives that are being obscured." (Hare-Mustin, p. 33) Self-reflexivity involves allowing oneself to create new visions to challenge assumptions of harmful and oppressive dominant discourses. It is a postmodern awareness and posture. Lastly, the role involves modeling and encouraging reflexivity in family members.

Conclusion

Practitioners who work with families will increasingly be working with some families too complex to characterize within language familiar either to them or the families. It is helpful to describe some of these families as postmodern.

With greater frequency, today's families live in unfamiliar situations that challenge many of the assumptions that practitioners have learned and practiced. Finding new tools by which to describe the complexities of these families and their contexts will further practitioners' efforts to create health outcomes meaningful to all members.

Those who prefer holistic approaches may best collaborate with families, in times to come, by virtue of their familiarity with postmodern strategies.

References

Allen, D. (1986). Nursing and oppression: "The family" in nursing texts. *Feminist Teacher,* 2(1):15.

Bellah, R. (1991). Bring along your compass. *Family Therapy Networker,* 15(5):53–55.

Bouley, G., von Hofe, K., and Blatt, L. (1994). Holistic care of the critically ill: Meeting both patient and family needs. *Dimensions of Critical Care Nursing,* 12(4):218–223.

Cheal, D. (1993). Unity and difference in postmodern families. *Journal of Family Issues,* 14(1):5–19.

DiNicola, V. F. (1993). The postmodern language of therapy: At the nexus of culture and family. *Journal of Systemic Therapies,* 12(1):49–63

Doherty, W. J. (1991). Family therapy goes postmodern. *Family Therapy Networker,* 15(5):37–42.

Eng, E., and Salmond, M. E. (1992). Community empowerment: The critical base for primary care. *Family and Community Health,* 13(1):112–123.

Fish, V. (1993). Poststructuralism in family therapy: Interrogating the narrative/conversational mode. *Journal of Marital and Family Therapy*, 19(3):221–232.

Gergen, K. J. (1992). The postmodern adventure. *Family Therapy Neworker.* 1992; 52–57.

Gergen, K. J. (1991). The saturated family. *Family Therapy Networker,* 15(5):27–35.

Guba, K. G., and Lincoln, Y. S. (1987). The cournernenances of fourth-generation evaluation: Description, judgement and negotiation. In D. I. Palumbo (ed.), *The Politics of Program Evaluation*. London: Sage Publications.

Hare-Mustin, R. T. (1994). Discourses in the mirrored room: A postmodern analysis of therapy. *Family Process,* 33:19–35.

Larkin, D., and Zahourek, R. P. (1988). Therapeutic storytelling and metaphors, *Holistic Nursing Practice,* 2(3):45–53.

Minuchin, S. (1991). The seductions of constructivism. *Family Therapy Networker,* 15(5):47–50.

O'Hara, M., and Anderson, W. T. (1991). Welcome to the postmodern world. *Family Therapy Networker,* 15(5):19–25.

Rorty, R. (1989). *Contingency, Irony and Solidarity.* New York: Cambridge University Press: 12.

Rosenau, P. M. (1992).*Postmodernism and the Social Sciences: Insights, Inroads, and Intrusions.* Princeton, N.J.: Princeton University Press.

Stacey, J. (1990). *Brave New Families.* New York: Basic Books.

Wright, L. M., and Leahey, M. (1993). Trends in nursing of families. In G. D. Wegner, and R. J. Alexander (eds.), *Readings in Family Nursing*. Philadelphia: Lippincott.

VOICES THREE

Family Rituals

Carolyn Brown wrote this poem to her husband on his 53rd birthday.

My Love at 53

Hello, my love of so many years,
of pleasures and pains,
of joys and sorrows,
of ups and downs,
like quicksilver changing,
life is like that.

In a moment, the flood of tender caring and cherishing and enfolding
with laughter and joy
joined.

And torn asunder the next
by anger and fear and frustration as
seeing self and you,
all of a piece,

I see myself in you,
in us,
and sometimes not a pretty sight,
and sometimes a time of celebration
and beauty,
with all that we have become . . .
and can be.

I see us, and you,
in our son
struggling so hard to become
who he is,
striving to be like you . . .
acting like you,
loving you and
treasuring each golden moment
of your love and positive regard . . .
and the next moment becoming opposite to all that you hold dear,
and the pain in your very center is clear to me.

I see your hands,
wide and capable,
holding with tenderness
stroking with gentle firmness,
calming my roiling soul
with warmth and strength.

I feel your voice,
concern touching as surely as hands laid on to heal,
arms encircling
with feather firmness.

I know your eyes,
pulling me into your self,
gray green brown,
golden flecks of sunlight
sparkling with the warm fire
of your pleasure,
dulled by the pain of oppressive,
depressive moments,
glowing in a moment of tenderness,
crinkles at corners,
pulling me into your love.

I sense your mouth
warm, soft, gentle is a kiss,
then razor-sharp line containing your being,
your thoughts, feelings, anger in a prison of self,
keeping close within,
letting no secret out,
protecting.

And then, in a moment,
open with laughter,
quirky, lurky smile on all the corners
opening your love.

Who are you my love?
Do I know who you are?
The secret parts of yourself are closed off
in Scorpio darkness . . .
The free, open parts hint at an expanse of self
unknown
to self,
to me.

I love you in the dance that is us . . .
moving together
apart
ascending and plunging
striking the balance
of our love.

Happy birthday
my love!!

i love you
november 16, 1991
carolyn brown
wife, lover, friend, partner

CHAPTER 8

FOOD AND MY FAMILY

Joan DiPasquale Davis

Your nutrition can determine how you look, act, and feel; whether you are grouchy or cheerful, homely or beautiful, physiologically and psychologically young or old; whether you think clearly or are confused, enjoy your work or make it a drudgery, increase your earning power or stay in an economic rut.

—C. W. *Suitor and* M. *Crowley*

FOOD

If there is any truth in that statement, then how, when, and where do we develop these nutritional behaviors? As we enter the 21st century, I wonder if anyone really takes the time to reflect upon what food means to them or their families.

When I think about the meaning of food to my family, it brings back memories of my childhood in the early 1940s. I was only 3 or 4 years old, but I remember my father coming home from work with some kind of sweet treat for me in his lunchbox. He would always whisper to me, "If you have been a good girl, I have something special for you, but you can't tell your sisters." Sugar was scarce during the early part of World War II, so this was really very special. I guess that's why I still feel the need to reward myself with something sweet now and then. By the way, years later when my sisters and I discussed the "hard times" of the war, I found out they had treats in their lunchboxes as well!

FOOD AND ITS MEANING

Food, then, was a treat and made us feel special. I remember the good foods, but most of all I remember the meaningful time the family spent at dinner sharing and discussing the day's events. All was usually quite pleasant as long as my middle sister and I didn't break into uncontrollable giggles about something and get sent to bed without dinner. I recall that the foods we ate were quite varied. In her younger years, my mother had worked for a Jewish family and had learned to cook many of their cultural dishes, as well as American and Italian foods. Naturally, with my father being from Alabama, we also had a lot of good old "down-home cooking." Breakfast and lunch were different. We were all pretty much on our own, since we all had different places to go at different times.

When I married, I took many of the family food traditions along but tried to make holidays even more special than I remembered. I baked cookies, candies, and special dishes and invited all my siblings and their families to celebrate with us. As someone with a sweet tooth and a history of constantly watching my weight, I always found that baking and cooking served as a labor of love and self-control therapy for me. Although all of our children thought the "goodies" were the greatest, to me it was the togetherness that made the foods so special.

Today, with only my husband and myself at home (he is retired, but I still work), we eat out most evenings. Breakfast is our special meal at home where we share the day's agenda. My food choices today are also quite different from what they used to be. My husband tells everyone that I'm "fat-free" and he's "fat-full." To me that's the way the world in the 21st century appears to be heading, toward a healthy awareness of what food means to the body. Family togetherness, love, and sharing do not appear to be as important to people as they once were.

Other Opinions

To uncover the meaning of food in other families today, I spoke with several people who represent various cultures. Here's what they had to say.

Thomas

Thomas is a 65-year-old family man of Welsh origin and the father of three. He remembered family meals as being eventful, talking about the family business and all, but his family "lived to eat."

His mom was a very good cook. She cooked nourishing foods, sometimes food they actually liked to eat. He stated that back then there was no such thing as low cholesterol, low fat, low sodium. Thomas's mom made a lot of goulash, meatloaf, hamburgers, potatoes, and things of that sort. He really doesn't recall eating much fish or lobster because the family didn't live near good fishing locations. Of course, they always had dessert!

Eating out was the real treat for the family. Sometime they drove 40 or 50 miles to a restaurant. Everything on the menu was pretty much made with ground beef. They didn't call the sandwiches hamburgers but that's what he thinks they were. It really didn't matter to Thomas—just being together was wonderful.

After he married, things changed. He worked late so many evenings that his wife fed the children early and then ate with him later. The family didn't get to eat too many meals together, except on Sundays. When the children were all grown and gone, his wife either ate early by herself or waited for him to come home, which was sometimes rather late. He states that now he "eats to live" and that's probably why he has never had a weight problem. When he's going to eat out, he thinks more about food because eating out is still a special occasion for him, especially visiting other countries and experimenting with the different foods.

Thomas believes that times have really changed. According to him, foods that are fat-free, cholesterol-free, sodium-free, and so forth are definitely not the foods he prefers, but he does try to watch his sodium and cholesterol. He states that the 21st century probably will bring a lot of health consciousness about food as well as changes in the food itself.

Things have changed so much from his childhood days. There are more fast foods and less family time together.

Jane

Jane, a 45-year-old Irish-American woman, is married with two children. She commented that food to her family means sustenance, a necessity of life, and, unfortunately, pleasure. Jane considers herself overweight. Her family enjoys eating but the real meaning of food is in the togetherness.

Meal time is a time of love and sharing. Sadly, according to Jane, they don't get to enjoy too many meals together since the children have gotten older. The children are all pretty much going their own way, but she and her husband still take time for dinner together.

When Jane was growing up, meals were very stressful for her because her mother always demanded that everything on the plate be eaten whether she liked it or not. She recalls one time when she stared at her plate for three hours because she didn't like the food. Her mother said she could not waste food because people were starving all over the world. For Jane, mealtime was an unpleasant time with food being a form of punishment, for what she did not know. She believes now that her mother may have had a pretty rough childhood.

Jane raised her children quite differently from the way she was raised. Fortunately, her children both liked vegetables, so she didn't have that worry. Her daughter still only eats half of what she takes, but Jane feels that's all right. Jane believes that she herself is overweight because of the meaning of food her mother instilled in her as a child. Today her feelings about food have certainly changed from those of her mother's, and the meaning of food to her children in the 21st century is likely to change as well, since nothing seems to stay the same. After talking to Jane, I realized that I may have been a mother like hers. I wanted my children to eat healthy, balanced meals, so they always had to eat a small amount of everything that I put on their plate. That's the way I was raised. I also heard all the stories about the starving people all over the world and passed that on to my children. Now, when I observe how my children are raising their children, I wonder how much I contributed to their strengths and limitations regarding food. There are not too many family mealtimes in their homes except on holidays. Family members just eat whenever they feel like it.

Rosa

Rosa is a 50-year-old divorced Mexican American with two grown children. One child lives at home and the other one lives close to her and is planning to marry later this year.

Rosa stated that she absolutely loves food so much that her mother used to say, "Rosa, most people eat to live, you live to eat." Rosa loves to cook and is constantly planning meals. She remembers when she was young, her mother would be cooking dinner and she'd be asking what they were having for the next meal. Her mom would laugh and say, "Let's get through this meal first, Rosa."

According to Rosa, no one could cook like her mom, and while the rest of her family liked to eat, none of them liked to eat as much as she did. Rosa recalls that even though her mom worked, she'd always have eggs and homemade breads or something ready for breakfast so that everyone could help themselves. Rosa generally came home from school at lunchtime and fixed herself something to eat, but it was always so great to come home after school and find her mom cooking dinner.

Dinner was always a special time for her family. They would talk and share the daily happenings. When Rosa got older, her mom still kept the old Mexican custom of the family eating Sunday dinner together. She enjoyed that because her mom always cooked special Mexican foods for the family. Rosa states that food meant a great deal to her growing up in the 1950s and 1960s.

Raising her girls was not the same experience. It was difficult to cook for them. They wanted none of the traditional Mexican foods. Her daughter Rial had food allergies, so Rosa would cook hotdogs for her one week, hamburgers the next week, toasted cheese the following week, and so on. Rial seemed to enjoy eating even if it was only one particular favorite dish at a time.

Lolita, her other daughter, was very fussy, but Rosa didn't argue with her; she just cooked whatever Lolita would eat, even if it was only half of a hamburger. Lolita still eats like that today. She probably wouldn't even eat if she didn't have to stay alive. Rosa stated that she and her girls don't get to eat as many meals together as when she was growing up, but she insists that they all eat together on Sunday evenings.

Her mom is dead now but her dad and his fiancée come to dinner. Rosa believes that family togetherness is very important. She does like to go out to eat occasionally, but she is very particular about the food she eats. When she goes out to eat, she wants good food. Rosa states that because she's Mexican and so short, she has to watch her weight constantly. She refuses to allow herself to go over a size 5. She states that when she pushes the limit, she cuts back. Her sisters eat everything, and although they aren't fat, Rosa believes that they need to start watching because it's harder to lose weight when you're older.

Rosa believes that it is unfortunate that food has lost its meaning for many people. Mothers don't have the time—or don't take the time—to cook anymore or to preserve their culture and special family times. She thinks that food in the 21st century will mean even less than it does today.

Steve

Steve is a 20-year-old single white American man. To him, food means nourishment for the body. He grew up with working parents, so he did not experience family meals and discussions of "the problems of the day." The only time he remembers any real family meals was when he visited his grandparents on weekends and on holidays in the early 1970s. His grandparents died within a year of each other in the mid-1970s and so did his experiences with family meals.

Steve recalls many times when his friends couldn't go places with him because they had to be home at mealtime. He thought this was completely ridiculous. Why would anyone want to miss a baseball game for a family meal? That was something he could never understand. Now that Steve is grown and working himself, he sees even less of his parents. As always they leave something in the refrigerator for him or he eats at his girlfriend Mary's house.

Mary microwaves frozen dinners for them or they just grab a pizza or something. Mary sees even less of her mom than Steve does. According to Steve, food is only important because people need it to live. He believes that everyone will be popping food pills in the 21st century, and this will save time to do other more important things.

Sylvia

Sylvia is a widowed 67-year-old Italian-American woman with three grown children. When she met her husband she had just moved from Italy to the United States with her family. It was love at first sight for her. Her family wasn't too pleased with Mike, though. He was of a different racial background. Interracial marriages were not very common in 1948.

Mike loved her mom's cooking, though, especially her spaghetti, which bonded him to her for life. Back then, Sylvia says that she cooked everything, all the Black cultural dishes that Mike liked, such as hog jowls and chitlins, as well as pizza, spaghetti, and rigatoni.

The young couple lived with Mike's parents for the first few years because Mike worked for the railroad and was gone much of the time. When their first child came along, they got their own place. They went from "precise" sit-down meals to a swinging-door kitchen. After her next two children were born, Sylvia tried to have set mealtimes like those she'd had when she was growing up because she wanted her children to know some stability.

Mike came from a large family. They ate together on Sundays only. He used to talk about how he hated mealtime on Sundays. His dad was an alcoholic who was seldom present or drunk when he was. His mom tried to be a positive presence, but with eight children to feed, it wasn't easy for her. The children fought a lot and even threw food at each other. For Mike, mealtimes were unpleasant and meant arguments and conflict within the family. Sylvia said that she would have been hung by her ears if she acted like that at the table. Mike liked mealtimes with Sylvia and his children once he got another job and could be home more. Sylvia tried to make mealtimes special for Mike and their family. They all laughed at the multicultural dishes she served. Her children said she could feed the League of Nations and everyone would feel right at home.

When Sylvia's children began to leave home, it broke her heart. It was just Mike and her most of the time. Mealtimes were different without the kids, but she and Mike always tried to eat together. With tears in her eyes, Sylvia stated that Mike is gone now and she is all alone.

Two of her children are in Atlanta and the other seldom visits. Sylvia doesn't cook anymore since no one is there to enjoy or appreciate her effort. She states that it's funny how much she misses all those good mealtimes with the family. For Sylvia, mealtime used to mean a time for happiness within the family. Now that she's alone, the meaning of food has changed. She feels sad for those who never experienced the wonderful memories of mealtimes in the "good old days" because, according to her, those experiences aren't likely to ever occur again in this world for anyone.

George

George is a 60-year-old married American of Scots-Irish origin. He remembers dinnertime as being a real "circus time" for him growing up. His mother was Scottish and his father was Irish. His father had a hearty appetite, which his mother refused to feed. George recalls her saying, "I won't be a party to his gluttony and demise." And she meant it.

According to George, you would have thought his mother was another Jenny Craig. Nothing she cooked had any taste according to his father. He and his sisters used to giggle constantly at the table when their parents argued back and forth about who would die first. His dad swore that his mom was trying to starve them all to death.

For George, mealtime was not a fun time at his house. Instead, it was a time of constant contention and frustration. However, George does remember some rare happy mealtimes when his family went to his paternal grandparents to visit. Those times were few and far between, though, because his mom would argue all the way home that Grandma was trying to poison them all with her gluttonous cooking. Of course, his mom always had to tell Grandma about her sinful cooking, and that upset his dad. George stated that even though mealtimes were sometimes frustrating, he and his sisters knew that their mom and dad loved each other and that things never got too far out of hand. So for him mealtimes were still a time for togetherness and sharing. Today, he compares those times in his youth to the very quiet times he and his wife now have during meals. He misses those good old days.

George had one child, who died young. He doesn't know if mealtimes might have been different if there had been a family. He only knows that it sure is different now. His wife doesn't go to extremes one way or another, so mealtimes are just a time for eating and not much more.

George believes that his mealtimes today are quite typical for people his age who don't have children, and even for many who have children. He believes that families do not have time for one another today, and that just might be why so many children are in trouble. He predicts that with television, computers, and fast food taking over, family mealtimes in the 21st century are going to be few or nonexistent.

Maria

Maria, a 62-year-old Italian-American woman, stated that food to her family means love, appreciation, and sharing. She raised her kids like she was raised, to appreciate the little and to share with all. Every payday she and her husband took all five of the children grocery shopping to teach them the value of food, money, and nutrition. She recalls that she would tell her husband what was on the menu for a particular day and he would name a meat and the children would yell out all the trimmings such as, potatoes, beans, and applesauce—whatever went with that meat. They went through every day of the week planning their menus right in the grocery store. It was great! Everyone had his or her job in the family kitchen as well; buying, preparing, eating, and cleaning up were all part of it.

A lot of heart and soul went into her family's meals. Later when the children all left home, Maria never really enjoyed mealtimes. She believes that it's not really the foods we eat that have meaning but the loved ones we share it with and the love, care, and attention that go into mealtime. Maria envies families who have small children and hopes that the 21st century will make love, togetherness, and mealtimes as special for them as they were for her.

Discussion of Conversations

Most of the individuals I spoke to believe that the 21st century will mean more fast food and fewer family meals together. Those who have positive feelings about food expressed certain common themes: Mealtime is a very special time for love and sharing. The meaning of food for the older adult seems to begin with memories of childhood when Mom's schedule was apparently less busy. The family is at the heart of what we feel about food today. Food means soul. Food means nourishment.

Those who have negative or no feelings about food gave such reasons as split families, mothers working, conflicts in family schedules, food used as punishment, and arguments and frustrating situations at mealtimes for their feelings.

What was obvious from the conversations was that, as individuals, we eat for different reasons: Some eat to live, while others live to eat. What was even more obvious was that the culture, the stage of development, and the situational time in the life of the interviewees had a great deal to do with their feelings about food and nutritional habits.

Theories

Suitor and Crowley (1984) contend that eating behaviors are unique and culturally influenced by the family throughout the life cycle. They view the early years as the opportune time to teach children good eating habits. The developmental stage of the family plays an important part in the meaning individuals held for food. Duvall and Miller (1985) established eight stages of family development:

1. Newly established couple (no children)
2. Childbearing family (oldest child birth to 2 1/2 years)
3. Family with preschool children (oldest child 2 1/2 to 6 years)
4. Family with school children (oldest child 6 to 13 years)
5. Family with teenagers (oldest child 13 to 20 years)
6. Family as launching center (oldest child gone to departure of youngest)
7. Middle-aged family (empty nest to retirement)
8. Aging family (retirement to death of both spouses)

Individuals in stages 1 through 5 with stable families and growing children placed a great deal of meaning on food. In the conversation with Maria, she stated that a lot of heart and soul went into her family's meals—that it's not really the foods people eat that have meaning, it is the loved ones you share it with and all the love and everything else that goes into it. Maria hopes that young families will experience positive mealtimes in the 21st century, as her family experienced them in the 20th century.

Those individuals in stage 7 and 8 did not seem to place as much meaning on food as they had in earlier stages. For instance, Maria commented that after the children left, she and Joel never really enjoyed mealtimes unless the children were visiting. Sylvia stated that when her family began to leave home, it broke her heart. She saw no use in cooking anymore because there was no one at home to enjoy or appreciate the food. Sylvia believes that families have changed too much with so many mothers working outside of the home today. She does not believe that the 21st century holds much hope for family meals and togetherness.

Most of the individuals with whom I spoke see mealtimes through their memories as children. Meals seemed to have more meaning to them then. According to Staab and Hodges (1996), physiological changes associated with aging, psychosocial changes in the living environment, the loss of companionship of a spouse, children, and friends, and altered socioeconomic status all profoundly affect appetite and nutritional intake. All of these changes may make eating less pleasurable and meaningful than it was at an earlier age. This is indeed unfortunate, since quality nutrition benefits the majority of adults over age 65 who have chronic diseases (Spradley, 1990). All of the individuals' origins and cultures seemed important to them. However, some of them admit that they have become so Americanized that they no longer adhere to the customs and the good nutritional behaviors they learned through their families as children.

Living Vicariously

Vicarious learning (Bandura, 1977) means that we learn through observation and imitation of others. In other words, we learn through modeling what we see others do or say, whether it be good or bad. Television is one of the greatest vicarious influences on food choices. Many television commercials promote junk food or less nutritional foods.

Consider, for instance, the Betty Crocker commercial for the double chocolate cake and butter-cream frosting. It is so inviting that viewers may salivate reflexively. Such a commercial stimulates thoughts of cake and other sweets. Such thoughts stimulate the impulse to eat. While it would be more prudent to eat a carrot or celery stick, the cake commercial strongly reinforces the impulse to eat a sweet dessert.

There were traditional television programs where mealtimes were portrayed as being very special times for family togetherness: *Father Knows Best, Little House on the Prairie*, or *I Love Lucy*. These programs modeled traditional families, where the fathers came home, meals were on the table, and everyone calmly sat down to eat and discuss the daily happenings (although with Lucy, it may not always have been calm). Such scenes are not common in today's programming.

Mom and Food

Mom plays a part in the vicarious meaning of food. Tannen (1994) states that, "Since moms are significant role models for daughters, very often they learn the language of eating from them." Relationships are drawn between mothers' eating habits and food and eating influences on their daughters. Eating habits are like a mother tongue that you learn as a child and never forget. Often you pick up your mother's bad habits, copying the ones that are less than ideal. Mothers didn't have the information or education about healthy eating they do now. Serving wholesome foods like red meat, whole milk, and buttery cookies and cakes baked from scratch showed they cared.

Gender Differences

The meaning or relationship we give to food is influenced by gender. Boys are taught to be tough and generally show anger or frustration through physical expression, whereas girls are taught to show more emotional expression. Food can become their comforter and emotional outlet.

As a woman, many times I have taken comfort in sweets. However, I have great difficulty in blaming my mother for my bad eating habits and weight problem. It's easy to blame mothers for being overweight or for food hangups. But adults are responsible for their own personal behavior.

Soulful Meaning of Food

One example of 21st-century thinking contends that food feeds the soul as well as the body. Food is simply food without meaning if it doesn't feed the soul. This is not a new concept, as many references of this nature can be found throughout the literature. Moore (1996) states that when we prepare a traditional dinner, it becomes an experience with the magic of everything we think, use, and do in the preparation. Therefore, a true dinner experience is one that not only brings the family together for sharing and togetherness, but one that also fulfills the needs of the soul.

Food for the soul is not just the chemicals and nutrients that we put into our bodies but also anything that promotes intimacy, "a hike in a nature park, a late-night conversation with a friend, a family dinner, a job that satisfies deeply, a visit to a cemetery. Beauty, solitude, and deep release also keep the soul well fed" (Moore 1996, p. 61).

Shopping for food can be a soulful experience. Consumerism can be defined as disenchanted shopping, while in soulful shopping we are profoundly aware of the wealth of culture that surrounds food: its seasons, national varieties, natural characteristics, and recipes.

Americans have gotten away from traditional meal preparation and replaced it with bland, overprocessed, tasteless food that does not nourish the soul. Food is an implement of magic. Only the most cold-hearted rationalist could squeeze the juices of life out of it.

Worldwide Meaning of Food

Musalger (1991) sees changes in the meaning of food throughout the world and these changes are not necessarily for the good. Many of the changes started during the two world wars, when men went to war and women went to work. He contends that "Women have a major influence on dietary habits in any culture. All over the world, women take care of children and are responsible for the preparation of food for their families" (p. 21). However, these same women who once stayed home, took care of the children, and prepared food for the family are now working outside the home and depend on fast foods for meals.

Many changes in food traditions have been initiated by the younger generation who view such traditions as outdated. Unfortunately, in developing countries, traditional foods made up of fiber and complex carbohydrates are now being replaced by foods high in fats and sugar, resulting in an increase in chronic disease.

People are aware of the meaning of food when it comes to good nutrition but oddly, they don't seem to practice what they know. For example, Parks et al. (1994) reported that the same people who said they wanted healthy menu items in restaurants did not choose the items marked as nutritious when the time came to order.

The meaning of food to all of us is important, not only for all the fond or not so fond memories we hold from childhood, but for the joy we experience when we nourish both body and soul.

References

Bandura, A. (1977). *Social Learning Theory*. Englewood Cliffs. N.J.: Prentice-Hall.

Duvall, E. M., and Miller, B. (1985). *Marriage and Family Development* (6th ed.). New York: Harper & Row.

Musalger, A. (July 1991). Not all change is good. *World Health*, (Report No. Z36.8WHO.3:W156, pp. 20–22).

Moore, T. (1996). *The Re-enchantment of Everyday Life*. New York: HarperCollins

Parks, S., et al. (1994). Changing consumer eating habits create new opportunities in commercial food service. *American Dietetic Association*, 94 (8):908–909.

Spradley, B. (1990). *Community Health Nursing: Concepts and Practice* (3d ed). Glenview, Ill.: Scott Foresman.

Staab, A., & Hodges, L. (1996). *Essentials of Gerontological Nursing: Adaptation to the Aging Process*. Philadelphia: Lippincott.

Suitor, C. W., and Crowley, M. (1984). *Nutrition: Principles and Application in Health Promotion*. Philadelphia: Lippincott.

Tannen, N. (1994). My mother: My weight. *Weight Watchers Magazine*, 27 (5):38–43.

CHAPTER 9

THE WEDDING: THE TRIUMPH OF HOPE OVER EXPERIENCE

Lynne Hektor Dunphy

AT THE CHURCH

They had been living together since 1986. And so it went—and then it was 1996. The bride wore an ivory dress, lace and tulle, with a silk flower wreath on her head, satin ribbons and little clusters of pearls dangling in her blonde hair. She was 48 years old.

The groom wore a tailored, dark, pinstripe suit. "No tux!" he had groaned. He was 49 years old, had ash-colored hair, and beautifully blue, unclouded eyes.

Her attendants were a mix of ages and types. The maid of honor was over 60, but certainly appeared younger. A Filipino by birth, she had a shiny, dark cap of hair and wore a violet off-the-shoulder dress, taffeta.

The "little girls," as they were referred to, were 9 and 11, respectively. They had matching dresses of lilac and pink and flowered barrettes in their hair. "What are we supposed to do?" they shrieked upon arriving at the church.

The reality of the people gathered, the organ music playing, the garlands of flowers galore, all of the wild flowers, Queen Anne's lace, and the solemnity of the moment finally sunk in for all of the participants.

His best man was his brother. It was the second time around in this role for the brother, and he dreaded doing the toast and having the responsibility for the ring. The ushers were old friends.

The wait, as before in his last marriage, was insufferable. And, of course, his mother was late. The ceremony was not to start on time.

She walked in alone. Her father was dead. It seemed and felt appropriate. She was far more nervous and more excited than she had anticipated. She was told that she looked pale upon entering the church.

The cloudiness of the day outside made the church especially warm and glowing within. That's what she remembered. And the heads of her family and friends all turned in their pews as she walked down that aisle, slowly, as instructed. She smiled. This was truly fulfilling. In the end, they agreed, they were happy that the traditional church service—definitely not their original choice—had been used. It seemed to give a stamp of authenticity to the whole endeavor. Their childhood memories and associations resonated within them. It seemed that, after all, their presence here was appropriate, meaningful, and real.

The Wedding

Then there was the exchange of vows, the exchange of rings, the kiss. They turned to the congregation. They announced themselves as "Mr. and Mrs." Back down the aisle together they walked, hand in hand. They were happy seeing everyone, greeting them, hugging them, and kissing them as they exited the church.

There was the traditional spray of birdseed as they exited the church. Rice was no longer permitted. It was what they wanted.

A Wedding and a Wedding

Family norms are shot, I reflected recently. Well, if not shot, certainly irretrievably altered. The occasion for this reflection was the planning and execution of the celebration of my own recent marriage vows to a live-in partner of 10 years.

He is one month shy of 50 and I am two years short of that momentous life marker. Nonetheless, or perhaps precisely because of this, we elected to wed. We woke up one morning and just *did it*. Actually, we had attempted it two weeks earlier but had trouble finding the right place and had had a big fight. I (the potential bride) was ambivalent about just "*doing it*" without fanfare and friends galore and celebration. So we returned home.

Planning was not one of our mutual strong suits. Suddenly, a week later, a close friend, single and 49, was found dead. He was one of my partner's closest "buddies." We were shot up. Life was shot. A week later, on a Friday morning, September 1 (we liked the first day of the month), we got up and finally did just *do it*! We found the city hall this time. The officials were pleasant. It was early. We were the first ones there. No, we didn't just want the license. We wanted the whole shebang, the whole enchilada. We exchanged vows beneath some paper wedding bells at the counter. A local contractor awaiting a permit was next in line; he was our witness. Our wedding "breakfast," our current favorite meal of the day, was eaten in a small, local luncheonette in the small Florida town where we had found the city hall. We told no one. We reflected on the fate that had befallen other friends, longtime couples who had finally married only to separate shortly thereafter. We watched and waited. What was in the nature of this official acknowledgment of wedded status that could cause ostensibly placid unions to suddenly rupture and break asunder? We shuddered. Would the same fate, unimaginable at present, befall us? Would the act of concretizing our relationship, bestowing upon it an official status, cause it to break into pieces? So we kept our secret. Gradually, however, word seeped out, like a leaking faucet. First, a close girlfriend. Then a boss—the insurance, after all. Then, a close sister. And then, the final and irrevocable step: our mothers.

Oh, they were happy to be sure. But, they hadn't been there! They hadn't been present! After all these years, all this time, they hadn't seen it happen! Thus, was it even "real"? We toyed with ideas.

In a generational reversal, they lived up north and we lived in sunny Florida. Should we have a celebration up north, near our families, or down south, near our friends? How should we do this? Should we even do this? There were obviously no rights or wrongs anymore—everyone did it "their own way," did "their own thing." What did we even want? (The quintessential question for our quintessential baby boomer generation, looming especially large with 50 on the horizon.)

In the end, we settled for "blood," we decided to reaffirm our vows with our respective families. What the hell, we decided. You only live once. Let's have a "real" wedding. It'll make our families happy, and maybe, as an aside, we told ourselves, maybe even make us happy too. Why not have another wedding? (Of course we had both had other weddings—first youthful, heated unions, marriages long ago abandoned and by now largely forgotten.)

Another opportunity for a party; certainly a better opportunity for a family to gather than a funeral! An occasion for the families to gather and "meld." It would keep my mother, the hostess-to-be, busy all winter, I reasoned. (We had already decided on spring. After all I had two busy semesters ahead and a book contract!) We had already decided on the where—the small country town where I had spent childhood summers, where my parents (after their Florida sojourn) had ultimately retired to, equidistant between the branches of my partner's significantly large and extended Irish Catholic family, and known well to my entire side of the family. The small, Protestant church (Lutheran, to be exact) that I had intermittently attended since birth was there. My father was buried in the graveyard there, beneath the rolling hills of Pennsylvania, split by the nearby and ever-present Delaware River. I knew the minister; he might reaffirm our vows in public, in church. So far, so good. It all seemed far in the future, back in the fall when these plans began. We weathered the selection of invitations rather easily, amazed at the similarity of our tastes. They were scripted in pink, bordered with pastels and spring flowers. The romanticism of our youth was triumphing; the traditionalism of our upbringing began to appear in new and sometimes startling ways. Would this be a trend? Would it begin to grow like the unstoppable weeds in our tropical Florida garden, to choke out and stifle the blooms of our respective independence, carefully nurtured in our 10-year relationship? We wondered. We stayed vigilant and watchful. Would we truly escape unscathed the potential land mines and booby traps that surely must lie ahead?

The months wore on. Showers were given for me, the bride. Professional friends and acquaintances enjoyed a break from middle age to revel in a ritual essentially intended for young and new womanhood. Christmas came and went; we celebrated our first "married" Christmas in our first year of residence in a new home. Wedding presents came throughout the winter, sporadically, and then in bursts. These gifts included household items, coupons for massages and oils, wines, books of poetry, bridal etiquette, wedding preparation. Cards came also. Big cards, glossy, with wedding bells, cakes, champagne, couples entwined and young! We wondered at what we were doing. Had we gone mad?

The calls from our mothers came with increasing frequency. There were decisions to be made regarding disc jockeys, for heaven's sake, and wedding reception sites, and the food, and the liquor. The guest lists, done and redone, the music for the church service, the organist, the rings, the dress, the headgear, the phone calls, all details that made the pace quicken.

We seemed to be on a hurtling train we couldn't get off. What was there to do but enjoy the ride?

We went to my mother's the week before the wedding. Our spirits flew. We were very excited. There was a lot to be done. Mother had told us that she needed us there. After the initial happiness of our arrival, tensions increased. The name cards and seating arrangements were particularly difficult. How could Aunt Helen really sit with that Gilbert and his new blonde girlfriend?

My mother's hand and voice and body were everywhere. This is what you get, I told myself, for not having done everything yourself. Every independent move I made demanded from my mother a countermove, or at the very least a comment. My long-suffering partner retreated into a head cold and a visit from out-of-town friends.

Rain

It rained all week before the wedding. The air was chilly and damp, and the green fuzz on the newly emerging buds were everywhere. We felt the rain sprinkle, the robins gaily hopping about, with the twinkling of white flowering dogwood trees, and the full pink and fat blooming cherry blossoms, crowned by the full purpled azaleas and yellow forsythia dotting the landscapes.

New Views, Old Views

In anticipation of the arrival of the hordes of family and friends, our anxiety heightened. Our meeting with the church pastor was particularly symbolic of the week. We found a wedding service that we liked. Again, to my amazement, we immediately and easily concurred. It spoke of God freely and of the sacredness of commitment and of the need to voice that before family and friends. It spoke to the need for reverence in life and of commemoration, of marking passages, and sharing. It did not, however, mention Jesus or the formal church. According to the pastor, it was new age. Well, yes, I suppose it was. So we are also of a "new age." We were, it was explained to us, receiving the Church's (with a capital C) blessing by having a service in church to reaffirm our vow taken earlier.

Old worldviews, long abandoned by my partner and myself, reasserted themselves all week. It reminded us again of our mutual abandonment of our families' spiritual roots and of the traditionally defined practice of religion in which we had been raised. We were surprised at the number of family members who actively practice their religion in traditional ways.

These newly revealed feelings mingled with the old and stimulated feelings of guilt in us. Guilt became familiar to us once more and we felt it deeply. We thought guilt had been put away long ago.

When I pondered these theological questions I was unable to reconcile beliefs with the traditional teachings of the Church. Because I am a child of the postmodern world, I seemed destined to stumble through life bare and bereft of the traditional spiritual comforts such symbols of certainty might afford me.

But interestingly, the trappings of religious ceremony, in this case a blessing on our marriage, provided a shell of some comfort: familiarity, tradition, symbols each gave us comfort.

Rituals were fundamental parts of my memory of the day. The music, the lace, something old and something new, something borrowed and something blue.

We forged on. I realized anew who I had grown into as a person, as an adult. No, I didn't believe. Would we exchange vows in a church, with blessings? Yes, we would. Perhaps our mothers could then die in peace. As for ourselves, we held a mutual disbelief, a shared skepticism, a heightened (postmodern?) sensibility, temperament, and disposition.

Any attempt to declare who we really were in the presence of our families was thwarted. We remained oblique, obscure—and, I would venture, wisely so. We had each other, after all, and have become a small and exclusive family for each other. We loved and love each other.

Our Families, Ourselves

Family tensions and dramas played out within us and caused occasional spasms. In our maturity we were more tolerant of diversity and more forgiving of differences. Our youth had us only see the absolute and have passions and hatreds. Now, such battles seemed barely worth it. Such games had been played out in our first marriages. Truces had long been declared with our birth families.

We are now in the active creation of the "postmodern" family. We seek unity, yet honor the differentness of two persons sharing day-to-day struggles and triumphs. Sharing the day-to-day ordinary boredom and tedium. And we share with our extended families. We glared and we harmonized. Isn't this what families have always done? So, our wedding proceeded. The residual bones of long-deceased fathers were all around us the entire wedding week, scattered in unexpected places in a particular song we selected to be played, a certain food dish we served, a shared piece of my father's jewelry passed down. I was reminded of the immutability of the family unit. It was stamped in every action.

As I age, I become more conscious of the generational imperatives that we are heirs to.

The balance of one's place in a generational cohort. In my maturity I ask, "How much do we truly control?" Less than we think, I am convinced, as my life goes on. And yet, less is also more. This was the stance I selected for the week of the wedding. The planning moved ahead.

Me and My Postmodern Family and I

A dialogue continues between the family as biologically determined variable and the family as chosen. Childless at 50, we chose to marry, against all odds. We deconstruct the family. We take a stance of family as freely chosen, emergent, and evolving.

My husband and I are emerging from our matrix of genetic and biological structure. We are moving on from our historical circumstance and emotional bonds. These bonds that both free and constrain us. These are the family ties that both impinge on and delight us. And they condemn and forgive us. Our family contains elements of our immutable "sameness," yet help us to stand apart as different and unique.

We are the family as it stands at the beginning of the 21st century. Our wedding was in keeping with the times.

Each person is invited to construct a personal family and to create a ritual, unique and filled with celebration of the family you choose. Wherever and however these connections are to be celebrated.

VOICES FOUR

Constructing a Family

after all

your blood becomes you
your lineage
a ladder
climbed through the times
your family the ones
you reach for
in the night
mothers fathers
sisters brothers
the rungs
steadying your ascent
or tangling tired feet
sometimes snapping
falling
asunder
but your family
the ones you hold dear
& keep near
your family
you can't live
without.

—Daniel R. Collins

Chapter 10

A Single Woman Adopts Catherine

Claudia Hauri

I cannot recall exactly when I decided to adopt; perhaps I was tired of kissing frogs in hopes of finding a prince . . . so I decided to get a princess instead. The event has been karma. Somehow Catherine was meant to be mine and I was meant to be Catherine's mom.

I was married at 25 and divorced at 28, two and a half years of a wonderful marriage and six months of hell. I moved out in 1971 since my ex said he had never had a home and my home is wherever I am because I am at home within. I threw my energies into my career—nursing—developed as a teacher, obtained my master's in 1974, and then became a family nurse practitioner and faculty in a university. I did some consulting in South America for an American school in Peru, for the Chilean Pediatric Nursing Society, and for the Red Cross Nurses in Colombia. I bought a larger house in 1977, published, began the doctorate, and settled in.

Then in 1984 I met a prince who was also divorced. We shared some fun times and some sad times, and quite a few depressed times. Prince eventually moved to Arizona to escape his ex-wife's wrath and I eventually healed. I guess this was the point that I thought about adoption. I remember going to a church to attend an adoption orientation program with another single friend also interested in adopting. I remember looking at the book of children available for adoption: singles, siblings, older than 3, of mixed race, and beautiful. Forms were taken home which somehow got to the bottom of the pile of things to do as I grappled and wrestled with the dissertation. During the next few years, I talked with friends and family about which gender should be a priority: first choice, a girl; age: 3 to 6 years since under 2 years was not my favorite stage; race: caucasian or mixed; and I would consider a handicapped child except for mental retardation. Some of my part-time practice as a nurse practitioner is as a consultant to the Association for Retarded Citizens (ARC) in maintaining the health of adults with developmental disabilities living in

---

Adapted from: Munhall P. & V. Vitarmuns (eds.). The Emergence of Women into the 21st Century, National League for Nursing. New York 1995.

group homes and monitoring the health of children 6 months to 3 years of age in an early infant stimulation program. So I am well aware of the limits for some children. I eventually completed the forms and, after a home visit, was cleared for adoption in September 1988. I was at the end of my rope attempting to finish my dissertation, so I really did not pursue the adoption further.

When the doctorate was obtained in 1989 I was free to be me again and was asked to be a consultant to the public health department. There was an abundance of infants and children being placed in shelter and then foster care and I was to do the initial intake physical, and if a court order had been obtained, I was to start immunizations in anticipation that someday the child would be attending school. The summer was an eye opener as to the culture of HRS (Human Resource Service), one of chaos and the system that was a web of intricacies and offices that reached far and wide through something similar to going through a dense rain forest. I'll never forget the siblings that stirred again the feeling in my heart about being a mom. Susie was about 6, and her brother 4. They had traveled to this country with their parents, who were apprehended at the airport for transporting cocaine into the United States. The children were placed in HRS custody and I did the physical in the shelter where they were placed. The children had no idea what was happening, I talked to Susie and reassured her in my rusty Spanish that she would be going "home" soon; her brother looked at me with empty eyes. As I kept in touch with their status, I did intakes on children who were abandoned by parents too drunk on alcohol and high on cocaine to care about their children, left in the streets with a name tag but no other identification and a note that the parent was unable to care for the child any longer, or left at the hospital after a premature birth. Some children were "normal," others infested with lice, others full of scabies and impetigo, others developmentally delayed, others with blank stares and no ability or desire to hug and respond to human touch.

I was touched and amazed at the love, tenderness, warmth, brightness, cleanliness, teaching, and caring that the majority of the shelter and foster parents gave to each and every child. As I made the rounds, talked with the parents, and told them of my intent to adopt—to give a child a chance at life—I was advised to become a foster parent and, at the appropriate time, express my intent to adopt, depending on the status of the child placed with me. In fall of 1989 I was given my license as a foster parent and was assured that I would have a child by December—to go ahead and buy a ticket for the child since I was planning on spending the holidays in New Hampshire with family and doing some cross-country skiing. The fall semester at the university passed. I made phone calls to the placement office but each time was told no, there really is no child to be placed at this time. A week before flying I obtained a bogus medical letter that explained to Pan Am why "Johnny" Hauri could not fly and to please reimburse the ticket without penalty. I had fun skiing and doing aprės ski activities and remember a conversation with my brother,

But Sis, how can you be a foster mother? What if "they" take her away?
Well, Ted, I look at it this way—HRS could take her away after a year—or a higher force could take her at 6 years to leukemia, 16 years to a drunk driver, 26 years to childbirth, or 36 years to whatever—when I lose the child is not for me to say. I just want to give her the best chance to be . . . for as long as I am allowed.

In January 1990, I was at a clinic in the center of town arranging for a clinical rotation for a student after which I found myself with some time to spare before the next appointment. Hm-mm-m I thought—HRS is around here somewhere. I found the building, found the placement office, found Carin, the placement officer, and introduced myself.

Hi Carin, I'm Dr. Hauri, licensed foster status, and was assured that I would have a child placed with me since there was such a need.
Well, the only thing I have a need for right now is an 11-month-old girl, mixed race, Hispanic, I think.
Tell me yes or no.
Can I think about it?
Sure, but I really need to place her by tomorrow.
I'll call you before the end of today and give you my decision.
OK.

That was it. No identification, no nothing. I went to the university and called my mom but she didn't answer. I called my best friend at work, but she was in a meeting. A faculty member was in her office so I told Louise about the transaction so far. She was reassuring, saying things like, "If it's meant to be it's meant to be—go with your feelings—listen to your heart and your gut—you can do it." So I talked to myself, "Claudia, this is your decision, you need to make it. This is your life and you are a grownup—and if you don't try you will never know." So I called Carin and said, "I'll do it" and she said "I'll tell you when to pick up the child." This was Wednesday, January 18, 1990.

The next morning I had a golf lesson with a friend at 8:30 A.M. which lasted till 9:30 after which I went to the university. Carin had already called and left a message to come to an office in the city where the child could be picked up at noon. I nearly panicked. I had nothing, not even a car seat, let alone supplies and food. So I asked Melba, a wise grandmotherly-type faculty woman to come with me to get "the child." We arrived at the office and I remember seeing an infant in a stroller in an empty room with an elderly person watching her. I signed some papers and received two blue folders, and was taken to and given the child known as Maria. (I later renamed her Catherine.) She was given to me with all her personal belongings: a large shopping bag containing a blanket, a bottle empty of milk (I was told she had thrown up at 10 A.M.), a change of clothing, a diaper, and a small stuffed lamb. As I held Maria I felt a warmth of heart, but her flaccid body was pale and white and noncommital. As Melba and I walked down the stairs we said to each other how beautiful she was, and how cute, and alert and oh my gosh! am I really going to be a mom? The memory brings back a smile and goosebumps as I sit here. Once in the garage, I put Maria on the trunk of my car and gave her the quickest, but probably the most comprehensive neuromuscular and developmental physical she had ever had. And off we went!

Melba held Maria in her lap enveloped in seat belt while I drove to the nearest second-hand store. There we found a car seat, playpen, and some clothes. Next was a discount store where I purchased a playpen mattress, two sheets, some more clothes, and some toys. The next stop was a supermarket, where I asked another shopper what size diapers I should buy, and where I bought enough staples to get me through the night and next day. The final stop was the university by 2:30 P.M. where I was greeted by faculty with open arms and champagne and lots of questions. Maria finally settled down and took a much-needed nap. I reached my mom and told her "we" were coming for dinner. Then I taught class from 4 to 5:30 and headed home with my foster daughter in the midst of rush-hour traffic. Maria cried on the way home and I sang to her to soothe her tears and discomfort. I also talked to her and reassured her that she was in good hands and I would stand beside her no matter what. My mom was delighted and loved her from the moment she saw her and has been a strong support and mentor ever since. I took Friday off to find child care and buy some more supplies and order diaper service and contact friends for a crib and other items. Over the weekend, I picked up a crib, changing table, and high chair and began to put our life back together. I introduced Maria to neighbors and we began to get to know each other. From the beginning, Maria slept through the night and happily entertained herself in the morning for half an hour to 45 minutes after awakening. The shelter home in which Maria had been for nine months was home for six to eight infants under the age of 2 years. Thus Maria, already a survivor, learned to entertain herself in her own world. This was a godsend to me, because it gave me time to shower, fix breakfast, and get the morning together before I became a "mom." I soon learned not to dress until after breakfast. This way I wouldn't have to change clothes because of stains and drips and drool and crinkles in the clothing. The same rule applies six years later. That first weekend was wonderful and I shall never forget it.

Maria and I had bonded within the first month—she was such a happy, smiling, bubbling baby. She needed time getting used to being in the stroller, and a new home with new faces, and new food and tastes (during the first week she had enough garlic and parsley to last her a lifetime) and new toys and everything. Prior to this, Maria had been at the county hospital for two months after being born 2 months premature and septic, then the shelter home, which was subsequently closed by HRS, and this was where I stepped in at the Placement Office. I familiarized myself with the two blue folders—one was the social work record, the other the health care record. Maria was being followed at a university-affiliated facility, a center for child development, for developmental delay and I needed to maintain the appointment schedule. There were no other notations of health problems, although according to the DDST-R, Maria was delayed in physical development. Personally I thought she was on target for mental development after watching her for a month. Whatever drugs she got during her prenatal period had given her extra pizzazz, as far as I was concerned!

The months passed by and we enjoyed each other and settled into a new routine for all. The first major event was a judicial review that was held in the summer of 1990. A panel of professional volunteers with legal training would hear the cases for the many children in shelter and foster care and make decisions about their future in order to relieve the burden of cases for the judges who, backlogged with cases, were months behind. The panel recommended terminating the mother's rights after hearing testimony from HRS and from me and from my mom who was the foster grandparent (duly fingerprinted and processed for misdemeanors and felony records!). Maria's records should have been transferred directly to Adoptions, but were not and so ensued another 15 months of agony and a tug of war with the case workers and subsequent case workers and judges and hearings and talk of visits and commotion that would have turned me off to the process except for the fact that I reminded myself that I had earned the doctorate through tenacity and perseverance and this was another excellent opportunity to apply what I had learned about those qualities toward a worthwhile cause.

I have notes about that time in my life: the times I was trying to reach a caseworker or a supervisor and the phone rang 52 times only to be answered (?) and then a disconnect. Then the phone would be busy when I redialed. Or the time I was talking to the case worker and he gave me the biological mother's address thinking he was talking to her—and I wondered if he had inadvertently given her my address and should I install an alarm system. There were moments of humor, when Judge Lewis asked what kind of doctor I was after I introduced myself as Dr. Hauri, and I replied a doctor of education. "Where from?" University of Florida was my reply as I made the gator jaws with my arms and the judge laughed and smiled and wished me well in my pursuit of Maria. He once again directed HRS to obtain the signature and move the case along to Adoptions.

That day finally came. I was nervous in many ways—this was a serious step I was taking as a single woman. I wondered briefly if I could manage, but then reminded myself that with my mom's help and the help and support of my friends I had coped quite well so far. I had experienced many of the normal fears and doubts a biological mother has—should I take her to the doctor for an antibiotic for the cold (no); is the temperature because of teething? (yes); the tears when I was tired and wondered whether I could keep this up? (yes). Friends asked if I wasn't tired when I went to bed at night and my usual answer was, "Yes, but it's a nice tired." I mean I was tired before, but this is different, it's a rewarding tired. I still feel that way today, only more so because of the light and love my daughter has brought into my life and the way she shows me the world through her eyes as I lead her through the world by the hand with all the knowledge and love I have to give. Hey, sure we fight and we argue and yell at each other sometimes in the morning, but we get over it, talk it over, and give hugs and kisses and eventually say goodnight at the end of the day. In retrospect, I was 47 when I was a foster mom for Maria—she is now 6 and I will be 53 this year. I started going through menopause when I was 50 or 51 and I remember clearly one night making an entry into Maria's memory book that we were certainly on the outs that day—she was in the terrific three's and practicing being independent, and I was in a hormonal swing that left me frazzled and intolerant to the little snit, saying *No*! all the time. The year my career was in the pits and I was growling like a bear, I taught Maria to say "Hey Mom, stop growling like a grizzly bear" or "Chill out, Mom, I love you."

It worked. I would look at her and a smile would creep across my face and I would have to admit to her that she was right and then I would give her a big teddy bear hug. And hugs have always been one of Maria's strengths. I taught her to jump up on the count of 3 when she wanted "uppy-uppy" and she would fit onto my body with a snugness that is uncanny—like we fit together. And she still hugs that way—morning, noon, and night. My friends will vouch for that because they are recipients of her love and hugs also. And now I really have to laugh at times because Maria will explain to me why I can't do something with the same reasons I gave her for something she wanted and the principle applies and I can't refute the logic I preached and so I admit—you're right.

And then I hear "Yes!" and her thumbs are up. My frazzles are becoming less and both of us are becoming older and wiser together. Because I will be 65 when Maria is 18 I took out the Florida Prepaid Tuition Plan. That was so I don't have to work to get tuition benefits; we can go wherever Maria wants to go and room in the dorm or a trailer or a condo and Maria can be a freshman and have her college life and I can go to Elderhostel and have my life. And then we can be together again when we want to be.

I mentioned the memory book. When I became a foster mom I joined the Foster Parents Association and I was told to start a memory book for Maria so she would have memories of the past. I did and to this day make entries although they are less often than previously. There are articles about the scandals in HRS and the children being abused and neglected because of the ills of society and the drug problem, the stories about the ups and downs I had while fostering, and times since then when I have felt the need to reflect and leave Maria a message about a time in our lives that has recently been experienced and lived in a very precious way. . . . My eyes get teary as I write this. Maria has taught me more about my life, our life, and life on earth than I would have ever learned had I not adopted. We used to look at the pictures in the memory book, but then I started pictures in albums since I knew someday that Maria would be reading and I did not want her to read certain items surrounding the foster time until she and I were ready to read and talk together. I have no record of her first 11 months except for some discharge papers from the hospital and some appointment slips for the Developmental Clinic. I wrote only what I could piece together and surmise and project from bits and pieces of information I was given. I would recommend a memory book for any mom. There are many times I would like to ask my mom about certain times or events or reflections on something, but the time is short and hurried when we are together and sometimes tense and the vibes I get are not always positive.

The adoption day came. October 20, 1991. I knew a lawyer in the neighborhood who would do the adoption for $475, which was later reimbursed by the state. I chose the name Catherine Marie so Catherine would have the same initials as mine. Her ethnicity is Hispanic/French—which ties in also with Catherine Marie. The social worker had done a complete job and all went smoothly in the judge's chambers. The only testy time was when the judge asked how much I made as a single woman—I was about to answer when the lawyer said that item had been cleared with HRS. Then I planned the party at a local restaurant so everyone who had been supportive and encouraging and helpful and worried with us could now celebrate with us. The memory book was there for signatures and an album of pictures records the good times and tears of happiness experienced.

Over the years—5 now—I have become friends with other single moms and other sets of parents through child care and now school. The support that comes through these friends is priceless. Susan and I had a real good thing going for a while . . . I would keep Jose in the morning (we had a back yard and they lived in a condo) while Susan would do her errands; that afternoon or another Saturday, Susan would keep Catherine (the condo had a real pool whereas we had a plastic one) and I could do my errands in peace. Susan's son was a year older and during the ages of 3 to 5 this worked very well. Since then Catherine is "all knowing" that boys are yuck to girls and do boy things that aren't cool. So there. Now I have moms and parents that have girls and the same tradeoff is accomplished to the delight and sanity of both parties. That's the physical side. The mental relief is also needed and received from longstanding friends I have known as long as 20 to 40 years. These are the friends who are willing to be a guardian should I die and my mom is no longer living. And these are the friends who listen to my complaints, and if they have had children they commiserate and understand very well, and if they haven't had children they still listen and give support in many different ways. I do not hesitate to ask for help if needed. Caring for myself keeps me healthy in more ways than one. Sometimes I pay $5 an hour for the same service when I get a sitter for Catherine. A long dinner and a movie with a friend can work wonders for an adult mind that has had too much 4-, 5-, 6-year-old talk and activity. When I first started with the sitters I started in the neighborhood and when those teenagers went off to college or university I asked a mom with three or four children who she could recommend. I figured that mom had a list for sure. I was given four and then some more, from the church she attended. Enough! I said, but Liz said you can never have too many. And she is right. Moms always know best. Frozen dinners come in handy on sitter nights—but I have to explain that concept. When I first got Catherine, I had to practice what I taught.

Over the years, I had taught parents to cook foods as naturally as possible—broil, bake, sauté, steam fresh veggies, salads with fresh herbs. No salt in cooking or at the table, use lemon or garlic and parsley as my mother taught me. . . . Then blend the leftover meat with the juice from the steamed veggies and freeze in ice cube trays. When frozen transfer the cubes to plastic bags, label and freeze. This can be done when the child is an infant and first learns to eat solid foods. On "sitter" days or "frazzled" days I would take out four cubes of chicken, four cubes of squash, and add a dessert, usually a fresh fruit compote that my Mom had made. The Junior Oster was used quite often in those days. Today, I don't have to blend the food, but I still cook enough on the weekends to make two or three frozen dinners for the future.

I remember some weekends in the beginning when my mom was out of town or we were on the outs and I was faced with caring for this much-loved person. I would have moments of panic—how am I going to survive? What shall I do? 48 hours? Two whole days? When Catherine was 2 or 3 and Deanna's son Andrew was 3 or 4 we supported each other and spent four or five hours each packing up supplies, meeting at the transit station, going for a ride, getting off, seeing the sights and the boats on the bay, and the people, and having an ice cream cone, and getting home, and both children and moms tired enough to have a two-hour nap. So six to seven hours were gone already. . . . Even today I think, here I am, 52 with a 7-year-old running around the house . . . life is real and this is really living.

The state provides Medicaid and a monthly stipend, both of which are invaluable. Although I have not really had to use Medicaid except for public health department visits, knowing that I have insurance for my daughter is great. To have her as a dependent on my insurance through the university would cost me about $300 per month. The monthly stipend was used for child care and is now used partially for afterschool care and money for college. Soon I hope the balance can be used to defray the cost of a babysitter to watch Maria after school; I think the daily pickup and piano practice overseen by my mom and two nights a week for dinner and to our house is taking its toll on my mom. And since I won round one and have had a break, I think I am ready for round two and another princess to hold Maria's hand and mine and join us in our journey through this life on earth . . . or maybe I will get that prince after all. . . .

CHAPTER 11

THROUGH THE EYES OF CATHERINE AT 7

as told by Catherine Marie Hauri to Claudia Hauri

ME

It's been seven years now that I have been a part of the family: an immediate family of my mom, me, and two animals, and an extended family of grandmother, uncle, cousin, aunt, and countless friends and cousins both here and abroad. I'll be 8 this month, but seven years ago I would say was when this family was born.

The first few months of my life were rough. I was born prematurely and was left in the hospital by my birth mother. Two months later, I went to a shelter home for seven months. I was then briefly placed in a foster home for four days and then went to another foster home, which became the house of my family. My then foster mom, my real mom now, was as pleased as punch to have me. She says we bonded within the month, whatever that means. Within two years the adoption was official, which made us an official family. I was soon in child care since my mom is a single professional woman. I was at this time floppy and underdeveloped for my age, but with homemade baby food and love and stimulation, I began to thrive.

At 3, I had caught up and was discharged from the child development clinic where I was being followed. By then, I was making friends at the child-care center. In fact, one of my best friends, Kalina, and I are going to fly together and be away at camp this summer for two whole weeks without moms, and this weekend I'm going to spend the night with my other best friend, Chelsea.

Life is kind of great right now, my grades in school are mostly A's after a miserable first grade of C's and D's. But then my mom had aspirations of a magnet language program for me, which was just a little too much for my right brain to handle. I'm a lefty and prefer creativity and imagination, gymnastics, ballet, and acting to reading, writing, and arithmetic.

This was written in 1997 in response to the preceding piece as written by Claudia Hauri. This is Catherine at seven.

Kindergarten was great, lots of fun things to do and songs to sing and stories to listen to. Then life got serious and it just wasn't my time. To complicate matters, Mom got this au pair from Germany to live with us for three months. She had limited experience with children and was learning English herself, so how could she teach me the words, even though they were only three and four letters long? Sonja was a trip all right, although we did have some fun times at the park and a couple of camping trips with Mom. I guess I never worried about what to do after school was out. I just tried to remember if this was a pick-up day and then ballet with Nana, or a pick-up day by Sonja and homework at home, or whatever. The days of the week, if I can remember which one it is, seem to go by so fast I hardly have enough time to play.

Mom

Mom sure worries about the schedule though. I even ask her at breakfast why she has that frown on her forehead and she says she's thinking about the day and the time schedule and what to cook for dinner that night and when was my hair washed last and did I return the book to the library and were the sneakers we bought a couple of months ago too small already and whatever else is in her mind. That's when I remind her to take her vitamins and drink her coffee.

Other times Mom has this blank look on her face and I am talking and all of a sudden I realize no one is listening to me, so I say "Helloooo!" and Mom responds at last. Maybe she is thinking about "life-before-Catherine time."

My mom won't tell me how old she is; she only says she's 50-something. I mean like I'm going to tell all my friends or something! So now I am in second grade and doing fine but I gotta keep my grades up, Mom says, otherwise there's no Disney World this summer and university. Mom has already prepaid for me to go to university because I told her I want to be a doctor (teacher-doctor not medical-doctor) and a nurse just like Mom. I love my mom and I'm glad she's my mom and my other mother was too sick to take care of me.

The mornings are the best, especially on the weekends when we have time to sleep late and snuggle in and talk and plan the day and tickle and talk serious sometimes. Mom really gets upset some school mornings when I get distracted and find something in my room that I haven't seen in a week and forget to brush my teeth or get my shoes on and walk the dog. She tells me on the way to school when we aren't doing the spelling words, that the nagging to get into a routine in the morning is all a part of her trying to teach me responsibility in life. There's always time for that. Geez, I just get some actions down relatively pat (like taking my shoes off before going on the rug) when others are added before I have had a chance to do a cartwheel. I wonder sometimes if Mom really wanted this "job" of raising a kid. I think that because there are times when Mom has scolded me and taken away TV or play time or some privilege that she says she is getting tired of all this discipline and stuff and that I had better shape up or else! That's when I tell her I hate her and she says that's

OK, she hates my behavior too at times, but she still loves me very much and always will. Then I say I love her more than she loves me—to infinity and beyond. And then we have a great big hug and talk or I do whatever it was I was supposed to do in the first place and Mom does whatever was on her mind.

Our Family and Neighborhood

Our family—my mom and I—lives in a neat neighborhood with all other kinds of families. First, there's Charlene next door who must be as old as Nana because she has white hair and doesn't walk so fast and hardly ever comes out in the garden except to put the garbage out or leave the litter from the cat boxes on the trash pile. Charlene was in the hospital last week and Mom took care of the cats with Betty, another neighbor. Charlene keeps TuTu, a white cat, in the house, and Patches and Tommy on the porch, and our Smokey in the yard. Mom sometimes asks Charlene, "How are things in the cat house?" and Charlene laughs and they talk some more. I get bored and jump on my trampoline. Or if we are at Charlene's house, I see what is in the candy dish and then ask if I can have two. The house next door to Charlene has a family of three parents and a son but I don't see them much and don't really know much about them.

There's Bobbie on the corner who has a son with a boat and a neat backyard with trees to climb and a humongous pool. I see Bobbie in the mornings when I am walking Roxi before I go to school. Across the street on the other corner is an Italian family with a house that has two stories. Mom tells me the kids are grown and live somewhere else. I'm always going to live with my mom and we will be together forever and ever. Then there's Betty and Nolene and their beautiful but pushy dog, Jasmine, who scares me because she's big and jumps up all the time. Betty says that's because she loves me. They have a pool where we go swimming sometimes. Mom has a picture of us at Betty's pool where she says I fell in when I was about two years old.

Things I Know

The house next to them belongs to Robert and Beatrice and their son Martin. He's adopted also, and is the same age as I am, except I am older, even if it is only three weeks. Mom says they aren't really friendly, but when I ask why she won't really tell me. She says some day she will, like when I will understand better. Like I don't understand things now. I understand a lot—including sexy things. I asked Mom if I could talk about my privates with her and she said of course, that there was nothing we couldn't talk about forever and ever, that families, big or small, share in everything until eternity.

Then comes another two-story house that I know nothing about. Then there are some houses but they have an office in them—Mom says they are residential-professional.

On the other side are two more of those houses. Then there is Rita, who I have never seen, who Mom says is also old. She has the best gardenia bush on the block! Next to us is Jeff and Carol, who are Asian and share their papaya as we share our carambolas and bananas. But the best neighbors are out the back gate and down the back street, where my friend Helen, who is 6, and her sister Clara and their parents live. Helen knew me when I was a baby and she was a baby, says my Mom. We play a lot and go to the same school. And then there are more friends and families in the neighborhood, but I don't play with them as much. A teacher at my school also lives out the back gate and down the back street. It's hard to get together with my friends sometimes—with Chelsea, my best friend, for instance. Her mom and dad are divorced and so every Saturday Chelsea spends time with him till Sunday, and that doesn't give us enough time to play even when I spend overnight on Friday beginning at 7 P.M. after gymnastics. I used to play with another friend who was in ballet with me, but now I don't take ballet anymore because it was too boring, and so I don't see Katarina either because she spends the weekends with her dad.

My mom and I took Roxi for a walk yesterday and went by a house where Mom said she saw a girl my age playing. Her name is Rebecca and she will be 8 in April and she spends every other weekend with her dad, but we can play sometimes, I hope. And then there's Ashley, who lives around the corner and who is 7 1/2 and has two sisters, one 11 years old and the other 2 years old. She has a mom and a dad and a swimming pool, but I have a trampoline. Helen has a mom and dad, and that's cool.

My mom says she was married once but is now divorced. I asked her if I had a dad and she said yes, and when I asked her where he was, she looked me right in the eye and said, Catherine, I don't know, I honestly don't know. I believe her 'cause Mom tells me she will always tell me the truth even though I may not like it and it may hurt. How can truth hurt? Oh well, maybe someday I'll understand.

NANA

I love my Nana best next. She is kind and quiet and gentle and beautiful and a terrific cook. But she is also strict, being from Germany and another generation. The worst is having to put on a dress and stockings and shoes with a bow when I go with her to the ballet. Nana gave me a beautiful pair of opera glasses to see the ballerinas better and I do love going and being there, it's just the getting ready and all fancy part that I don't like. My Nana is 80-something, but Mom told me not to tell a soul, including Nana. I don't have to tell Nana. I'm sure she knows how old she is. She might not hear so well, but she can do the math problems quicker than I can.

It's interesting and also boring to watch my mom and Nana together. They look alike in some ways but not in others. At times my mom cares and does things for Nana like she does for me, and then other times she gets angry when

Nana wants her to do something, especially in the morning when we have to leave the house at 8 A.M. and get to school. Mom says she feels like a piece of ham sandwiched between Nana and me. There are times when I think Mom wants to explain more to me about how she was raised and what her family was like when she was growing up, but Mom doesn't share that yet. I guess I'm too young or Mom thinks I might tell my friends and all. Aren't secrets for sharing with someone else to make another secret?

My mom's brother and wife and son—my uncle and aunt and cousin—live in Boston, so we don't get to see them much. One of these years Mom says we are going there for Christmas to see and ski in the snow. I've only seen snow in pictures. I've seen a koala climb a tree in Australia when Mom was there on a sabbatical and I was 4 1/2. We also rode a camel. And I've tried snorkeling this past summer in Costa Rica. Traveling is fun. I like American Airlines the best, although I'm just as happy at home with my Barbies and swing set and trampoline and my dog Roxi.

PETS

We got Roxi after my mom said I showed enough responsibility (that word again) taking care of PigNut, a guinea pig we had for about a year. Phew, cleaning out that cage was a stinky mess! Maybe a rabbit would have been better. Mom had two cats when I arrived on the scene. One, Cat Ballou was a "soppy old affectionate puddy cat," as Mom says, but she had to be put to sleep because she was old and had tangled with a racoon or something in the yard and had hurt her jaw. The other cat, Smokey, is still around, but not for long once Roxi came into the family. Actually, she never was very affectionate and was always happier outside than inside and now lives in Charlotte's yard next door where she is safe from Roxi by virtue of a fence. Sometimes, I see her looking over here in our yard and I call to her and give her some food on a plate on the other side of the fence. I love animals but not bugs and spiders and roaches and mosquitoes. My mom is the same. Of course—she *is* my mom.

A SISTER

Mom and I have talked about adopting a sister but for the past two years there has been no one coming here to be a part of our family. I sure would like a sister to play with. I heard Mom talking once to a friend, saying she thought it would be great too for the two of us to go through life together as sisters. I know there is a 6- or 7-year-old out there that needs a family. Just because there's only two of us doesn't mean we're not a family. Families grow bigger and families get smaller. I'm going to adopt when I become a mommy too, so that I have a family just like ours.

CHAPTER 12

Reflections on Becoming and Being a Mother

Sarah Selen Steen Lauterbach

My Baby

From the moment I looked into my baby daughter's eyes, lying on my chest on the delivery table, I knew what my mother, her mother, my father's mother, and mothers in my family for generations had experienced.

Speaking at my parents' 50th wedding anniversary 11 years ago, I was remembering the powerful realization when Marlow was born that I would be a mother forever. Even though I had carefully planned becoming a mother and had chosen it completely, I had not fully understood what being-a-mother would mean. I had not realized that the decision to become a mother would completely change me forever.

Since Then

Since that moment, I have had many reminders of what "forever" means. Marlow is now 23, and after years of experience and mothering, I am still very engaged in being-a-mother. Held now as a mother in captivity by my almost-grown children, I have been a single mother for five and a half years. During the last 12 years I have resumed an academic post and tried to combine the two carefully.

Life is much more complex than when I was a new stay-at-home mother. But mother work remains the hardest, the most complex work that I've ever done. It is rewarding if things are going well, but when times are difficult, I have questioned my choices, as many mothers have in moments which test one's patience.

My children, like my work, have enriched my life more than I can describe. I have strived to be a loving, effective, fully present, but not always stick-in-the-mud mother. Being a mother has been so much fun. My children often inspire me.

Jared once made a Mother's Day card right before my doctoral graduation, and his words still sing in my heart. He said, "Happy Mother's Day. I can hardly wait to sit under a tree and read your dissertation." He was 14. Alexandra recently shared that she might do research on siblings' and twins' experience of having a baby die. She thinks that the experience and stories of siblings needs to be told.

Even though I look forward to having an emptier house one day, my children continue to be central in my life . . . along with nursing work and being a member of a large extended family. Nursing, motherhood, and family have each informed the other.

My philosophy of life and optimistic spirit were fueled in my childhood and have been validated by my experiences as a mother. Optimism at times has kept hope alive. Interestingly, mothering and teaching are similar. Motherhood, in addition to providing me with a human science and understanding of children, has informed me and my understanding of nursing as a discipline, as a human caring spirit, art, and science.

Art

I am drawn to the art of two women whose work reflects sentiments about motherhood in the late 1800s and early 20th century. Henriette Wyeth painted a beautiful work entitled "Death and the Child." I discovered it during my investigation of the creative art and literature surrounding infant death for my doctoral research. The painting hangs in a Pennsylvania school in the Delaware Valley. The beautiful impressionist painting depicts a child being lifted up to heaven, lovingly, by the hands of a woman. Mary Cassatt's paintings of mothers with their children in nurturing day-to-day activities convey the sentiments and themes of motherhood during the late 1800s. Though her paintings were of upper-class friends and mothers, whose servants performed most of the nurturing, she preferred to paint simple folk who had primary responsibility for the care of their children.

Donohue's (1996) book of nursing portrayed as "the finest art" has many examples of the idealism and reality of maternity. Mandette's "Desert Mother and Child" (1994) and Munch's "The Sick Child" (1907), as well as the cover of Donohue's book, are examples.

Munch, who lost his mother when he was young and his sister when he was an adolescent, used a variety of mediums to portray his intimate relationship with death. Fragonard's "The Happy Family" (1769) conveys the theme of mother as pivotal in the happy family, caring for everyone.

Some of the most meaningful moments in my own experience came from day-to-day nurturing and caring activities. Bedtime rituals of baths, stories, and songs in my home were reminiscent of my childhood, where my mother read to us five children from the living room each night. Our bedrooms adjoined that room. With almost-grown children in my home today, I find ritual and celebrations are still important. My children have always appreciated good food and love a special meal, which they now often help with or prepare themselves.

Rituals and small celebrations, having meaningful day-to-day experiences, building memories all became a focus for me as a mother. Jared, at 3, wanted to visit the camel daily, so for several months many of our daily outings included a drive by and quick stop at the Philadelphia Zoo. The parking lot happened to be positioned perfectly, right outside the camel lot, and we would say, "Hello, Mr. Camel."

Steichen's *The Family of Man* (1955) and Mason's *The Family of Children* (1977) combine photography with selected literary passages and depict universal sentiments concerning the meaning of life. Carl Sandburg's poem highlights the universal themes of the human experience:

> *There is only one man in the world and his name is All Men.*
> *There is only one woman in the world and her name is All Women.*
> *There is only one child in the world and the child's name is All Children.*

Human Experience

Many women share the experience of motherhood. Each mother interprets and lives experiences differently, within the multiple contexts of her life. One woman's story may still contain universal, as well as unique, sentiments and themes. Combined with a current interest in a postmodern view of family, and thinking about the future, narratives of mothers hold truths about experience.

The photographs, along with my personal story, contain reflections of motherhood, which are not completely represented by postmodern views of women and life process, but nonetheless, may be representative of many mothers' and families' experience.

However, the postmodern view of bereavement as *moving through*, leaving the dead behind, is not consistent with experiences of mothers who participated in my doctoral research. These women experienced death of infants in late pregnancy or shortly after birth.

They described poignant experiences of just the opposite phenomenon. Through memory, symbolic memorials, and rituals, mothers in my research *brought their dead infants into continuing life process*. This was found to be not only during the intense period of grief following the baby's death, but was interpreted as being-a-mother to the dead child while caring for live children.

Some Stories

A mother, at a small family dinner with her son and daughter-in-law, upon hearing that I had experienced the death of my second twin baby girl in my last pregnancy, said that she had a 4-year-old daughter drown in a small pond in her backyard many years before.

She said that this child had required as much mothering as her living child. She described that a primary occupation in the years that followed the death was helping her family deal with the death. She went on to say that she had often needed to cry and experience her loss with loved ones, but that she had not been able to do so.

Her family needed to know that she was all right, and that she was not preoccupied with the child's death. She had never discussed the loss with anyone outside the family, and only rarely was the dead child referred to by anyone. She had never voiced her occasional feeling of total despair. She asked if it was all right to share this with me. We talked softly with tears in our eyes for several moments. Then we wiped our eyes, rejoined the dinner conversation, and finished eating.

The conversation had become more hushed as everyone became aware of our interaction, but as we composed ourselves, we resumed our social roles. (I had actually known that the husband of my friend had had a sister die in childhood, but had not really ever connected it with my research.) When the friends were leaving, this woman hugged me and expressed how grateful she was for the opportunity to share, and that mothers in my research were very lucky to have an opportunity to be understood.

Daily Living/Mothering

As I write this, it is 6:00 A.M. on a Saturday morning in November and my thoughts return to my present experience of being a mother. I had hoped to sleep past my 3 or 4 A.M. awakening period. Today Marlow has to be at work at 6:00 A.M., so her alarm went off at 4:00. She seems not to be able to get up without help. Finally, she crawled out of bed. In bed with me at that time was my youngest daughter, Alexandra, who had come into my room when she got home around 1:00 A.M. She had an argument with Jared and since he is her best friend, she was very upset.

While I was calling out to Marlow, trying to stay in the warm bed, hoping to go back to sleep, I thought how totally involved with my children I remain, in spite of their ages.

Finally, Marlow got up and had a shower in my bathroom because it is where our makeup and shampoo are kept. At 5:30, while I was still in bed with Alexandra and our cat, Elvis, both of whom were sleeping soundly, I asked Marlow to awaken Jared to get up to go to his lifeguard job. She made him coffee and as they talked pleasantly, I got up to join them. Moments like this are so wonderful. I made coffee for myself and Marlow left, with "I love you." Jared and I sat talking about his and Alexandra's argument. He finally left, but not without giving me a hug. I was up now and began writing about being a mother.

Reflection

Two months later, I have begun to work on this story again, and I am struck with the above passage, how perfect a scene it paints. It is important to correct the picture. We have had very excruciating moments and years as a family. I'm thinking particularly of the times when something was discovered to be wrong with my children, such as Jared's bout with epiglottitis when he was 2 months old, or his falling on a tricycle and knocking out his front incisor when he was 3, or of Marlow careening down the mews driveway on a bike. She was learning to ride a bike at 4. The perfect twin pregnancy with Alexandra and Amy and perfect midwife delivery of Alexandra, were followed by the traumatic birth of Amy, who died nine days later.

In the couple of years before we moved to Mississippi, I experienced much worry and anxiety about the safety of my children on Philadelphia streets as they navigated their way to three different schools in different parts of the city. We moved away from Philadelphia to Mississippi three years ago.

The culture of small-town Hattiesburg and the distance from Philadelphia make it seem like a different world with many lifestyle changes. Leaving the children's father and the city was difficult. "This is my town," stated Jared during the time he and Alexandra played baseball in the Fairmount Little League, on the fields beside the parkway, near the art museum, with Philadelphia's center city and skyline as backdrop. I was reading fiction during that spring and I found the incredible amount of time that baseball required to be perfect for becoming immersed in narratives.

When we moved, it was hard to leave our family of friends and life in a complex urban neighborhood. My intention was to move us away from the complexity of Philadelphia, away from the temptations that had beckoned to each child so that I could launch my children nearer to where I eventually plan to live.

Three years later, each child has become more focused, gained in impulse control, is pursuing goals, but still misses "home." It all may have happened in Philadelphia too, but I also moved as an adolescent. Some issues had continued to be exacerbated after my husband moved out of our Victorian home in University City two years earlier. In accepting a job offer in Mississippi, I moved closer to my childhood home, the farm where I grew up in the backwoods of northern Florida, where my mother and four siblings are now only six hours away.

More Reflections

Our present home and family life is not always the ideal picture painted in the narrative above. But we care deeply about each other's feelings and actions, almost always talk about decisions and choices, enjoy each other's company, depend on each other for help and support, and deal very openly with conflicts and issues. Many of the small rituals and experiences are repeated in this almost-grown family.

Participation in decisions, making choices about how to live and be, has been very important in this family. Even though I made the decision to move, the children made choices. Originally, Jared planned to live with his father, but circumstances developed that precluded that choice. The children decided initially to support the decision to move, even though Jared and Alexandra were in great conflict about it.

The first year we alternated between adjustment and missing our old life. Three years later, the missing continues, and each may eventually choose to live in Philadelphia. The children are stronger for the experiences surrounding our move, or at least they appear to be, and they voice this occasionally, now.

The structure of family life, though, even in our family with two parents and younger children, included the children as active participants in decision making. It is a very different structure and process from my childhood family, which was more patriarchal and authoritarian.

However, the importance of family rituals in my family has been singular. My mother was a school teacher, and a teaching school principal for several years. My dad, in my early years, lived away from the family, as he was in the Army. By necessity, children in my family had to participate, work, and help with household tasks and activities.

Back to the Future

Two months ago when I first began this story, I was at a conference and I had many conversations during the three days I was away, because I call my children at 6:30 each morning to get them up for school. (I even called from England a couple of years ago while presenting at a conference in Bournemouth.)

Late the night before I left for the conference, Marlow had a fainting episode after she hurt her finger. Medics came and checked her out, and I asked a friend to call a neurologist with whom she has worked. Edith was unable to arrange a medical appointment, so Jared and Alexandra agreed to stay with her, not let her drive, and call me if anything else happened. Also, I planned to call mornings and nights.

I am feeling very much the mother here, too, and beginning to feel the need to assume a primary role with my mother and sister. At the same time, my professional life, teaching, research, and professional activity are in full swing. I have about 15 years left to make a contribution. I am having similar feelings to those when I finally decided to become a mother, that of a biological clock ticking. This time the biological clock is ticking in terms of work.

When my children were young, I pushed my desire to make a professional contribution aside. It was necessary, because of my choice to become a mother, not just once but with each pregnancy, delayed education, and professional career. The biological clock demands that choices to have children or to work be made. Some women choose not to be mothers, but to devote undivided time and attention to career, but I suspect that they too experience a similar clock. Work and motherhood share some of the same meanings. For me both require creativity and discipline and are helped by an optimistic spirit.

The career clock ticking has other meanings that are potentially very painful, personally. My mother is advancing in age. I am getting older and experiencing some physical and energy changes. The power of myth (Campbell, 1988) offering the idea that the dead support the living is very comforting to me as I look to the future. My grandparents were pivotal people in my early and adolescent years. They and the many adults, teachers, aunts, and uncles helped my mother care for, guide, and support me and my siblings. I think they were missed very much by my mother, and I feel certain that they continued to support her after they died. It has been hard for my mother to not have them in her everyday life as she has continued to care for her adult children.

My relationship with my mother has been *key*. Even though she has not always agreed with me in all I have done, she has given my siblings and me unconditional love. It is hard to think about a time without her human presence.

At the same time, this is the most exciting time of my life. My children are becoming more and more OK, and as they mature, they seem to be reflecting the tremendous commitment and work that has been invested in them.

My son is currently considering becoming an English teacher. Alexandra is planning to follow her dream to combine art and English in working with handicapped children. Marlow is working in sales and does not yet have a clear career trajectory.

My children all value money, but it is becoming less of an incentive in their choices. Interestingly, my students and work require a similar motherly care and commitment. The results of teaching, research, and professional activity, I hope, is reflected in my students' education and the nursing discipline.

In the End

Finally, not sad or depressing to me at all, I am the mistress of my own destiny. I do not share my house, space, bed, or bath, with anyone but my children and my cat Elvis. I left behind a lot in the move away from Philadelphia.

I am not divorced yet, though I have been separated for over five years. But, essentially, I am free of what became a very difficult marriage. Still regretful that I wasn't able to "bring him along," the separation from my husband has given me back my life.

I am beginning to be interested in relationships, but doubt that I'll ever be in another committed relationship. My children have lots of advice and want to develop an Application to Date My Mom. My brother has made up an Application To Date my Daughter for me to use when the time comes. An interview that accompanies the application has questions about grade point average, legal entanglements, and seat belt use, objective tests such as IQ, drug panel, ACT and SAT scores, and college plans, and experiences with family chores, laundry, yard work, cooking, and cleaning. But most important is whether the person can interact with and relate to our family. Interestingly, this has also been articulated by my son, as a criterion for friends.

This is a most wonderful place to be with my children. I am still a parent, and each will be quick to say so. They have a formidable mother, yet I dressed in costume along with them this past Halloween and visited several of our friends.

It was such great fun. Marlow and I sat outside on New Year's Eve. We had a glass of champagne and talked about life, the new year, our hopes and dreams.

My parenting philosophy has included insisting that each child do stuff for him- or herself but also do chores for the family, such as vacuuming, laundry, and yard work. It has almost always required my presence and participation. I have expected that each learn to fix meals, clean house, and be a full participant in family events and rituals. Dinnertime is important and money is tight. I think we are stronger for the move. I love the collegial relationship, but I am fully the parent. My children will each attest to the fact that I will go *nose-to-nose* with them or their friends, if necessary and in a heartbeat. Being a single parent has required that I learn assertiveness, and sometimes tempering this new skill is difficult.

I would do almost anything for my children, including going to the ends of the earth to rescue, help, and just "be" with them. In spite of my work, which is challenging and wonderfully rewarding, I am still mother—but I'm also an academic nurse. In addition, I am a daughter . . . and a sister, a friend, a colleague, and a neighbor.

When I became a mother, I had lots of advice from friends and colleagues about how I was not superwoman and that I needed to come to terms with it. I have always struggled for balance in everything that I have done. I have made many mistakes, but my concept of *intentionality* has helped.

I had the luxury in my children's early years, because I was married and had the intention to be fully involved in rearing children, to stay at home with my children. Each child had some issue that I was not willing to turn over to a caregiver.

It has been wonderful and I am very glad to have done it.

REFERENCES

Breeskin, A. (1979). *Mary Cassatt: A Catalogue Raissonné of the Graphic Work*. Washington: Smithsonian Institution Press.

Campbell, J. (1988). *The Power of Myth*. New York: Anchor Books Doubleday.

Donohue, P. (1996). *Nursing, the Finest Art: An Illustrated History* (2d ed.). St. Louis: Mosby-Yearbook

Lauterbach, S. (1992). In Another World: A Phenomenological Perspective and Discovery of Meaning in Mothers' Experience of Death of a Wished-for Baby. Doctoral dissertation, Teachers College, Columbia University, New York.

———. (1999). In Another World: Five Years Later. (Research in progress.)

Lindbergh, A. (1955/1983). *Gift from the Sea*. New York: Pantheon Books.

Mason, J. (ed.). (1977). *The Family of Children*. New York: Grosset & Dunlap.

Meryman, R. (1991). The Wyeth Family: American Visions. *National Geographic*, 180(1):78–109.

Steichen, E. (1955). *The Family of Man*. New York: Museum of Modern Art.

CHAPTER 13

BECOMING A MAN IN A GAY FAMILY: DIALOGUE AND REFLECTIONS

Edward M. Freeman

The title of this chapter is a reference to Paul Monette's autobiography, *Becoming a Man: Half a Life Story*. Monette tells the story of half of his life, presuming that he would die from AIDS before he reached his 50th birthday. Indeed, in 1994 he succumbed to the disease before he turned 50. He adopted the perspective that becoming a man was not simply a matter of coming of age, but of coming out of the closet. Monette lived for many years out of the closet as a gay man. But his life out of the closet was preceded by a long period of time of furtive and sexless affairs. During these closeted years, he denied the goodness of his attraction to the same sex. He played the roles that he believed would make him acceptable to the so-called straight world of Ivy League schools. Thus, he depicted his life as becoming a man even as he gradually left behind his closet of shame and secrecy.

Monette opens the first chapter with a central debate of the autobiographical voice, which I will pose as a question: Is my experience entirely unique to me or do I share some part of it with others?

> I speak for no one else here. . . . Yet I've come to learn that all our stories add up to the same imprisonment. The self-delusion of uniqueness. The festering pretense that we are the same as they are. . . . Such obedient slaves we make, with such very tidy rooms. (p. 1)

Monette maintains the view that, in reference to the closet of secrecy, all gay men and lesbians have experienced the "same imprisonment." Enslaved by their heterosexual masters and left to feel unique by attraction to the same sex, they must tell their stories of life inside the closet in order to build their tribe's culture. This is to say that lesbians and gay men join a tribe, their tribe, when they retell and recollect their memories of isolation from one another, of a time gone by when they felt coerced to pass as straight.

The legacies of life inside the closet could be called their cultural fodder. The closet unites them afterward just as much as it isolated them when they were inside. United by the memories of pain, lesbians and gay men learn to laugh at the closet, at that Monette called their years spent in the practice of "ventriloquism," which is his metaphor for trying to pass as straight.

I am a gay man, and was a ventriloquist. I have many stories to tell of coming out and can identify with others in my tribe who have been subjected to hatred turned inward. But I wish now to make the point that I did not live in just one closet but many. As my self continues to open like a rose, I recognize that while one closet door was slammed shut and bolted behind me, there are many more closet doors through which I still must pass in my opening.

Such closet doors include new work settings, new relationships—indeed, any circumstance that will require my attention to become myself in the new circumstance. One of my stories of coming out involves becoming a parent long after identifying myself to others as a gay man. Therefore, my intent in this chapter is to tell not just my story but "our" story. As I see it, our story as lesbians and gay men is that we have always been parents, but have more often neglected coming out as such.

Roland, my nephew by birth who later identified himself as our "son," joins me in telling the story of our family. We lived in San Francisco for five years before he graduated from high school and left for college, and I accepted an employment position in a distant city. Major life events during these years included the birth of a business, selling and buying a home, completing a doctoral degree, graduating from high school, student exchange with a German family, typical teenage transitions, including a brush with the law, and travel. San Francisco was both foundation and foil for our family, because the city offered liberal vistas from which to view our nontraditional experiences.

Paul and I met in San Francisco in the mid-1980s, soon after we had moved from Boston and Dallas to the City by the Bay. It was to become our second or third significant relationship. Paul was employed by a major Silicon Valley firm, and I was a nurse researcher involved in developing new instruments in self-care theory and supervising clinical drug trials for experimental agents in HIV/AIDS. We lived from the start in one of the city's gay neighborhoods.

Roland was 13 years old at the time. He was the oldest of my sister's children. Roland's mother neglected him after his father died in an alcohol-related motor vehicle accident. The neglect was so great that the courts had appointed social workers to intervene. Roland learned to distrust his mother, and lived sometimes under the same roof and other times with my mother. He and his mother grew apart. When few options for reconciliation remained for Roland and his mother, he came to live with Paul and me in San Francisco.

Roland had been aware since early childhood that I was gay, but he did not face the issue until he came to live with me. He was sexually naive at the time of his arrival and experienced pubescent shame in reference to talk about sex.

So discussions about sex in the first six months after his arrival, when they occurred, were left to Roland to initiate.

Roland entered the eighth grade in September following his arrival in August. His preference was to study in a public school, so he entered a middle school of the San Francisco School District. He was a committed student in the first two years after his arrival, but later turned to teenage passions, seeking peer approval. Thus, the sophomore and junior years of high school brought him few academic achievements. In the summer between the sophomore and junior years, Roland went to Germany where he lived with a family near Munich. The following two summers his German "brother" visited San Francisco for extended visits.

In the following dialogue, Roland (RB) and I (EF) discuss the family life that we shared over the course of five years. We are reminiscing, because we have lived in separate and very distant places for the past two years. Roland is now a junior in college on one coast and I live on the other.

The context for our dialogue is the rearing of a child in a gay home. Therefore, the dialogue will revolve around the themes of sexual orientation, such as coming out of the closet, secrecy, shame and guilt, feeling different from everyone else, teenage sexual exploration, and religion and sexuality. The themes are intertwined in the dialogue.

EF: I think back to the time that you first arrived. I knew that things were not going so well for you, but I knew that I wanted to be a parent. It seemed like an ideal arrangement. It was ideal until it came time to start paying for everything, like braces for your teeth, new clothes every three months—you grew like a weed right from the start. But even harder for me was coming home every evening after work. I had been used to dining out and working late at the office. That pattern had to change if I was to parent you well. I didn't know more than one or two gay men who were raising children, but I was acquainted with at least five lesbian parents. I idealized their work as parents. Little did I know about the realities that lay ahead.

RB: When I first arrived in SF, I was stunned to find how strong the gay community really was. It consisted of a tightly woven network of companions and friendships. Because you were a nurse at a hospital that specialized in treating AIDS patients, I volunteered there for a short time just before I started the eighth grade. It was in the first month after moving to SF that I came to understand how the gay community operated, which, in turn, influenced how our home was governed.

EF: Sometimes I can't see the connection between living in a gay community and its influences upon the family. I mean it's all too close to me. So when you say that the gay community influenced how our home was governed, I don't know what you mean.

RB: I think that I had more freedom than most kids. I kind of saw your sexuality as freedom. Oh yeah, I had to go to school, do my homework, stay active in school things like sports and the newspaper, but I came to understand something about freedom deep down that I never had learned before. I could bring up any subject, discuss just about anything, and I knew that it would be OK. Our home was governed by this inner sense of freedom that I learned.

EF: I am interested that you call it freedom. Coming out of the closet can be one of the most challenging experiences in any gay person's life, and it was no different for me. When the coming out process begins, a gay man might not call it freedom but bondage—a kind of bondage that he must overcome from within. I can remember being really scared about my attraction to men and wanting to hide it from myself and everyone else.

Later I put my inner sense of self into perspective and moved to San Francisco, where I consolidated my gay identity. Then you joined me, and I faced another coming out. This time I needed to learn how to be gay as a parent. So I was back to the start of another coming out. In a sense I had formed my personal identity within certain limits that no longer suited me as a parent. Unwittingly, I needed to become unshackled from what had been my personal identity. I wasn't only a gay man any longer, I was a gay man and a parent.

RB: Coming out was not so easy for me either. I had this friend named Andre, who was a classmate at school. I made a friend out of Andre when he was in trouble with the cool kids at school. I always was part of the "in" group, so I kind of stood up for Andre when the guys decided not to hang out with him.

Andre and his father lived in a tiny one-bedroom apartment in another San Francisco neighborhood. They didn't have much contact with gay people (or, at least, they didn't acknowledge their contacts), so I wasn't about to tell them, and especially Andre, that you were gay. I made up this lie that your companion, Paul, was really your fiancée named Paula. I came out with the truth later. You told me that it was OK not to tell the truth about this until I felt that I was ready. I felt like a coward and didn't like to lie. I look back on this experience and laugh about it now. But it was no laughing matter at the time. I wanted to be like my friends, you know what I mean—it was all so complicated . . . maybe that was my prison, sort of my hell, if you can call it that . . .

EF: I remember that there was a honeymoon period with you after you arrived. I tried to put a good spin on everything that you did. And, in fact, you really didn't do much that bothered me.

There was the time that your algebra teacher called to say that you were not turning in your homework. But even then I told myself that you needed to find your new boundaries and that this would take time.

You concealed a lot, but it was all so natural to your stage in development. You were suddenly starting to look like a man, but still felt like a child. You shut the door to your room, and I knew that you needed privacy. I suspected that you must be dealing with your teenage need for privacy. But, just as important, you were hiding the private world of pain that you endured during the years after your father's death, when your mom and you moved from place to place.

RB: I didn't want to piss you off when I first arrived, but it was really a shock to be going to school every day and to stay on top of things at school. Your life and home were so quiet, nothing like what I was used to.

In your house I could hear my thoughts—and sometimes the silence was deafening. So I kept lots of noise going on the radio. Do you remember I was scared at night, especially in that neighborhood where the Spanish-speaking kids didn't want any boys like me—you know, real white?

EF: Prejudice comes in all forms, and sometimes it's more straightforward to experience it when it's a matter of skin color. I mean that a gay person can stay in a closet, but you can never—well, almost never—hide the color of your skin. I knew that you were scared to be in a new place, where you had to learn new languages and become an outsider looking in, at least for a while. After all, Roland, you were raised in a suburb of Dallas. Talk about being an outsider in San Francisco.

RB: Outsider is right, you said it. I was outside the gay community, at least sort of. I saw all of your friends as different from anyone I ever knew. They were so much fun to be around, and didn't have all the hangups of straight people about sex. I wondered if they were for real, so I just kinda watched them until I could understand the whole picture.

EF: I remember one of the first Halloween celebrations that you attended with me on Castro Street. You and Andre were walking down 18th Street when you saw a couple of men making out in a car parked on the street. Later you told me that you and Andre talked about this scene, and you both came to the conclusion that everyone has to make decisions about what he wants to do in life, and who's to say that one person's decision is better than another's.

RB: Yeah, I guess that I was starting to get easy about everything, in fact it started to become sorta fun for me to be part of something that was not like anything else that I had experienced with my mom and dad back in Texas. It was about the same time that I asked you about how I could start a relationship with a guy if that's what I wanted to do. We talked about it, and you told me to stick with kids my own age. Then I went to Paul to ask him the same question, and he was, like, surprised, I mean he wondered what was I thinking—I had always talked about girls. I suppose he just didn't want to talk about the idea that I might like it both ways.

EF: Well, Roland, you didn't like it both ways. But I understand you to say that Paul liked the idea that you were a straight kid in a gay family, that kids like you couldn't be recruited into what the religious fundamentalists call the "gay lifestyle."

RB: Paul was really proud of me being straight. He sorta lived the straight life through me, ya know, all that talk about girls and how to make them happy. Paul didn't date women, but he sure told me how to date them.

EF: Paul was so happy to be a parent, to be your parent. He didn't have much chance to warm up to the idea of parenting. Suddenly you were there in San Francisco, an adolescent and ready to be a teenager—if you catch my drift. He needed time to get to know you. I, at least, shared many memories with you and of you prior to your move to San Francisco.

RB: Maybe Paul had to come out about being a gay parent, and it was easier for him at first to stay in the closet of straight parenthood.

EF: Nothing was easy for him or you. Everything was new for all of us. I want to talk about your troubles in high school, when you experimented with drugs and had a run-in with the law. I remember that you changed slowly as you grew older, and you were not the same person that I had always known. Your secrecy increased as you started to spend more hours with a classmate who grew pot at home.

RB: I tried pot several times and didn't really like it. Then I met this guy and his mom—she was a school teacher—and they grew pot at home. I figured what have I got to lose. Pot never tasted so good, but the buzz was great. I was going every afternoon to their house, and got stoned just about three out of five afternoons every week. It was like *Tales of the City*. (*Laughs*)

EF: What a bad memory those days were for all of us. I knew that things started to get out of control when I saw your eyes every evening. But I was home so late that I didn't see you over dinner as I did when you were in middle school and earlier in high school. Could have been that my career was just too consuming for me. And, to be honest with you, you started to get really tiresome. We were following different values and incentives for personal growth. I thought a lot about your mother during these months and thought that you were fulfilling her destiny to be addicted.

RB: I wouldn't say different values, I'd say different ways of having a good time. Come on, you're just too serious sometimes. I know what I've got to do to make it in the world. You made sure to teach me that. So I was going to have fun, and I did it big. You went to college at 16. How's that for too serious?

EF: OK, maybe you're right. But bailing you out of jail one day and answering the calls from the counselor at your high school were scary for me. I was scared that you were not the same person that I knew and loved.

RB: It took time for me to understand your fear, and now I know that I might also be afraid if my kid did what I did. Hey, you weren't so stupid after all! (*Laughs*)

EF: I wanted to know you, Roland. It was this desire that held me together in some dark times. I was always sure that I loved you, and love for me always finds a way to forgive.

The dialogue between Roland and me provides images of life in a gay family with a child. These images are colored by the environment of the family, and, therefore, may not be a reflection of gay families in other less gay-friendly cities. San Francisco provided them with a place to become men and to grow in love, without many of the constraints of Dallas, Topeka, Savannah, or Cheyenne. In many ways San Francisco is true to its name. It's the city of Francis and cloaked in his grace.

"I speak for no one else here," Monettte contends, as do I. However, Roland and I talk about his experience as a straight man coming out of the closet, which leads me to wonder if coming out is experienced only by lesbians and gay men. Surely Roland's experience of the closet is shared by many children raised in gay and lesbian families. He laughs now, but I remember the pain that I saw in his eyes when he asked me not to tell his friend, Andre, that Paula was really Paul. He tidied his closet in these early months together with Paul and me, as did Monette once, as did I once. "Such obedient slaves we made." Social shame has its way with all of us.

The dialogue offers a view of the transition of one child, who, just as he was to enter his adolescence, left a straight family and entered a gay household. He faced his own entrance into sexual manhood in a foreign place. In reference to Roland's transposition, I often thought of the psalmist who asked, "How can we sing the Lord's song in a foreign land?" He could not turn to his father, then deceased, to translate the meaning of attraction to women or, more importantly, how to become a man. Instead, he turned to his gay uncle and his mate for translations and interpretations.

Translations and interpretations will never be easy for teenagers, as adolescence confounds the best intentions of straight and gay parents alike. The dialogue presents themes of growth and development from the life of this teenager that are similar to the life of any teenager. However, there are differences to be noted, as well. In particular, Roland was faced with different reasons to keep secrets than are faced by teenagers in straight families. He was a member of a gay family. North American societies still inhibit widespread acceptance of homosexual behavior and the public openness of gays and lesbians as persons in the society. Roland was faced with the closet of adolescent sexual desire, even as he entered what might be called an emerging but not widely accepted depiction of family.

Others may develop enhanced understanding of gay families if they understand the forces that shape societal rules of sexual identity and familial enclosure. The dialogue between Roland and me provides images of a gay family for nurses to consider as they study the experience of adolescence and family life. The challenge for all of us is to discover how adolescence, as lived in a gay family, is more like than unlike adolescence in other family units.

In my view, becoming a man is made more perilous when hidden behind closet doors. Becoming a man in a gay family, therefore, might mean less peril for the adolescent, because the parents have already wrestled with the demons of the closet. Gay parents are in a psychological space of understanding the teenager's need for privacy. Disavowed of the "pretense that we are the same as they," gay parents remember what it is to become a man.

Reference

Monette, P. (1992). *Becoming a Man: Half a Life Story*. San Francisco: HarperCollins.

CHAPTER

14

A NORMAL FAMILY: FROM THE PERSPECTIVE OF A 21-YEAR-OLD YOUNG MAN

Daniel Collins

WHERE IT'S ALL AT

I believe that the microcosm reflects the macrocosm, undeniably, uncontrollably, and inevitably. Assuming that there are motions—cosmic phenomena—that exist on an infinite, universal level, how can one put forth the proposition that the motions of smaller units of interaction within that universal plane do not respond directly to those larger motions? All religions are based upon it, as are all sciences. After all, what is science if not the religion of fact?

Astrology, for instance, is based on the idea that personality, destiny, prosperity, and so forth are all determined by motions in the stars, that human interaction is directly influenced by larger motions. Darwin's theory of evolution states that beings either adapt to fit their surroundings (which are controlled by the larger motions of the ecosystem, essentially) or fail to survive. Even basic laws of physics insist that smaller objects are inevitably propelled along a path by the gravity of larger objects, that the earth revolves around the sun, the moon around the earth, the oceans toward the moon, vacationers toward the ocean (you see, I'm onto something here!).

But seriously, change on the larger scale effects change on the smaller scale—the trickle-down policy of the cosmos. Is it so unnatural, then, to witness a shift of priorities, moral or formal, in the smaller system called family in light of the massive, brewing paradigm shift overtaking the larger system called Earth?

OF ATOMS, FAMILIES, AND WAVES

The traditional structure of the family is changing. It is no longer defined by name, by location, even by blood. It does not exist within the guidelines placed upon it by our ancestors or our parents or our stepparents or whatever.

In this age we have managed to split the nucleus of an atom—so why not the center of the nuclear family? *The Third Wave* by Alvin Toffler explains the history of society by dividing it into three levels of development: agricultural, industrial, and informational.

His premise is that all aspects of society and culture develop more or less simultaneously within these "waves." Human interaction (the sociosphere) develops in conjunction with technological progress (the technosphere), which is fueled by knowledge (the infosphere). All aspects of culture are interdependent.

During the "first wave" of widespread agrarian society, the conventional family consisted of a farming father, a meal-making mother, and numerous chore-tending children. The average life span was shorter, the educational possibilities were fewer, the technical knowledge was simpler than it is today. The form of the family fit the function.

With the increase in knowledge and technical know-how, the industrial revolution occurred and the form of the family changed again. The nuclear family of the mid- to late 20th century was the physical embodiment of the culture it existed within at the peak of the "second wave."

Now, at the dawn of the "third wave" of American society, with the period of industrial boom, prolific expansion, and colonization reaching its end, we are facing yet another change in the structure of family, only this time it seems to be taking everyone by surprise (or at least every political speech writer since Jimmy Carter).

When politicians speak of "the family," however, they typically do not mean the family in all its luxuriant variety of possible forms. No, when the authorities urge us to "restore the family," it is this second wave nuclear family they have in mind. By thinking so narrowly, they not only misdiagnose the entire problem; they also reveal a naiveté about what steps would actually be required to restore the nuclear family to its former importance. Thus, they frantically blame the family crisis on everything from smut peddlers to rock music.

Some tell us that opposing abortion or wiping out sex education or resisting feminism will glue the family back together again. If we truly wish to restore the second wave family, we had better be prepared to restore second wave civilization as a whole, to freeze not only technology but history itself.

Where I'm Coming From

Perhaps some people are clinging to a bygone definition of family because they are alarmed by the tremendous increase in the rate of change. Perhaps it doesn't threaten me because I had the unique opportunity to grow up in a family that some people would consider perfect.

I was raised in a handful of small towns in rural Maine, most of which had more cows than people, but never more than a few hundred of each.

My parents were both born in Hoboken, New Jersey, and fled the chaos of city life for more tranquil surroundings in order to raise children in relative peace and quiet. My mother was one of eight children, and decided that eight was just too many. I have nowhere near the capacity to understand the complexities of her relationships with her parents or siblings, but I know that she wasn't satisfied with the family that she was raised in, and she chose not to model her future family life after that of her past. I know that her consistent lectures on the dangers of drug and alcohol addiction are a reaction to watching loved ones struggle with it. It breaks her heart when I smell like cigarettes, and in return she breaks my eardrums (constant advice echoing off my soul saying "She's right, you know, she's absolutely right").

She has done everything in her power to improve her life without losing track of her goals. Financial success has never been as important to her as emotional success. "A good education is the most important thing in the world!" she always says, and has had a fine education herself.

It's funny how objective knowledge and subjective behavior sometimes differ. There's something you gotta love about a woman who has been racking up degrees in developmental psychology since about the time that you were learning to breathe who still tells you that your hair needs washing five seconds after walking through the door after three years of living 500 miles away. There's something about still being a duckling 21 years after the fact.

Don't get me wrong. She knows her objectives well, and we have a much more sophisticated level of interaction now than I ever could have imagined while freaking out at 15 when the nearest movie theater was 45 minutes away.

Son of Two Shrinks

You should try being one of four children of two psychologists. I grew up eating Rorshach stew and WISC-R for dessert. On any given night the table conversation could have gone like this:

Tom Sr.: So what's new with my sons, ah?
Little Kathleen (age 2): How many bones are in my body?
Kathleen: Sons *and* daughter . . .
Tom Jr. (age 19): I've gotta get out of here. Can I have the car?
Tom Sr.: We'll discuss this later . . .
Me (age 18): He automatically gets the car just because he's home from college? I want to go out tonight. (*Remember, even the nearest coffee shop is half an hour away, and we only have one available car.*)
Patrick (age 14): Can I go with you guys?
Kathleen: Nobody's going anywhere right now . . .
Tom Jr.: But Dad said I could, Dad, you already gave me . . .
Me: Since when is age an acceptable substitute for experience? You can't just give him the car because he's older, you can't justify that decision, you . . .
Little Kathleen (seizing her opportunity in the ensuing chaos): Can I have cookie?

Tom Sr.: This is not the time to debate the rationality of quantitative decision making. We're eating dinner.

Patrick: Can I go to Joey's house?

Tom Sr.: What is this, an auction?

Kathleen: How will you get there? When are you coming back?

Patrick: Tom can drive me when he goes out.

Me: But you said I could go out! Can we debate this affront to my rights?

Tom Sr.: I can have you all committed if this keeps up.

THINKING

I was never allowed to make any statement without thoroughly backing up my intentions, nor did I allow my parents the luxury of statements like, "I'm your father and I *said so*!"

From an early age I was taught that along with speech, along with thought, along with anything, there came the responsibility of consequence, and eventually the wisdom of forethought and careful intellectual calculation.

I taught myself to respect thought and action, not titles and popular concepts of right and wrong. My views have always been at odds with incompetent authority figures whom I disrespect. This is how I know when I am on the right track.

DAD

My father has to be one of the most intelligent, yet down-to-earth people that I know. He has always listened to my thoughts as though they were coming from the mouth of a colleague and given my ideas the same credit and importance as anyone's, even at a very early age. He admits to learning from me, which is not a popular concept among most adults when you're, say, 7 years old.

When I was 13 and refused to be confirmed in the Roman Catholic Church, he simply told me that I'd better be able to tell him why. "Religion is a smile on a dog," I said, quoting Edie Brickel. He never mentioned it again. In past years he has confided in me that he stopped going to church because the company wasn't very good, and that he really believed more in the idea that all creatures are part of the earth's spirit more than God's. I've recommended books and essays on the Earth Spirit to him ever since.

Most of my friends who tried to opt out of God's grace in a similar fashion got a slap on the forehead and a dozen Hail Mary's. My father was one of those kids who was left-handed until a nun and a ruler convinced him otherwise.

It's amazing how easily my generation has managed to do away with traditions that don't hold any meaning for us. Unfortunately, I don't think that enough people know why they break these traditions. They have no plan for developing new ideas once the old ones are erased. This goes back to the responsibility of consequence. I was lucky enough to be encouraged to think before I jump.

A Minority

My family is part of a rare minority. It is the last stand of the nuclear family structure with the first inklings of third wave ideology. This is largely because of the philosophies that my parents believe in and have applied to their lives.

Both of my parents work outside the home. They work mainly with their minds, although they value being able to work with their hands. They are both employed in the field of education, in the realm of information and psychosocial communication (the trademarks of the third wave).

Their work is not something that they leave in the office, but a way of thinking on an everyday level. I was never grounded or pounded for my misdeeds. I was questioned and lectured, investigated, advised, explained to, and heard out. I didn't get money when I made the honor roll—I received intellectual praise and honest respect. I will not necessarily copy the structure of my family if and when I have my own (I have some complaints just as anyone does), but I will definitely try to emulate the phenomenal level of communication, love, and intellectual and emotional support that they have managed to maintain throughout the last 21 years of my life.

Where It's All Going

Third wave civilization will not try to stuff everyone willy-nilly into a single family form. For this reason the emerging family system could free each of us to find our own niche, to select or create a family style or trajectory attuned to our individual needs.

Indeed, this is not the end of the nuclear family—simply the end of its reign as the prevailing norm. (It is already evident that very few people currently exist within its confines.) Eventually, when the inevitable change in family structure becomes apparent to even the most hardheaded traditionalists, discrimination against alternative family systems will end. As of now, homosexual marriage is still illegal in nearly all of our 50 United States. Many people still think that it is somehow morally wrong to be homosexual.

In my hometown (you remember, the one with all the cows and education cuts), people call you crazy (in so many words) if you *allow* your wife to hold a job. It's amazing how violently some success has been achieved, more or less by ignoring certain fundamental problems (the relative reality of instability) that permeate the world.

It is easy to base future family plans on the idea that the safe (if unfulfilling) haven of middle-class television-inspired consumerism will actually last, while remaining blissfully ignorant to the social condition of the majority.

Who is to say that we will have the luxury of raising children in a relatively risk-free environment when we are rapidly pursuing ideological goals that spell certain doom not only for our *way* of life but our actual lives themselves?

Toffler's theories that society keeps changing, and my own ideas on the relationship between microsystems and macro-systems, lead me to believe that by working with other aspects of society, we can not only better understand but also actively change the social implications of raising a child in the 21st century. education reform, for instance, is a necessary step in social change.

If new ways of thinking about the family are introduced through education, new acceptable forms are sure to follow. The rerouting of technological process, and the ideologies involved, greatly affect the path of social progress, and therefore the acceptable definition of units of interaction within that given society.

This goes back to the concept that the function follows form. If the function of a family system is to work cooperatively toward the common goal of spreading information and love (as opposed to producing sons to carry on a business), then who is to say that it is wrong to include two homosexual parents, a few resident aunts or uncles, adopted children, live-in spiritual guides, and a few working artists?

If it takes a village to raise a child, then I'm not too surprised that so many are left to raise themselves. The values of community interaction, of shared burdens and common goals, have all but disappeared in our high-energy technological society.

Ideals Revisited

Consider the decentralization of society as an option for our future. Imagine the common good taking priority over the individual rat race in the form of cooperative living arrangements between groups of families. It is true that most of the communes formed in the 1960s and 1970s rapidly fell apart, suggesting that communes as such are inherently unstable in high-technology societies. A closer look reveals, however, that the ones that disintegrated most rapidly had no economic base and saw themselves as utopian experiments. The communes that have succeeded over time—and some have—are those that have had a clear external mission, an economic base, and a practical, rather than purely utopian, outlook.

So What's a Society to Do?

It is not necessary to disregard our current social model altogether in order to survive this age and fashion a responsible, interactive system of communities for the future—only to rearrange the priorities involving "progress" and humanity.

To develop further the beneficial aspects of informational technology and to move away from the current paradigm of no-holds-barred expansion at the cost of human concern and environmental stability could be the external mission that glues successful future communities and various types of family systems together.

Imagine a group of families (of various structures) living in close proximity, managing and responsibly using an area of land, communicating and working through computerized workstations within the home and all taking part in daily functions such as the maintenance of the land and houses, the cultivation of food, the raising and education of children.

It would be a combination of the best aspects of all waves of society, all forms of family. Imagine being unhooked from the intravenous needle of centralized society, mainstream media, and the like. Obviously it is much easier to imagine such an ideal existence than to make it a reality, but imagination is the necessary beginning of change. I believe that I will always be an educator, whether as a professor, an activist, an artist, or a parent, and I will always try to teach children what I can about the importance of individuality, responsibility, and cooperative effort, whether they are mine or not. Hopefully, I can use my educational opportunities to figure out just how to convert my mental revolutions into social evolution.

CHAPTER 15

THE FUTURE OF THE FAMILY: FROM THE PERSPECTIVE OF A 21-YEAR-OLD WOMAN

Christine Fitzsimons

CHANGE

The future of the family depends on our ability as a culture to accept change. I am not a scientist, so I cannot quote facts and graphs concerning the family, but I can give an honest opinion.

I have learned a lot through my own experiences and the experiences of others. When it comes to family life, what I see around me is a lot of pain and misunderstanding. As a junior in college, I am making decisions that will affect the rest of my life. And some of these decisions are consciously pushing me away from family life.

When I was asked to write about my feelings and experiences with the family, I wasn't sure I had the right. I felt as if I was too critical of the family, but I soon found that I was not alone in my views. While people talk about the future of family, their main response is skepticism.

I know that change is imperative if the family is to succeed, but challenging traditional values seems an overwhelming task. Few young people grew up in the ideal nuclear family, but the experience of being on the outside has given us the strength to fight for change. If family is to be a positive force in the 21st century, now is the time to break down the obstacles that have held us back.

FINDING MODERN ROOTS

Coming from an immigrant Irish family has been a wonderful experience for me, but it has also brought challenges. Both of my parents are first-generation Americans, and their ties to their roots are strong. They grew up in crowded neighborhoods in Queens, where their best friends were often their relatives. When a holiday or special occasion comes around, these are the people they want to share it with. Extended family was always easy to find when they needed help or advice. I understand and respect this connection they have to bloodline, but I find that I cannot incorporate their close ties into my life.

Suburban Life

Because my parents chose to raise my brother and me in the suburbs, we do not know the tribal closeness they associate with family. Because of distance, I do not know the people that I am expected to put first in my life. Instead, the people I hold dear are others like myself, who understand the feeling of rootlessness.

If it were not for my strong mother, I would have been lost. It was a dream for my parents to be able to send me to private schools and then off to college. But while I was living their dream, I lost the benefit of their family role models.

Many young people feel that their ties to family have been severed, and something needs to make up for that loss. I believe that young men and women should be taught to seek out positive role models, regardless of family ties. When there are problems in school, a teacher will typically ask to see a parent or family member. Today's children can't always honor this request. Divorce, abuse, and abandonment plague us in the home. A child can no longer be expected to have a "real" home life. I was lucky enough to have a strong and independent mother as a role model, but she couldn't make up for the lack of a father. Because my own father was an abusive alcoholic, it has taken me years to accept the possibility of such a thing as a good man. If we allowed children to have role models outside the family, there might be a chance for some relief. My mother became a surrogate mom for a few of my friends, but this was not considered normal. I really believe that if we shared the resources that positive adults have to offer, we would create a much healthier young population. Why should it have been considered strange that my mother was a mentor to my friends? I wish I could have known a man who was as willing to share himself as Mother was when I was a child. I highly value the passing on of culture in a family. But I believe that if a family is going to choose to leave its clan, it must also adjust to the needs of its children. A child cannot learn from an unknown relative 200 miles away; there must be someone they can go to for support at any moment.

Family Values

When I brought up the phrase "family values" to my group of friends, their first response was laughter. Everyone is talking about family values. Liberals and conservatives alike claim to know how to reinstate these values, but nobody seems to look at just what kind of life these values direct one toward. From my point of view, the family values of yesterday perpetuated much of today's unhappiness. They might sound good, but in practice they hurt. Family values have done so much harm because they represent intolerance.

For me, the supposedly wholesome family values that permeated my hometown were the cause of much of my unhappiness. When my mother divorced my father—and saved our future—I was in second grade and I was humiliated. My grade-school principal told me that she would pray for my soul, and some of my friends were told not to play with me. All of a sudden, I ceased to fit into the happy-family mold, and this was unacceptable. Having this experience with being the outsider has given me an understanding of what it is like to be different in our society. Because of high divorce rates, I'm actually "normal" again, but I will never forget what made me strong and independent.

I believe that family values are being used like requirements for an elite club. They promote oppression by encouraging overzealous support for one ideal family model, and the results are repeated over and over again. When we are treated badly as children, we learn how to treat others badly at a later point in our lives. We learn the art of mistreatment and become very good oppressors the older we get. A child who is told that it is wrong to be different holds in the pain until it can be put onto another.

Homosexuals, single parents, and many others feel the brunt of this pain because they are considered different in our society.

Loving by Example

My vision of the future is based on teaching love by example. So many aspects of family life can be painful, but I do believe that one thing can make a huge difference, and that is the couple at the heart of the family.

When parents are loving toward each other, the children will learn to love. Growing up, I saw so much lying in relationships—parents who obviously hated each other "staying together for the children." I wish those parents realized that children see everything. I wish they could hear the child they "spared" 10 years later. Children are born mimics; it is up to the parents to choose the material they use.

Like many young people, I was taught how to be self-sufficient, how to succeed, and how to protect myself. But no one ever thought to teach me how to share my love. How does a tough young woman learn to meld independence with companionship? I learned how to hate a man, but not how to love one. Men and women have been through so many changing roles in the last 30 years. It is time to start respecting each other.

A friend gave me this poem a few years ago. I do not know who the author is, but I believe that it shows the struggle we go through.

For Every Woman and Man

For every woman who is tired of acting weak
when she knows she is strong,
There is a man who is tired of appearing
strong when he feels vulnerable.

For every woman who is tired of acting dumb,
There is a man who is burdened with the
constant expectation of "knowing everything."

For every woman who is tired of being a
sex object,
There is a man who must worry about
his potency.

For every woman who feels "tied down" by
her children,
There is a man who is denied the full
pleasures of parenthood.

For every woman who is denied meaningful
employment with equal pay,
There is a man who must bear full financial
responsibility for another human being.

For every woman who was not taught the
intricacies of an automobile,
There is a man who was not taught the
satisfaction of cooking.
For every woman who takes a step toward her own liberation,
There is a man who finds the way to
freedom has been made a little easier.

Power and Kindness

Men and women have been battling for power for too long. A family is hopeless if the parents don't respect each other and do not treat each other with kindness. I have again gone against family values recently by living with my boyfriend, but I believe that I have learned much from the experience. I am finally learning to share myself without giving my self up. I have also learned what it takes to earn respect from a partner. Because I have done this, I will not go into a marriage blind and naive, only to end up resenting the surprises that pop up in my partner's character.

A Future Vision

It is likely that I will be starting a family in the first decade of the 21st century. This idea both excites me and fills me with fear. I will not bring a child into the world until he or she is free to have choices. I want to be a mother, but not until I find a man who shares my ideals. And I want to show my children by example how to love, not how to hate. I want my children to have adults to look up to, so they never feel alone. So much work is needed before I can live as I dream, but I am confident that it is possible.

VOICES FIVE

Attempting to Grow a Family

Connie Vance wrote this verse upon reaching a personal insight.

Regret

Sorrowfully I wade through pools of deep regret,
Of irrevocable choices made, of dangerous paths mistaken for happy ones.
Succumbing to self-pity, I weep and rail against my weakness—
Prisoner to the ache of longing, desire, and defeat.
Why? The mystery of Fate *and* Choice.
Ashamed, I rummage through the hidden secrets of regret,
Then lifted by the call of Life*—the only moment that is* Now—
I sing a song of strength—of ecstasy for the days of Happiness
Arising from the death of deep regret.

Patricia Munhall wrote this poem upon reflecting about her father before his death.

A Want Unfulfilled

Down your market aisle today
I cried
To see grown, proud and aging people
On the floor chasing rolling pennies.

Proud man, painting walls,
Spraying grapes, apples and the floor,
Your castle's under siege,
Your wife has stolen your soul

Pathetic man, still a child of want,
of need,
Tired lines mark and cross your face,
Peeling skin scarred with pain

Shoulders stooped, spirit bending,
But not bent
I so much want to cradle you,
But you would never let me

Chapter 16

Infertility: A Neon Light

Linda Gonzalez

Miracles

I had always been fascinated by the seemingly miraculous events surrounding the conception and delivery of a child. My mother had experienced difficulty during my birth, and with tears streaming down her face, she had shared the story of our brush with death several times during my life.

My parents desired to have children and, considering the terrific difficulties my mother had experienced, felt blessed with their two daughters. My childhood was filled with love, and although we didn't have a great deal of money, I sincerely never noticed. My sister and I enjoyed a simple but very secure childhood filled with chocolate Easter bunnies, camping trips, and an occasional shopping spree at the local Sears department store.

My mother's love of children did not stop with her own. She frequently watched other children in our home and practically raised my cousin as her own. As a teenager, I was often embarrassed when she would stop and coo at a stranger's baby when we were out on a trip to the grocery store or shopping mall. She seemed to be everyone's mom and she certainly relished this role. As the years went by, I too developed her love for children and looked forward to having my own family, and I knew that my mother would certainly enjoy her role in their lives as well.

Life Proceeds

I soon went away to college, pursued a career, and eventually fell in love. Life was not idyllic. I seemed to frequently learn about life the hard way, but so did many of my friends. We were experiencing the world as young adults and truly searching for our own identities. I eventually married and began a new life with my husband.

Plans and Plans

Everything seemed to be working out fine and I looked forward to beginning our family. I had never considered a family without children. I thought we would be a couple until we had a child, and then, once the children arrived, we would finally be a family.

We were married for about a year when I began to want children in earnest. My husband was sensitive to my desires but neutral about starting a family right then. It was not that he didn't want children, but the how and when had never been a great concern for him. He even told me that he had considered not having children because he was concerned about raising children in the present society. It is not as safe as it was when we were children, he said. Kids can't even play outside by themselves.

Initially, I was hurt by his seeming indifference toward children, and concerned for our future compatibility. I could not understand how someone could entertain the thought of a childless life since I wanted a family so much. However, he reassured me that he would never stand in my way of becoming a mother and I was sure he would be a loving and supportive father. I concluded that things would work out fine and he was probably just having the natural concerns most people have before taking on the responsibility of parenthood.

The Beginning of a Beginning

Although we had only been married a short time, I was ready to begin a family. Once we began trying to conceive, I was nervous—filled with excitement but also a bit scared. I could almost visualize our beautiful child. I was hoping he or she would have my husband's dark curly hair and hazel eyes. If it was a girl we would name her Christina, and if it was a boy he would be named Peter after my husband.

We were both busy with our careers but I still managed to keep track of my cycle and made sure our timing was correct. I had never had any serious health problems and thought getting pregnant would be a relatively easy task. I didn't tell anybody because not only was it a personal matter but we had only been married a short while and friends were advising us to wait a few years before having kids. Regardless of what others thought, I was excited about starting my family.

Several months passed without any luck, although I certainly experienced symptoms of what I called pseudopregnancy. Every time I had a stomachache or a headache, I thought I was experiencing the symptoms of pregnancy. Nevertheless, I got my period every month. Frustrated, I realized it was going to take a little longer than I had anticipated, but I did not mind because I figured that it would give me a few more months with my husband before we had children.

Time Passes

The months passed rather quickly, and before I knew it, a year had passed and I still wasn't pregnant. Since I had never researched the medical definition of infertility, I did not realize I had officially fallen into that category. I knew my mother had a lot of problems with my conception, and I was beginning to entertain the thought that things might not go as smoothly as planned. I continued to mark my calendar and make sure we had sex at the right time each month. It was stressful, but I thought that the end result of having a baby would be well worth our efforts. Sometime between the first and second years of unsuccessful attempts at conception, however, I began to realize that the problem might be greater than I had initially thought.

The Search Begins

A friend of mine at work, Sally, was also having difficulty getting pregnant. She had done some research on infertility and sought medical treatment. I can still remember when she quoted me the medical definition of infertility: one year of unprotected and unlimited intercourse not resulting in a pregnancy. Since I had just spent the last two years unsuccessfully trying to get pregnant, those words echoed in my mind for several months. I had spent so much effort trying to get pregnant that I was emotionally unable to truly feel my experience of unsuccessful attempts at conception.

Once the denial began to disappear, a tremendous amount of pain began to set in. Sally shared her experience with me and the frustrations she had felt when her friends were conceiving and she could not. I truly identified with her experience, which seemed to help me get in touch with my own painful feelings. It was difficult because I did not know how to handle them. I had never felt such a deep sense of loss. I continued to try to conceive, although I was beginning to lose my dream of a family.

Sally conceived a couple months after we shared our secret with each other. It was difficult to watch her go through pregnancy and not be able to share the experience myself. It was during this time that I told my husband that we might be confronting infertility. It was difficult because my husband was on a completely different emotional level with this experience. While I was completely devastated and overwhelmed with pain and grief, he seemed to accept the situation and preferred not to discuss it with anyone, even me. It was as if he swept it under the carpet and continued to live life as usual. At times, I felt frustrated with our relationship as well as with just about everyone else in my life. It seemed that no one understood my pain, including myself.

The months continued to pass as I kept busy working and trying to hold onto my dream of motherhood. It was very important to me that my mother understand my situation and the impact it would have on her as well: My sister was not married, and I could not conceive; this meant she might never become a grandmother. I knew she was hurting for me, but I also knew she was suffering her own loss. Her dreams of grandchildren were slipping away, but she held on to the hope of a miracle. I turned to my family for emotional support, but only I could deal with the raging emotions within me. I felt punished and hurt, but my dream of a family did not disappear.

Dreaming

I could have two, three, or maybe even
I could have the pitter-patter of little feet running across,
I could spend endless hours rocking, cradling, and showering them with love.
I could have the pride of knowing they were sent to me from God,
I could share the joy of my children
I could feel complete in knowing my Irish and Indian heritage will not end.
I could be a mother, daughter, sister, wife
I could car-pool, play Santa, and read bedtime stories
You see, it would be wonderful because we will not just be a couple but a family full of love,
We would have children, laughter, tears, and hugs.
This is my dream,
Only a dream.

Reaching Out

It was during this time that I sought medical treatment. Deep inside, I knew the problem began within my body. I felt so awkward sitting in the waiting room of the infertility specialist among the many other women. It was a very busy office, and it did not provide the personal care I was seeking. My health insurance did not cover infertility and the treatment was very expensive. I could not help but feel guilty as I handed over our payment and knew our dream of a larger house was being set back further and further.

The doctor performed many tests and medical procedures without success. My desire to have children was still very strong, but I was beginning to lose hope that I would conceive. I kept my appointments and followed the doctor's advice, but as the months and years passed, I began to think that modern medical technology would not work for me. My options were limited because we did not have the financial resources to pursue all of our medical options. I would watch television shows about women who conceived after years of infertility with the help of medical technology and a price tag of over $100,000. My husband and I were a young couple who worked very hard; we had nowhere near that kind of money. It was so painful to know the medical community was probably able to help me conceive, but I could not afford it.

More Time, More Pain

Another year passed and I began to slowly withdraw from family and friends who had children. It was just so painful to see them with their children and the happiness they brought them. My friends and family did not understand my aloofness. There were times when I wanted to explain so that they might be more sensitive to my pain and understand why I was not attending their party or following up with social events. But I was afraid to open up to them.

My husband reinforced my silence, stressing the importance of not telling everyone our personal business, and I continued to suffer. I began to feel more and more isolated and lonely. It seemed as if everyone I knew either had children or was pregnant, and this just magnified my inability to conceive. My husband could see my pain and tears but could not do anything to help. I felt depressed because I was beginning to see the impact my infertility was having on most of the relationships in my life. I knew I was absorbed in my pain, but I could not get beyond it.

I met another woman, Emily, who was also experiencing infertility. She shared with me her feelings of inadequacy and guilt. Her husband had reacted somewhat differently than mine and he had given her an ultimatum. He told her either she should seek medical treatment or he would find someone else who would give him a child. I felt so sorry for her and the pressure she was feeling from her husband. I knew firsthand that it was not easy to undergo the sometimes painful medical interventions, and his added pressure made things even worse.

There were many times that I felt less of a person, or maybe even cursed by God. I would think about different things that had happened through the years and wonder what I had done to deserve this punishment. At that time I was emotionally consumed by my pain, and seeking any answer, rational or not. There were times when I thought had cried a river but still my tears continued to fall.

Tears

I saw a child running through the park.
Tears fell on my pillow.
My best friend told me she is pregnant.
Tears fall on my pillow.
Someone asked me why I do not have children.
Tears fall on my pillow.
Stayed home alone—tears fall on my pillow.

The Other Side of Pain

I started attending a support group. Initially, I felt nervous talking with the other women because I thought exposing my pain to strangers would make me look weak or vulnerable. Since my husband did not like talking about this issue with anyone, I had become somewhat used to hiding my pain. Because we seldom discussed my infertility, it was almost as if it didn't really exist.

However, sharing my story with others proved to be very beneficial. The other women were very sensitive to my pain because they had felt it themselves. The more I was able to openly discuss my situation, the more real it became to me.

This experience proved to be a stepping stone in helping me get to the other side of my pain. Many of the women in the support group focused on the medical or technical aspect of their condition; however, I identified with one woman in particular—Melissa.

Like me, she had gone to college, gotten married, and attempted to start a family. The phrase "start a family" is interesting because it implies that without children there *is* no family. Melissa and her husband wanted to have children but were unable to conceive. She sought medical treatment but to no avail. She felt frustrated by her husband's overly optimistic view of technology and feared he would be insensitive to her physical discomfort during the invasive medical procedures. Melissa also felt her parents' view that "a miracle will happen" was not realistic. She was afraid she would disappoint them. She seemed to carry the burden for herself and her family.

I was able to identify with her situation because I was also battling with my own frustrations—trying to accept my infertility emotionally while my family kept telling me to "be patient and it will happen." I was in a tug of war between hope and acceptance for years; my hope was preventing me from accepting my condition.

Anytime I verbalized an acceptance of not being able to conceive, my family and friends would tell me I was being negative. I used to get very angry at them, but I finally realized they were just too ignorant of my pain and suffering to really know how to properly console me. I also began to realize that there were no words that would help me overcome my suffering because my pain was just too deep.

I was truly in mourning for the child I would never have. My infertility had changed the way I looked at life. I had never had an extremely exciting or extravagant lifestyle, but I had a happy childhood, enjoying the simple things in life. My husband felt that his troubled childhood had prepared him for the difficulties in his adult life. Perhaps if I had not grown up in a loving family, I would not truly know my loss. This awareness of my infertility had changed me and I would probably never be the person I was before.

After four years I sought rather aggressive medical therapy. I had laparoscopy surgery in hopes of finding out what was wrong and possibly identifying a solution to my problem. The procedure was difficult because I had a reaction to the anesthesia, and although it was an outpatient procedure, it really frightened me.

The information obtained from the procedure gave me a name for my problem: I had endometriosis, a leading cause of infertility in women. The surgeon gave the good news that everything was lasered away and I should have no more fertility problems.

I was overjoyed by the news for 24 hours, but then I thought that I had better reserve my emotions until later in case things didn't work out. I was fearful of miracles and hope after four years of disappointment and pain.

It was during my fourth year that I began to release some of my internal pain. It was not a quick process, but I found strength through prayer, sharing my story, and offering my experiences to other women enduring infertility.

I don't know if I was entirely ready or able to help other women, but I certainly felt compelled to try. Several women I comforted went on to conceive and give birth to beautiful babies. This was difficult for me, but I still shared.

I eventually learned to hide my pain from my friends because I did not want to interfere with their happiness and I was getting tired of being depressed all the time. I wanted them to feel comfortable with me, so I learned to say and do all the right things. I had hurt and been hurt so many times over the four years that even though it was probably shallow to conduct myself and my conversation in such a rehearsed manner, it was necessary.

I had lost contact with friends and relatives because of my self-imposed isolation, and I didn't want to lose anyone else from my life. I would sometimes be so exhausted after having dinner with a pregnant couple that by the time I got to the car, I would just collapse. It is difficult to spend several hours saying the right things when you feel like your heart is going to jump right out of your chest.

I sometimes felt as if I had a big neon sign that read INFERTILITY over my head. However, after using this method to interact with other people, I actually began to feel empowered. It was a good feeling because although I may have felt like a woman that did not work, I still had the ability to be funny, personable, and a good conversationalist.

Moving through the Pain

The pain was still there but it was no longer in control. I was in control. I felt empowered by not wearing my heart on my sleeve. I still hurt and I still cried, but the tears did not flow as frequently and my painful emotions were not controlling my life any longer. It was still there, but in my own way I was learning to manage the pain.

My husband became more sensitive to my experience during this time, and I to his. I began to realize that even though he did not usually verbalize his feelings, he had endured loss as well. I do not know the extent of his pain, because I think it is his way of protecting me by not sharing. It is hard because I am sure there are feelings, and I hurt for his pain. But we began to grow together during this time instead of being separated by this wedge of pain.

Understanding

He realized we could not create a child regardless of how we tried, and he finally realized the pain it caused me. It was strange because I was initially frustrated with his and other people's attempts to console me. But when people stopped saying things to me, that made an impact as well. It was now not only real to me but also to my family and friends. We certainly had our share of ups and downs, but somehow we had managed to survive and hold our relationship together. I did not always understand his reaction to our inability to conceive, but I also respected him for not holding me accountable for our infertility. He may have not always been a great support, but he never pressured me—and in the long run that proved to be exactly what I needed.

He gave me unconditional love regardless of my ability to bear children. His initial concerns and neutral feelings about parenthood were rather soothing to me later in this experience.

Hope

Over the years, we observed many family members, friends, and coworkers have children while we stood on the sidelines waiting for our chance. I was truly beginning to feel our chance would never come. However, I still had a very small glimmer of hope deep within me. Infertility is not always a black-and-white issue; even if there is only a 1 percent chance of conceiving, you still hold onto it. I have strived to find a middle ground in which I could maintain a perfect balance of hope and acceptance, but I'm not there yet. I still find myself on an emotional roller coaster sometimes.

Action

We began to discuss other ways of becoming a parent, such as through adoption. My husband and I are very open to adoption, but it is not always an easy process. I have heard some heartbreaking stories, but I have heard even more stories of love.

A friend of mine was adopting, and she confided in me that even though she is excited, she was still dealing emotionally with the loss of the pregnancy experience. It was difficult for her to see pregnant women because it produced a lot of emotional pain. I assured her that once she had her child, it would probably relieve some of the pain. I hope I was right. Regardless of the outcome of this experience, it seems to steal a portion of your heart. I am sure my friend will have a happy and fulfilling life with her family, but her experience of infertility will be with her forever.

We Are a Family

Through this experience, I have realized that although I do not have children, I most definitely have a family. My husband and I have created a home and we are our family. I am absolutely amazed at the love we have in our home. We are no longer a couple waiting for children but rather a family facing the challenges of life with love and support. We enjoy each other's company and have established a lifestyle that works for us. Our dog also enhances our home with love and companionship. The shock of my infertility has dulled and I am attempting to establish a fulfilling life regardless of where I go. I cannot control every aspect of my destiny.

I eventually returned to graduate school in hopes of expanding myself professionally and intellectually. I work hard to grow emotionally. I spend a great deal of time with many other issues in my life, and my hard work and effort are rewarded. But no matter how hard I work, I cannot "earn" a child. My parents had instilled a strong work ethic in me as a child and I truly bought into their values, and thought that later in life, I would reap the rewards. I had been a good kid and tried to do the right thing. I had never had a problem with drugs, alcohol, or school. I put effort into laying a solid foundation so that when I got married and had children I would be prepared to care and provide for them. I had lead a somewhat traditional life and I wanted to continue to do so.

When most of my friends and family members were having their children, I felt betrayed. I learned that life is not fair and bad things happen to good people. Life does not discriminate. I decided that I did not want to feel that I was being punished anymore because I knew that if I did, I would live out my life in bitterness and anger. It would interfere with my spirituality as well.

I truly believe in a holistic balance. As long as I was angry at God for my childless life, I would never find peace within myself. I missed contentment and peace. I wanted to feel hope and excitement about our future together. I had been depressed for so long and I wanted to relieve some of it. I realized that I would probably never recover from my inability to bear children, but I still had to live my life.

I have heard other women who had lost their children to death say you never get over it, but you learn to adjust to the loss. My husband and I created a family and I wanted to contribute to our happiness, but I could not contribute as long as I was overwhelmed with grief. I also have a responsibility to other family members and I cannot function fully as long as I remain consumed by my pain. My concern for my family is a good thing because it shows that I am moving beyond some of my pain.

Since my fifth year, I have maintained my desire to have a fulfilling life with my family. I have probably even become a better person in that I am more sensitive to other people. I try to be cautious when I communicate with other people because I know firsthand the emotional pain insensitive comments can inflict on a person. I have spent the evening in tears or been sad for weeks because of things people have said to me. I am sure I was overly sensitive at times; however, I was trying to survive a devastating experience. I was not prepared for the experience, which seemed to come from nowhere and turned my world upside down.

Forgiveness

My desire to find peace led me on a journey of forgiveness. I no longer wanted to be angry at God for my infertility. I had so many things to be thankful for and it was important not to lose focus of that fact. I also wanted to stop isolating myself from friends and family members because they can have children and I cannot. It is not their fault, and I must forgive them for not understanding my pain. I had to recognize my pain existed, but it belonged to me. This is an unfortunate situation, but it is not anyone's fault. I knew I really had to let go of so many issues in order to grow. Who really knows the reasons for anyone's tragedy. It is sometimes necessary to stop asking "Why me?" and say, "If this is what I have to work with, let's make the most of it."

I had to redefine my life and my goals, and I know that the future may hold other detours that I'm not aware of yet. I cannot completely control my life, but I can try to control my reaction to it.

It is necessary that I take this experience and redefine my life. I had to let go of the naive and overly traditional person who dwelled within me and adapt to my new reality. I think that I am more real now than I have ever been. My pain killed a part of me but also made me feel more alive than I had ever felt before.

It Changes Your Forever

Unable to conceive but not unable to dream.
Unable to be a mother but not unable to give love.
Unable to push a carriage but not unable to climb a mountain
Unable to create new life but not unable to create new goals.
Unable to not know the pain of loss but not unable to survive.

POSTSCRIPT

One day my neighbor's 7-year-old son, who had lived next door for four years, asked me where my children were. His innocence did not cause me pain, but I realized our family is probably different from what his world has yet to reveal to him.

I have read that society may look upon childless families with suspicion. It seems that many people do not fully understand why my husband and I do not have children. They wonder if my career goals are my priority, or if we are too selfish to relinquish our freedom to a child, or why we are waiting so long to have a child. But my family functions much like any other. Our love makes our house a home, and our love makes a couple a family.

CHAPTER 17

THE QUEST FOR AN ALTERNATIVE FAMILY: CONFESSIONS OF A CHILD-FREE LESBIAN

Gabnella Rosetti

EXPECTATIONS AND EXPERIENCE

As with many early baby boomers who reached childbearing age in the late 1960s, I always assumed I'd have children. There was never any question. Properly tracked as a female child of the 1950s, I loved my dolls and nurtured them, even as I knew that in these times, according to both my parents, I could do or be anything I wanted.

By the time I was 16, I knew I'd have to clean things up from my childhood before I could have children of my own (notably, sexual abuse at age 7 by my stepfather and ongoing erratic physical abuse by an emotionally disturbed mother who refused to get help for herself).

In my late teens and early twenties, I was having fun experimenting with "sexual freedom." Motherhood and family were so far away that they didn't seem worth bothering about at the moment. Besides, maybe I wouldn't choose them after all. I was a budding feminist then, too, dabbling liberally in bisexuality, as I have continued to do throughout my adult life. Feminist literature on "the Pill" frightened me enough to stop taking it. I switched to diaphragm and spermicide, which were supposed to protect you from some venereal diseases as well.

Unfortunately, this form of birth control is only as effective as its user. When I became pregnant in my early twenties, I was in no way prepared financially or psychologically to care for an infant, and neither was the baby's father. I did what most hip West Coast women did in my circumstances in those days—I went to the women's clinic and made an appointment for an abortion.

I had absolutely no doubt that this was the right thing to do at the time, although I felt amazing gratitude and delight at realizing that I was indeed a "breeder." Good, I thought, and when I'm ready, I'll be able to do it. I had not counted on the hormone crash that precipitated an extended case of postabortion blues and vowed that if I was ever pregnant again, ready or not, I'd go through with the birth. Needless to say, I used my diaphragm religiously after that.

Later

More than 10 years later, at age 35, I had a solid career as an artist-educator. Feeling much improved from the depression, I thought I'd become pregnant, marry him, and play our family life "by the rules."

We didn't get pregnant. His sperm checked out satisfactory at the lab, so the doctor and I were really at a loss to explain my inability to conceive. And I began to doubt seriously that I could do anything in my life by the rules.

While on sabbatical in New York one summer shortly thereafter, I met a very simpatico woman. She was also a bisexual, also an artist, and also had just about given up on finding a man as a life partner.

This woman also wanted to be a parent. She said she didn't want to have children herself, but that she'd love to coparent. After many lunches and dinners over a 6-month period, we agreed to live together and make a nest for a family. We agreed that we would both remain free to be with men if we wanted to as long as we honored our relationship, the children, and a stable family unit.

We fell in love a few months later. Our relationships with men eventually atrophied, and we became a monogamous couple.

Creating a Family

Since I was the one who wanted to do the childbearing, I claimed responsibility for doing the research. I started with informal interviews with heterosexual single mothers and lesbian mothers. I discovered that many of these women had opted for artificial insemination. I interviewed women who had been products of artificial insemination themselves.

At one point I met the illustrator for the now famous and controversial children's book, *Heather Has Two Mommies*. Written for 4- to 6-year-olds, *Heather Has Two Mommies* concerns two lesbians, a physician and a carpenter, who move in together and decide they want to have a baby. The physician inseminates the carpenter with anonymous donor sperm, and Heather is the result.

The story follows Heather into kindergarten, where she shares the story of her alternative family with other children from alternative families. There are children with single parents of both sexes, a child being raised by grandparents, and a child who has two daddies.

Heather's illustrator lived in a colony of gay and lesbian couples in Ithaca, New York, where there seemed to be a small baby boom in progress. The story was based on a composite of lesbian "nuclear" families in Ithaca. Many of

Ithaca's lesbians had close gay male friends who were happy to donate sperm for the privilege of participating in the child raising, although the children generally lived full-time with the biological mother and her lesbian partner.

I also read a feature article about a similar baby boom in a gay community in New Hampshire, where in many cases both women in the partnership were inseminated by the same donor, creating half-siblings.

Artificial insemination (AI) seemed to be a good place to begin with our plans. I really wanted to keep the AI process as quiet and as personal as possible. The plan, a synthesis of fantasy and stories revealed by the lesbian mothers I interviewed, was to have the chosen donor abstain for three days before the projected time of peak fertility. He would stop by for drinks, dinner, and the donation on the most propitious fertile evening. He would masturbate into a veterinarian syringe. Yes, some of the women did use turkey basters, but I was afraid I'd laugh the sperm right out of me if my partner used one of those.

After the donation of sperm, my partner would do the "honors" in our bedroom in an appropriately romantic setting (candles, music, champagne, sensuous lovemaking).

In reality, not too many lesbians get pregnant this way. After the first or second attempt, the process is usually much less ceremonious. It tends to degenerate into a morning cry resembling "surf's up!" during the fertile period, followed by a mad rush to reach the donor of choice. He may or may not be home. Or he might have spent himself with three days of wild lovemaking with his own partner, thus lowering his sperm count. Or he might not even be in town, necessitating a quick plane trip to wherever he was and a frantic session in some inexpensive hotel room, sans candles or champagne. Yet, despite the changes in tactical details, the process remained a private act among friends and lovers.

Soon it became clear that I was probably not going to find a donor among friends. I did not have a large circle of gay male contacts. The few I knew, artists all, were HIV-positive and dying horrible deaths.

Within two years, nearly all of my gay male friends were dead and the remaining ones had been newly diagnosed. The ones who would not be tested were naturally out of the question as donors. Concerned that during the sporting phase of trying to become pregnant, I might have slept with Mr. Wrong, I was also tested. The result was negative.

Going Public

Now to go more public with the plan to become pregnant by making an appeal to a physician. It was daunting. It took me six months to work up my courage to seek an obstetrician-gynecologist who might be sympathetic to my plans.

I already had been vilified for being a lesbian by colleagues from the small southern town where I had been teaching. Apparently, bisexuality was accepted as a concept but not as a lifestyle. I was reluctant to reveal my lifestyle to any professional who might make a critical judgment, even in a big city like New York. When I did see a physician, I would offer a rational argument for becoming a single mother based on the limited chance I had at my age (now 42) of finding a life's mate before my biological clock ran out.

I was working as a temporary employee in a publishing house at the time. I asked the most hip-looking woman there if she could recommend an equally hip physician in New York City. She did, and he was, and after a few preliminary tests, we began the process for artificial insemination.

There was one drawback: live donors are illegal in New York State unless the donor is the woman's husband. Thus, we would be limited to using frozen sperm. I went back on the fertility drug Clomid and monthly fertility tests while he established contact with a sperm bank in California. I also researched a couple of banks, notably one with an optional disclosure contract that would allow the child to contact the biological father after age 18. My physician did not approve of that bank, however; his choice, he said, was impeccable in terms of donor screening and the quality and reliability of sperm.

Rule Breaker

I can't express what an exhilarating discovery it was to suddenly realize that I was living out a miraculous reversal of the dominant culture's rules. I was breaking the rules. Not only was I now outside the dating game, "refusing to be the goods that go to market"; I could also control the market through the selection of sperm and of the baby's sex.

I'd chosen to have a baby girl based on interviews with single and lesbian moms who were raising little boys. They all said it was tremendously difficult (but not impossible) to raise a son in a household without male role models. With what I already knew about child rearing, I anticipated difficulty enough within an alternative relationship; adding the Y chromosome and its attendant ruthless social pressures seemed sheer folly.

Catalogs of donor profiles rolled off the fax. I'd rush over to the office, picked up a sheaf, and rush home to go over them with my partner. We'd mark a few, get the long profiles, and begin the screening process. At first, I chose donor characteristics close to my own ethnic heritage, rationalizing that the strangeness of the process would seem less so if I recognized familiar features in the persona of the child.

However, my partner is not from the same ethnic background, and slowly we began to widen the range (mixed donors, including Eurasian, Native American, South Asian). The physician balked at my request to use African-American sperm. (Rationale: bad enough to bring a child into the world without a father, but then to add the burden of being biracial? I guess he wasn't as hip as I had originally thought.)

I knew from the interviews that an artificial insemination didn't always work on the first try. A woman who was herself an AI product (as were her two siblings) said that her mother tried three or four times for each child before she became pregnant.

My partner and I were prepared for this; we had already set aside a small nest egg for our future family. Each insemination cost approximately $800, about 40 percent of which was mercifully covered by health insurance for the first year (insurance did not cover the cost of sperm or shipment).

On the first AI attempt, my partner and I selected three donors, and I called the physician's assistant to place the order. The sperm were flown in from California in liquid nitrogen tanks to be stored until the optimum fertile moment of my cycle.

On day 1 of my menstrual cycle, I called the office, set up an appointment for day 10 or 12, used home fertility testing until it registered a positive, then went in for "the procedure." It was icier and more clinical than I could ever have imagined it to be.

I was extremely nervous; it was much, much worse than losing my virginity at an early age. In the first place, I was really attracted to the doctor, who was handsome and brilliant and sexy. Of course, he'd have been a great donor himself, but I was interested in him as a lover. I don't know if he knew. My nervousness was seven-tenths trying to hide my attraction to him and three-tenths hoping this insemination would be a "take," though I suspected it might not be. I didn't want to go through too many repetitions of lifting my hips to this gorgeous guy knowing I could never have him.

I was also alone. My partner had to work, so I initially approached the project as if I were planning to be a single mother after all. After the exam, the doctor went to the lab where the sperm was quickly thawed, centrifuged, and tested for mass and motility. The doctor then returned to the exam room, inserted a thin plastic tube into my vagina, and injected one vial of sperm into the other end where it was allowed to flow (drip is more like it) more or less "naturally" into the vagina and hopefully up and through the cervix.

I was propped up on the table, feet in stirrups, under a relentless florescent overhead light more evocative of corpses than conception. I think I was wearing a light blue sweater and remember feeling as though I were completely disconnected from my body. I had to lie there under that sterile operating room light for what seemed to be forever.

I was sent home with the tube still in me, taped to my thigh. Out of habit, I took the bus home rather than a cab. Talk about mortified! I thought the turkey baster idea was irreverent and ridiculous, but this made me feel like a science project.

Of course, the AI didn't take. My period came right on time two weeks later. I was sad, but prepared for the result. In the meantime, I read a bit more about clinical AI procedures, and suggested that for our second attempt we skip the tube phase and inject the sperm right through the cervix. The physician agreed. He also wanted me to come in the very day of the positive home fertility kit reading to confirm the optimum time to inseminate. Confirmation of fertility was accomplished via sonogram. The machine appeared to be a dildo hooked up to a computer.

The doctor explained that he would place the sensor into my vagina, locate the ovaries, then move the head around searching for ripe follicles large enough to hold viable eggs.

The first time he did it my knees turned to water, collapsed outward then snapped back and I stopped breathing for a few seconds. He noticed my reaction and asked if it hurt. "No, not really, no, just a surprise," I responded, as my muscles tightened and then spasmed involuntarily around that damned "dildo." He smiled in a slightly conspiratorial way and went on. He must have known I was attracted to him, the slippery satyr. But then, he turned the computer monitor toward me. Even though it wasn't news to me that photographs of the body's inner space and of extraterrestrial space resemble each other, I was still awe-struck when I first saw the filmy nebula-like tissue, follicles like suns and planets floating in a milky galaxy of gasses and organ fragments.

He pinpointed follicles with the ease of an astronomer locating stars, then clicked on the computer. Out rolled sonograms from the printer, markings intact, noting the data he needed to confirm fertility. I asked for copies, which he cheerfully gave me. Watching the monitor during sonograms became my favorite part of the AI process. The cervical-bypass method was far superior to procedure number one.

We thought the first try at the new technique was a take. I missed my period—but it wasn't viable. Nine weeks later I began bleeding. I did some more reading. Maybe the little zygotes weren't attaching. Let's try progesterone suppositories. For the next attempt, we used progesterone. For future attempts we blitzed the exploding follicles with three and four inseminations per cycle. I would stay off my feet for days at a time, trying to hold the incipient conception each month.

Over the next two years, we'd get positive readings on home pregnancy tests, then weeks later, estrogen readings from the lab that negated the pregnancies. I suppose the longest one held about 11 weeks. We stopped telling our friends that we were trying to get pregnant.

Once, by accident, I stopped at the wrong office while trying to find a lab that would take an estrogen reading. I had been asked to remind the technician to send over the three vials of sperm he'd been storing for us at the lab. The office I had stumbled into belonged to a fertility specialist. He took a blood sample for the estrogen level reading, didn't know what I was talking about regarding the stored sperm, and when he found out who I was going to, suggested that I'd been going to the wrong physician.

He bombarded me with success stories and mentioned some high-tech procedures I thought I'd never resort to. This estrogen test, which was negative, proved to be a turning point in our family planning. Upon hearing the results of the test, my doctor reluctantly admitted that he didn't think biological motherhood was going to be possible for me after all, at least not with frozen donor sperm. He warned me against trying the more expensive procedures because they were even less reliable than AI, especially for a woman my age. I was devastated, but I appreciated his honesty and ethical concern.

My partner and I discussed what to do next. Move on to the fast-talking fertility specialist? Procedures like in vitro and GIFT started at five figures, or so we understood. We had exhausted all of the set-aside funds and half of my retirement account on the AI attempts.

Grief and Loss

My partner said she would support me if I wanted to keep trying. I was emotionally exhausted and quickly sinking into a depression that lasted nearly three years—not exactly the best climate for a newborn. I felt deeply, irrationally, that my body had betrayed me—worse, that some power (call it God) had betrayed me. I wanted to experience biological motherhood; I wanted to carry a pregnancy to term, give birth, breast-feed, experience every precious moment of creating a nurturing environment and watching an infant develop.

This was the first time since I'd entered adulthood that God had said no to me. During the years that I tried to become pregnant, especially the last two, I meditated, prayed, took care of my body, kept my professional skills and career going. I'd regressed to toddler behavior—bargaining, pleading, "behaving" myself in the best way that I knew so that whatever intelligent power existed would smile on me and bless me with what I wanted: a child.

I even dabbled in pagan practices, performing elaborate rituals on the beach at dawn with candles, watermelons, and shiny new dimes. I consulted psychics, who told me that they saw the baby coming, to have faith. I even had dialogues with the voice of what I believed to be the spirit of the unborn: when I asked the spirit where she was, she answered, "On the long journey of forgetting," which seemed a perfectly logical answer from a spirit seeking reincarnation.

My partner and I bought children's books and toys. During one of the longer pregnancies we shopped for baby furniture. I'd started keeping a chronicle of the pregnancy in the form of a letter to the unborn baby. With each successive failure to hold a pregnancy, I became less productive, less effective in my work.

After the last failure, when I stopped taking hormones, I believe I was about as close to a serious mental breakdown as I have ever been. I undermined any chance I had toward social or professional progress. I felt guilty because I knew my partner could feel and must be affected by negativity emanating from every pore of my body. I chain-smoked and drank heavily. I made secret plans for suicide.

Before I succumbed utterly to depression, my partner and I discussed another option for creating our family: adoption. Unfortunately, the physical effects of hormone withdrawal had already set in, and I was beginning to harbor dark thoughts. If the point was biological motherhood, what did that say about me as a potential parent? That I was only interested, selfishly, if the child were my own flesh and blood? Would I feel less "maternal" toward an adopted child, and if so, what business did I have bringing a child into my life at all?

I tried to block these thoughts and reviewed my notes of interviews with single and lesbian mothers, finding reasons why artificial insemination and hit-or-miss sport sex were not the best methods of creating a family after all. A bisexual friend who'd had a child during one of her heterosexual phases told me I was completely irresponsible to consider having an AI baby with an anonymous donor. Children need to know who their fathers are, she insisted. Well, yes, I mused, my half-sister's abandonment issues might have been exacerbated by the fact that she was never allowed to see or know much about her biological father. But could that parallel an adoptive situation as easily as one of artificial insemination?

Another friend, who was an AI baby herself along with a younger sister and brother, said she had no problem with an anonymous father (she was also an artist and felt that "not knowing" freed her to create the other half of herself, *herself*) . She did say that her brother had a more difficult time with it and was now a dysfunctional adult (drug user and homeless), although she said he'd had problems before he found out he was an AI baby. Another lesbian mother said she suspected that the gay friend who was the donor for her two children was sexually abusing them on weekend visits. Still others, who became lesbians after having children, had their children taken away from them by the biological fathers or their families. Another lesbian mom who used an anonymous donor for her AI child said that her own family took the baby away from her because she was a lesbian.

So while adoption meant going even more public with plans to create a family (not a pleasant prospect for me), being open certainly seemed to carry extra emotional baggage that neither my partner nor I wished to take on. The second successful adoption by gays that I was most familiar with was accomplished by a professional male couple. Their housekeeper appeared at their door one day with an infant boy and begged them to raise him. She already had six other children whom she could barely care for.

The couple adopted the baby privately. The child turned out to be mentally retarded, a result of the mother's state of malnourishment and lack of prenatal medical care. The two men devoted themselves to the boy, giving him the best education and environment they could afford. He was apparently a very well adjusted young man, performing well beyond expectations, when he was taunted by some neighborhood youths one day as he was coming home from school. He tried to escape by running away and was struck by a car and killed. The tragic ending of this story is, of course, in no way related to the homosexuality of the boy's parents; it could have happened to anyone.

Perhaps it was the depression that caused me to remember this story at the time I was considering adoption; perhaps I identified with their grief, having lost several unborn children by the time I met the bereaved parents.

I've come to accept depression and creative blocks as part of the fabric of an artist's life. Aside from short-term therapy, I tend to deal with these episodes by trying to separate from the feelings and find rational causes for the circumstances that precipitated them. And I try not to take on any new projects until the depression subsides. Losing unborn babies was an experience I had not expected to deal with, and I weathered this depression with a less than rational approach. I am convinced now that losing a child creates a void that is never filled. Like depression itself, the experience must be woven into the fabric of who I am. At any rate, my partner and I have put our quest for a family on the back burner for the time being. Rational thinking about the situation has led me to an adjustment that includes renaming my current state as child-free rather than childless. Being childless suggests bereavement and lack; being child-free suggests that there are options open to me, that have always been open to me, that I haven't considered. I have also found myself reflecting on parenthood, and the Western notion of family in general, with a jaundiced eye.

A recent experience illustrates: I had just spent one of the worst Christmases of my life with my dysfunctional family of origin. As it happens, we are a family of women (one mother, one half-sister seven years younger than me, and myself). As a partnered lesbian who wanted to establish an alternative family either by bearing a female child (sex selected) or by adopting one, the single-genderedness of my family of origin would seem to be significant. However, I cannot say that being raised in a fatherless and brotherless home made my family neurotic, nor did it make me a lesbian, although that would undoubtedly make the proponents of traditional family values absolutely ecstatic. Not at all: there is no formula to explain our particular misery; to paraphrase a famous Russian novelist, my family is unhappy in its own way.

Parenthood might be considered an act of heroism: thrust upon some, pursued by others. I used to believe that there would be a magical year in my life when I would be ready to raise a family (including being financially stable, having some training and knowledge in parenting skills, and having worked enough on myself to heal my own childhood wounds). Now I suspect that none of us is ever truly "ready" for parenthood at any time. We all think we'll raise our children differently from the way our parents raised us (particularly if we're from unhappy families). Some of us do manage not to make their mistakes, but inevitably we make our own.

Parenthood is "heroic" because it inherently embodies conflict. There are high-water marks that seem to be common to the experience, notably during a child's adolescence, when most parents can expect their children to hate them, or at the very least to be embarrassed by them. Anyone who chooses to spend eight to ten years of their lives in that kind of open conflict must be either heroic or completely crazy.

The holidays this year thrust me back into my own adolescence. After several days of being manipulated and micromanaged by my family, I became the rebellious teenager I was at 15: raging, screaming, and otherwise behaving in a most uncivilized manner, much to the shock of my mother and sister, who usually reserve that behavior for themselves.

Around and around we went, trying to force each other into acting as negative mirrors for an energetic game of "Who's the Biggest Martyr of Them All?" I returned home exhausted and emotionally vanquished, not quite ready to enjoy the negative humor of the clichéd dysfunctional-family holiday scenario.

Instead, I wondered: If I did have a child, what would our Christmases be like in 30 years? What wounds would we reopen against our rational will? What shared traumas will have scarred us for life? After three years of unrelieved heartache, a glimmer of rational thought seemed to be making a welcome appearance. I thought about the sacrifices my partner and I would have to make to raise a child. No more last-minute decisions to head to the beach for the weekend. Nix on the exotic food deliveries on nights we didn't feel like cooking. Forget the impulse buying of expensive toys for ourselves. Our nest egg was depleted; how would we afford infant care when we both had to work? And what about those rules? Wouldn't we be copy-catting the nuclear family structure and its attendant discontents, except for the fact that our child would be raised by two parents of the same sex? Positive considerations soon refaced the negative. As child-free adults, couldn't we contribute more to the emotional health of children in the role of the nonparent, the significant adult in whom children confide, who acts as a safe testing ground for children's notions of how the world works? That's a role both my partner and I have tended to fill in the lives of our students and our friends' children. If we were parents ourselves, would we lose the objectivity of women who have spent most of our lives dealing with the world on adult terms?

For the first time in my life, I began to see being child-free as a special gift to ourselves and to the world. We've given away most of the toys and books to children of family and friends. We are not closed to having a family at this point. Should an opportunity present itself, we would embrace the parenting experience with all the love, energy, and skill we could muster. But it is no longer an obsession, a mandate that we are actively pursuing. If it happens, through some miraculous set of circumstances, it will most likely be thrust upon us, ready or not.

VOICES SIX

FAMILIES GRIEVING

JoAnn McKay wrote these verses to her daughter Suzanne, who died of cancer at the age of 28. In this poem she tells us how much she learned from her daughter.

I learned these lessons the hard way from my hero. She may have been only 28, but she was one of the most beautiful people I have ever had the privilege of knowing. A lot of grief and a lot of growing but what a gift all of us have received.

Yesterdays and Tomorrows

If there had been no yesterdays
There would be no tomorrows.
If there had been no rainy days
There would be no rainbows.
Because the sun comes up in the morning
There are sunrises to capture.
Because the evening shadows fall
There are sunsets to savor.
The road of life has twists and turns
That mold and create our being.
The ins and outs that shape our soul
Give us wisdom to give to others.
The gifts of life may last but a moment
But the beauty lives in our core.
Each day can bring a golden treasure
And can be missed if we close our hearts.
I have been taught with bittersweetness
To lead with the heart each day.

To live as if there were no tomorrow
Only the promise of this moment.
It doesn't take a million tomorrows
To leave a legacy of dignity and love.
For the touch we make this moment
Can ripple on through the ages.
The Father of fathers can bring a gift
When the days seem dark and dim.
In our daily lives it can be missed
If we run too fast to see.
Tell someone you love them
Remembering to give a gentle touch.
You're building your legacy for others
For tomorrow may not be.

The verse was written after she died—actually after I started talking to you (Tricia) about her. One time when Suzanne was in college I was taking her back to school and the song (by Bette Midler)"Wind Beneath My Wings" was playing. She had been having a rough time with school and relationships at that point and had needed a little extra TLC. I had to be careful to let her take the lead and let me know when she needed me. She was at a point in her life that she needed her independence, so I had to take her lead and trust her to let me know when she needed me close. She looked over at me with tears in eyes as we were driving (I even remember exactly where we were—we were just going onto Huger Street off Interstate 26) and said "Mom—that's exactly what you are—the wind beneath my wings. I don't know how I would ever get through life without you." Little did I know that those roles would be reversed and I would be the one saying "You are the wind beneath my wings." Needless to say, it made me cry and even then she didn't want me to cry. My heart just about shatters when I remember that. On the other hand it is one of the most precious memories I have.

Wind Beneath My Wings

There's a photo I've been holding close
Keeping the memories alive
I gently touch the face
But it's cold and I can't feel you
I look into your eyes with no response
I cherish the smile but it is fixed and still
I close my eyes and I can see your face
And the movement as expressions change
I see the wave of your hand
I can hear your laughter
I feel your warmth and remember
"Mom, you're the Wind Beneath My Wings"
But you allowed me to be there
You allowed me to love you
You allowed me to care for you
You honored my existence with your wisdom
A selfish wish was to keep you
But I had to let you go
The pain had to cease and
You needed to be free
To soar with the eagles
Through the clouds and the mist
So when I wake each morning
And when I slumber each evening
I feel the gentle wind blowing
I feel the warmth of your touch
I think of you and dream I can soar
You give me the strength I need
You are the Wind Beneath My Wings

I wrote this poem in July, a few months before Suzanne died. She couldn't read it, but said she would when it was time. She then asked to have it read at her funeral.

The Gift

For all the times you spilled the milk
As my reaction you looked to see
With eyes and smile to melt the heart
I felt the gift between you and me.

For all the times I spoke in anger
And tiny fingers touched my face
Taking away the stress and fear
I felt the gift of God's grace.

For all the laughter and happy times
With running feet and eyes aglow
Lifting spirits and living life
I felt the gift as I watched you grow.

For all the scraped knees
And nights with fever and pain
Stroking your hair till morning light
I felt the gift as my energy drained.

For all the mornings we left for school
Racing to meet the bell's ring
A goodbye kiss as you left the car
I felt the gift that each day brings.

If I had to prove deserving
I know I'd have failed the test
But I'm thankful for the grace
Of the gift with which I've been blessed.

Suzanne

Sometimes the tears begin to fall
From who knows where
Like a soft gentle rain
They appear from the darkness
My heart is so filled
With the love and the memories
Trying not to see the images
Of the times you were in pain
And hearing your sweet warm tones
Telling me to stroke your back
To ease the discomfort welling within
With each touch I wanted to take the pain
Pull the tumors from your sweet body
And make you healthy and whole
I prayed by your side
With eyes closed and aching heart
Letting a mothers' heart and love
Try to make it all okay again
But this time it was beyond me
I had to let you go
With all the dignity you possessed
You tried to touch my aching heart
Telling me you were ready
But you hated so much to leave
You said your good-byes to all
And left your legacy of love
For all of us to share
I owe you more than I can ever repay
You gave me a lifetime of joy
With a few growing pains tossed about
But we shared our time honestly
Whether painfully or playfully
You're always in my heart and mind
Most times without the tears
They are falling more freely now
Cleansing and renewing my spirit
As if you sent them to touch me
Telling me to live and share love
Keeping your legacy alive
On this day we talked about
That we both knew may not come
I'm holding you in my heart
And touching those you wished me to
I love you with all my heart.

—*Mom*

Amanda wrote this poem when her little sister died from cancer. Amanda was 15. Her sister was 10 years old.

Long Ago

Long Ago I met you in my dreams.
Long Ago we danced to a sweet tune under the moonlight.
Long Ago we kissed in a sweet embrace.
You were an angel sent from up above.
You were always there when I needed you the most—
But where are you now?
I'm guessing that when the wind blew that day, it took you with it.
Maybe one day you will come back and my dream will be peaceful again.
But until then I will remember not too long ago when I first met you in my dreams.

Patricia Munhall wrote this verse many years after her father's death, because it calls into question the belief that time heals all sorrow.

Timeless Wounds

I'm most ambivalent about snow.
There is little hope for me.
I can't seem to grasp knowing in a little bit of sure.

Loving you while dying, not till.
Red blood awash the body, the bed,
Then a song, then a cry, then a wail.

The day your father dies
One sits in stillness
The only movement, the tears falling
At the significance of it all

In the cosmos of the gone
I stumble
Through the disconnection of his leaving, then

Ten years later, and then another ten,
I poetize
In those same tears, the impossibility.

Chapter 18

Dedicated to My Tommy: Give Sorrow Words

Katherine Parry

Give sorrow words. The grief that does not speak
Whispers the o'erfraught heart and bids it break.

Shakespeare, Macbeth

Silence

My family had an unspoken collusion over my brother's death from suicide at age 18. I was 13. Following his death, it was tacitly recognized that my parents would not permit talk about his death. They would not express their feelings—love, grief, or sadness—in front of me or my younger sister, who, at age 7, was considered too young to be involved. There would be no talk about him, no memories or recollections about him. This implied that I was not to talk about him or express my feelings of grief about him in front of them.

And so, after my brother's death, we did not mention his name. His room was repainted and his things were given away. There was no funeral or memorial service. His body was cremated and his remains stored in a cardboard box in his closet. That box later disappeared.

What my mother would call "getting on with life," most others would term avoidance of pain. This was characteristic of both my father and my mother, who did not like to deal with feelings. However, according to my mother, most of this protection was for the benefit of my father who would not speak even to her about the death of their son.

Our Ghost and My Grief

It seemed like we were a family with a ghost. My brother's presence remained, unmentioned and unmentionable. Growing up in this dark atmosphere, observing it and suffering in silence within it, was part of my upbringing. I knew from past experience that to bring up feelings that no one wanted to hear would lead to criticism or personal disparagement.

The consequences of this silence, which has not really been breached among us 35 years later, has had repercussions that reached far beyond my teenage years, leaving me with anger and rage beyond the comprehension of most individuals.

The Grief Journey

It has taken me years to uncover my grief, to process the death and suicide of my brother, to recover from the years of censorship of feeling that is still imposed by my family. I am angry about many things now.

I am angry about all those times as a child, even before my brother's death, that I was told not to cry.
I am angry that I was emotionally neglected before my brother died, and that after my brother died, I mourned alone, in solitude.
I am angry that my parents' behaviors did not change and that the family pathology of prohibiting the expression of feelings continued in spite of such a significant warning sign of problems as the suicide of a teenage son.
I am angry about the lack of insight and sensitivity on my parent's part that led my brother to believe that disappointing them was a reason to die.
I am angry at their perception that I should be "over this," an opinion expressed by friends, ministers, and my family.
I am particularly angry that I'm not supposed to be angry.

The Theory

It is now understood that loss can often result in prolonged grief. The difficulties of recovering from grief can have adverse consequences for personality functioning. If childhood loss and mourning are to have a favorable outcome, certain conditions must be met. The child must have a reasonably secure relationship with his or her parents before the loss. It is best for children to be allowed to ask questions, to participate in family grieving, and to have the comforting presence of a parent after the loss.

If these conditions are not met, then "disordered variants" of mourning can occur. When the bereaved individual is not allowed to express yearning, anger, and sorrow, untold harm and psychological damage can be expected. I wish I had understood the causes and effects of lack of grief work that shaped my life.

Because of this lack of understanding of grief work, it has taken me many years to find the strength, the will, and the insight to read the professional literature about suicide. This blind spot in my reading has probably been part of my defense to keep the process of recollection and pain away.

How "It" Happened

I found out that my brother had died when I accidentally overheard the phone conversation between my mother and the dean of my brother's university. It was early in the morning and my father and younger sister had already left the house.

I heard a cry of pain from my mother that was unlike anything I'd heard from her before or since. I think I cried then, but I also felt puzzlement, numbness, and pain.

My mother came under control but was not quite sure what to do, so she told me that my brother was dead and then sent me off to school.

I had missed first period of school, and in second period I whispered to my best friend that my brother was dead. She just stared at me, not knowing what to say. I stared back. I wasn't sure what to say either.

Somehow the word spread that morning, and kids who had never talked to me before came up to me to say they were sorry. It felt good to be the center of attention. But I felt very guilty about it, because I knew that it was for the wrong reason.

Then I was called out of school. My mother had decided that I should come home. I was 13 years old and my sister was 7 years old. I don't remember anything else that day. I particularly don't remember seeing or hearing my father.

The next day I remember waking up and getting into bed with my parents, thinking that maybe it was all a nightmare, but it wasn't. I felt pain and it was real. I learned something frightening: that the secure, everyday reality we lived in and counted on was fictional. I realized that my life could be ripped apart and shattered suddenly and without warning in a way that I had not imagined.

Later that day, my parents left for California where my brother had died. My little sister and I stayed with a neighbor. My sister didn't know my brother very well. She was puzzled about the whole situation yet acted normally.

I felt like smashing her face. I wanted to know what to do and what to feel. I wanted someone to help me desperately. I must have dragged myself through the next few days. I was supposed to water the plants while Mother was gone, but I didn't. I didn't feed my pet bird either. I was letting it starve, but I couldn't stop myself. I looked at it every morning and turned my back without taking care of it. I knew that I was letting it suffer, but I felt like I couldn't take care of anything else but my own pain. I needed care and I couldn't function or give care to anything.

When my parents got home my mother was mad at me because the plants and the bird had died. I ran out into the yard and cried over my bird in a way that I hadn't cried over my brother. Then I buried it and wished I could run away from home. I felt I had been deserted and misunderstood, and I had been. No one wanted to see my tears or hear my grief or even talk at length to me about death and pain.

I still don't remember my father at all during this period. I think he became very withdrawn.

SUICIDE?

Several days later, my mother told me that my brother had killed himself while in a state of depression. That was a big shock because this possibility had not occurred to me. I felt unprepared to cope with anything more. But now, I became preoccupied with questions: Why did he do this? How could he have left me? Didn't he know how much pain and damage this would cause to me? Didn't he care about me?

It was like an entirely new twist on the whole event. I could not comprehend it, but I felt that I had to try to find the meaning in this, but I was forced to do this alone, without any help or support.

PROCESSES

Anthropologists have written that all societies have rituals and rites concerning death, the disposal of the dead, and the proper attitude for mourners. They state that these rituals are important because they help the bereaved give expression to their grief in public and private ways.

However, my parents did not want a funeral or a memorial service. My mother wanted to put it all behind her and "go on with life."

I never saw her or my father cry over this. We didn't cry together, hold hands, or share our grief in any way. No one inquired how I might be feeling—not my mother, my father or my older sister, who was no longer living at home.

There was no caring about how I might be thinking and feeling, how much pain I might be in, how alone and isolated and confused I must feel. I lived in a cloud of numbness and confusion, wondering what to feel and how my brother could have done this to us, to me. A few weeks later, Mother showed me my brother's suicide note. It was long but repetitious. He was killing himself, he said, because he was ashamed of having flunked his first semester of college. He did say goodbye to me in the letter. It was just a short sentence, but it has meant a lot to me. This was February. Tommy had come home for Christmas and he had not mentioned any problems to anyone. This was not unusual. I had learned early on that the expression of problems would be taken as a rebuke by my mother. He and I had fought a lot at that Christmas because I wanted his time and attention, but he was keeping to himself.

After reading this suicide note, I was very angry at my parents. I knew that they had not been aware of what really made him tick. Even though I was younger, I noticed that he typically kept all his feelings in. He was quiet, like me, but where I cried and slammed doors when I was upset, he just internalized everything. I doubt my parents even understood the idea of "internalized," although they were college-educated and well-read.

We grew up in an atmosphere where expressions of fear or unhappiness were ignored or disparaged. I was enjoined to "think positively" by my mother. This seemed to be another way of negating the life of emotion.

Bowlby states, "Children are quick to read the signs. When a parent is afraid of feelings, the children will hide their own. When a parent prefers silence, the children, sooner or later, will cease their enquiries." My mother had Tommy's room repainted and gave all his things away. I used to sit in there, missing him and feeling that they were eradicating him. It became apparent that my sister and I were not to talk about him or bring up his name because it might further injure my father, whom we were supposed to protect.

The Remains

We didn't talk about him or hear his name spoken aloud. I didn't know anything about my brother's body and, enjoined to silence, had no one to ask. But within a month, a cardboard box appeared in my brother's closet. I didn't know what it was and I pried a corner open. It looked like gravel, but I saw a sliver of bone and I realized that it was my brother's remains. I was numb. It was a horrible encounter with the physical evidence of death and I had no preparation for this. Further, I did not know who I could talk with about this. It was out of the experience of my friends, and my parents had made it clear in nonverbal ways that we did not talk about Tom's death. I could only wonder to myself: How could all there was left of my brother be in that box? How could they have just left him there, in a box, in a closet? Could he not have been given a proper burial and grieved over like the fine boy that he was? How could this be all that was left? It's so awful to see that this is all that is left of him and just sitting here, like a pair of old shoes. Why couldn't we have had a funeral like regular people? He was my brother. They should have more for him than storage in a closet in his own room. I wanted to say goodbye to him, not to his bones. There was so much to him and now he is gone and he has been reduced to this horrible graveyard gravel.

Pain

There was no one to go to about this. No one wanted to hear these feelings. There seemed to be no end to this. What would happen next? What were they going to do with him? I locked up many emotions about that encounter—horror and pain. It was many years before I was able to express the terror of that moment, and finally live those emotions and discharge them, as it was many years before I began to cry for him and over him. It was like carrying around a lump that I didn't know what to do with. It was like being haunted. I spent the next year in a sort of isolation. I went on in pain. I used to sit in the church on the corner of our street, hoping that the pain would go away.

My brother's remains disappeared from the closet. I wanted to know where they went, but there was no one I could ask. I couldn't cry because it felt as if I didn't know how. I had put my feelings God knows where, somewhere far away. I read religious books. Just reading calmed me. I wanted to believe that my brother's death had some meaning. I felt scarred and set apart from other kids my age. I did not believe that any of them had to endure something like this.

My friends could not understand this situation. They did not mention Tom's death to me, and I did not feel I could talk about what I felt, since what I felt was so confused. Truthfully, I don't remember those next few years well.

Life when on and I felt a constant low level of resentment and disgust that we would go on and on like this, never allowing feelings to surface, never mentioning my brother's name. The silence seemed full of silent grief and unrelenting pain for me. I nursed my resentments, growing further alienated and apart from them.

Studying was an escape for me. I could immerse myself in books and lose myself there. I was drawn to Buddha's admonition that "Life is suffering." I felt I had been embraced by death. I felt that death had taken me in and shown me the decay and dust of final dissolution. However, my parents wanted to believe that I was "coping" and "adjusting."

Reaction

> *Sorrow concealed, like an oven stopp'd,*
>
> *Doth burn the heart to cinders where it is.*
>
> *Shakespeare,* Titus Andronicus

As a teenager, I began to act rebelliously. When I was 17, my parents expected to control me and thought I should listen to their rules, but I would have none of it. I felt that I had to care for myself and my own emotional needs during the years while my parents were withdrawn, and I wasn't interested in what they had to say now, when I did not need them. I made my own decision about whether or not I should have sex with my first boyfriend.

However, my parents found this out and became very upset about it, threatening to lock me in my room. I was very angry that although I had been a good student and a compliant daughter, they were criticizing me for an act that involved my body, not theirs.

I had planned this, arranged for birth control, and as far as I was concerned, it was none of their business. Consequently, they sent me to a psychiatrist. I was happy about this. I had asked earlier to be sent to a psychiatrist, but my mother rejected this idea. I suspect that my request threatened her wish to have everything "back to normal" and her continuing denial that there were any problems.

Help

Although I was happy to go, I was angry that it was this incident that prompted their concern. After spending so much time in my head, I wasn't sure how to talk with this elderly gentleman and I didn't know how to express my feelings well, so we never did talk about my brother or his death. Instead we talked about my relationship with my parents and I was given antidepressants, which lifted some of the persistent feelings of gloom.

Even though I wasn't talking much, I was glad to be there. The psychiatrist convinced my parents to stop criticizing me. The secondary benefit was that it felt good to make my father spend the money on me for this. I believed it was the least he could do for me, and I felt he owed me a great deal for abandoning me when I needed help and support.

I believed more in my father's capacity to be responsive as he was more intelligent and introspective than my mother. My mother, I felt, was a woman of little sensitivity or insight who disparaged me in small ways, pushing away all my needy feelings and worries by telling me that I was "too sensitive."

I believed that my parents were partially responsible for my brother's death and totally responsible for the harm done to me by closing off the grieving process. Somehow I was expected to take care of all my feelings and my pain alone. How could my mother have expected me deal with this on my own? Where was my father? He had just disappeared into himself. How could they have left me alone?

I did not start talking about my brother to a therapist until my thirties, when I entered analysis. Until then, I discounted my feeling of numbness, my perception that I was being haunted, and my anger at my parents until graduate school. There I read a lot of Freudian theory, enough to make me realize a connection between my early experiences and my depression, anger, and unease.

I finally started grieving for my brother, crying over the pain he must have felt that made him take rat poison and knowing that he was lying down not to sleep but to die. What must that have felt like? I knew that he had died in the emergency room, vomiting, but unable to be revived. I finally let out the feelings of shock and anguish, crying and wailing over the memories.

Silence Still

My mother still does not want to talk about these years. In her mind, the way they dealt with this was "normal." When my father died, there was no funeral or service.

When I told my mother that I didn't want this to be a situation like my brother's death, she said, "What do you mean? What does Tommy's death have to do with anything?" I told her that we were all left to ourselves then. She said, "That's not true. I remember talking to you about Tommy." I said, "Once, Mom, once you spoke to me about Tom's death." She started to whimper and cry and said, "Well, I don't see what Dad's death has to do with Tommy."

Her response pissed me off because I was reminded of all the times when I wanted and needed to talk, but she or Dad would look like they were going to cry and the conversation would stop. It was as if their pain was something holy that couldn't be disturbed. They avoided their pain at my expense.

At Dad's death that year, I did not want to be removed from the process of death, burial, and grieving. Over my mother's initial objections, I insisted on seeing my father's body. I wanted to say goodbye to Dad in my own way. Later in the year, my younger sister and I scattered his remains. Because there was no memorial service, we had a "picnic" for friends and relatives.

Dad's death was a positive event for me because I had people to grieve with and I could fully experience and share my emotions. It helped too that losing a father is a common experience that most people can relate to. Now, I keep a picture of my brother and me as children together on my table.

After my father died this year, I began talking to my brother, telling him how I feel and the things that are bothering me. He fills the niche of big brother for me still.

Valuable Rituals

My experience that year as a volunteer in Vietnam helped when I saw the family altars with pictures of the beloved dead among the fruit, flowers, and incense. That made me feel that my way of living with Tom's memory was a human experience, enshrined in their culture although not in ours.

I now see another analyst who has encouraged me to face the anger instead of rationalizing or denying it. Other therapists have not wanted to see this part of the process. Hillman, a well-known contemporary analyst, has written, "It depends upon each individual involved in analysis to stand for his experience—his symptoms, suffering, and neurosis, as well as the invisible, positive accomplishments—in the face of a world that gives these things no credit."

An Ending

Let mourning stop when one's grief is fully expressed.

Confucius, The Analects

It has been a long journey, but now I feel I have the right to my brother's memory in my own way and the right to my anger. The grieving process has not been smooth or continuous. It feels as if there were several layers that needed uncovering, over and over, a little bit deeper each time.

I am 49 now, and the past two years, during which I have been seeing a psychoanalyst again, have been most intense. One very painful memory, which has been like a precursor to other, deeper pain, was how I let my pet bird die after my brother died. It is like a deep hole. As I start to go back in memory to those sad days, I fall into this memory first.

I have felt so guilty about this because I loved this bird, because I was responsible for it and it was the only pet that I was allowed to have in our family. I had trained it to fly around my room and to allow me to put it on my finger and put it back in the cage. The bird was like a wonderful friend that I was able to give my love and affection to, but in my rage at feeling deserted when I most needed help, I let it die.

My therapist has suggested that I transferred my anger from my parents to the bird or that I did to the bird what I felt my parents were doing to me, inflicting suffering, letting me hurt, deserting me. She has suggested that perhaps it is better that I did this rather than hurt myself. The urge to want to die too was strong because the pain was so great, so unrelenting, and it seemed like there would be no end to it. Perhaps that action was the only one under my control.

The most difficult memory to retrieve, experience, and process was finding my brother's remains. My first experience of this memory came during one session, among many, of therapeutic touch with a nurse practitioner. Unexpectedly and a propos of nothing related to this incident, in the middle of the session, I found myself feeling sad. Then I was immersed in the pain of that moment, sobbing "No, no, no" over and over. I couldn't even stop and explain my emotions to the therapist because I was suddenly so overwhelmed with all the feeling and emotion of that moment when I opened a cardboard box sitting in a closet and realized that the box I had just opened contained all that was left of my brother. In that moment, in the therapist's office, I finally felt the pain and horror of that discovery. And I could only cry "No." It was like the feeling in the poem that Fredrico Garcia Lorca wrote about the death of his friend:

I will not see it!
Tell the moon to come
for I do not want to see
the blood of Ignacio on the sand.
I will not see it.

Tommy, I wanted to say goodbye to you like a sister and a friend. I wanted to kiss you again and say goodbye and see your body laid to rest with my prayers and the prayers of everyone who loved you and whose lives you had touched. But look at what they made you! They burned your body to bones and gravel and put you in a cardboard box in your closet like an old appliance. God damn them! Here you are back in your room, but in a form I had never imagined, right in front of my face. It is so horrible to see you like this. I loved you and now I'll never see your face again.

How can this be a world where this can happen? How can Mom and Dad leave me to face death by myself? This is so painful and I'm afraid. I want to die too. It hurts so much to see that this is all that is left of your dear body. Just this grit that looks like dirt. How can this have been you? There is nothing recognizable left for me. How could they do this?

They took away the chance for me to see you or touch you again. I couldn't even cry over you. I have only this gravel to cry over, and it's not enough. God, they didn't even put you in a nice box or an urn. How could this be happening like this? Why did they just leave this in the closet of your bedroom? I didn't get to touch you or see you before they burned you. You are all gone, reduced. I'll never see you again. Even in a big house with two cars and a membership at the country club. I wish I had taken some of your ashes. I wish I could have eaten some of them so that you would be part of me, so that you couldn't be taken away from me again. I miss you so much, please come back. Don't leave me.

Something it is which thou hast lost,
Some pleasure from thine early years.
Break, thou deep vase of chilling tears
That grief hath shaken into frost!

Alfred, Lord Tennyson, In Memonam I

Pain to Anger

It was several months later before I could reach that pain again. I could talk about the experience, analyze and intellectualize it, but not really feel it. And again, more time passed in counseling before I could approach the feeling of that memory, letting more and more of these painful emotions and feelings out.

The second most difficult task has been to release the repressed anger at my parents. I have rationalized their role and pretended to myself to be forgiving but I feel an ocean of resentment inside. My own anger is frightening to me and I have avoided its expression. I have been aided in this by numerous friends and family who feel that I should be "over this" by now. After all, they say, it was a long time ago. Your parents were suffering too. It was a great loss for them. They came from a certain generation that was stoic. And so on.

I have learned not to express these feeling to most people because it seems to arouse a great deal of anxiety. People seem to want to hear that I've "moved on" or "let go"; that I am not being "negative"; that I am showing compassion, resolution, or other more cheerful and "mature" reactions.

I have found that these reactions only increase my anger and my frustration about sharing these experiences. I have, believe me, a shitload of anger and rage. I hate my parents for the neglect and disparagement that I and, I believe, my brother received as children. We were both the shy, introverted ones. In the pictures that I have of us as children, my brother looks frail and uncertain, while I look more robust.

When we were children, I worried for him because he kept so much to himself. I hate my parents because they abandoned me when I most needed help and comfort. *God damn you both*! I'm here too. Don't you abandon me. This death happened for a reason. This happened because you stay in your own worlds where there is no room for needy, scared children.

You pushed us both away and I hate you for that. He died for nothing. And nothing has changed. They killed you, Tommy, and now they are killing me. I don't exist as a person with feelings and emotions. I am like a robot now. I eat, go to school, come home, do my homework, and get up the next day and do it all over again alone. I'm dying inside. *God damn you*!

I am also writing as a therapeutic tool for myself, to help me better understand my own actions, feelings, and emotions during this period. Just reading the outline of this story astonished me. The whole time I was thinking, God, I was only 13.

All these things happening and my parents not saying a word to me about how I was feeling—it was a shock to realize how terrible this situation was, and how far from normal. Writing this has helped bring the pain to the surface where I can finally deal with it.

Sharing

Although I am almost 50 years old now, the pain is so acute and so fresh that it feels like this happened yesterday, and perhaps in my psyche, it did. Like the many other stories I read written by survivors of suicide, I hope that telling my story might help other families understand why grieving together, however painful, is important. And last of all, I write to honor my brother's memory, to give him remembrance, something which in my family he was denied. I want others to remember something of him. I wish I could do a better job of this, and perhaps in the future, I will find a way.

Chapter 19

The Holocaust Revisited: Protecting Our Families

Ellen Goldschmidt Ehrlich

Let History Not Be Prologue

"Never again" is the cry of the Holocaust that thunders around the world. Yet we see tragedies of equal barbarity continue in our modern world. How do we prevent this from happening? One way is to keep the stories alive for future generations.

Fifty years ago the stories of the Holocaust shocked the world. Then, the survivors went on to build new lives, new families. Silence about the past was often the rule for both family and the outside world. With time, and as more atrocities occurred in our world, the survivors and their children have been encouraged to speak out about their experiences. Remembering the Holocaust, keeping its stories alive for our families, is one way we can help to prevent this repetition so that we can truly say "Never again" for people in our world.

It is not uncommon to hear the statement, "History repeats itself." We cannot allow this to occur. We must tell these personal stories. Furthermore, it is well-known that talking or telling not only informs others but liberates those who have endured terrible secrets and have experienced or witnessed horrible abuse to humanity.

Children of survivors pass on stories from one generation to the next, but eventually, unless they are recorded, the stories are lost. Maintaining and recording our heritage is important to understanding the phenomenon of family in the United States.

This chapter pays homage to those we have lost, to those who are survivors, and to the children yet to be born in the 21st century. I will begin with my family's story and then share the stories of other second-generation survivors.

Tears

In front of a monument in northern Germany, something that happened over 50 years ago left this normally stoic person with tears pouring out of her eyes. I had come to Germany to learn more about my roots. Though I accomplished this, what I did not expect was the barrage of powerful emotions.

My story

My father gave me a family tree that dates back to 1525 in Germany, but even though I have grown children of my own, I know little of the people who were my family and where they came from. I have heard stories of how over a hundred members of our immediate family had been lost in World War II. After my mother died at the age of 90, I felt a powerful urge to find my roots, so last summer I took a trip to Germany with my oldest daughter, Beth.

Hannover

We were welcomed by the mayor's representatives in my parents' hometown. In Hannover, we were received at the town hall, served cold drinks, and taken on a walking tour of the old town. We were shown the site of the old synagogue, which is now a parking lot with a memorial erected next to it. We were also taken to the Holocaust Memorial. Here, I saw the names of my grandfather, uncles, and aunt who died in the camps. For the first time, I broke down and sobbed uncontrollably. I wondered about the lives of those I never knew.

Arrangements were made for us to meet with the town archivist to help find my grandmother's grave in one of the city's three Jewish cemeteries. I was struck by the double tombstone: one side inscribed with my grandmother's name, and the other side blank. I will never know where my grandfather was buried. All this sadness engulfed me, yet we could not have been treated with more gracious hospitality and kindness while we were in Hannover.

Lippstadt

The next day, already a day late, we arrived in Lippstadt, my mother's birthplace. We were greeted in the mayor's office with coffee and cake. The town reporter was there, camera in hand. The mayor told us that my grandparents' home had been torn down. The deputy mayor offered to take us on a walking tour of the town and show us the street where my mother grew up. The name of the street had been changed, and as we walked down the street, Beth said, "that looks like the foundation of Nana's house." My mother had her parents' house returned to her after the war and sold it for a pittance to the couple who had lived with my grandparents until they were forced to leave. The name plate on the door did not look familiar. The deputy mayor asked if we wanted to knock on the door. Beth said no, but I won. A carrot-topped teenager, munching on a breakfast bar, answered the door. We asked if the Steinbergs, my grandparents, had lived in this house. The teenager said she did not know but would ask her father. The present owner of the house came to the door and said that he had bought the house from the relatives of the couple my mother had sold the house to, and that he had been learning about the families who had lived in the house from the neighbors.

Inviting us in, he showed us the garden. When his wife came home, they showed us the brick in the wall inscribed "Steinberg 1917." We were invited for drinks in the garden. My first thought was that I did not want to impose, and then realized that I would be insulting them if I refused. So the best glasses in the house were filled, and we sat and talked about the house, and what they had learned about my grandparents.

They thought that the town had published a book with my grandparents' name in it but could not find it. We took photos in the garden and in front of the house. Later we received copies of articles from five local newspapers with the story of our visit and our picture in the garden of my grandparents' home.

Before we left, the deputy mayor suggested we check the town archives, though they might be closed. We went to the archives and they opened for us and found and copied the citations in the book on my grandfather and great-grandfather.

Earlier, in the mayor's office, we had been asked if there was anything else they could help us with. I responded that I would like to find the relatives of the people my mother had sold the house to. The mayor's deputy checked the phone book and said there were just too many people with that name to find on such short notice. Then, as we were coming out of the archives, we saw a man in the street coming toward us with great intensity. Heinz was the nephew of the people who lived with my grandparents, and he had brought the book with my grandparents name in it and gave it to us. After we chatted for a few minutes, the deputy mayor suggested that she show us a place for lunch. We left for the center of town and she said goodbye.

Deciding to try another place, we came out of the restaurant and were met again by the man who had given us the book. Heinz was my age, but he said he had a sister who was 10 years older and who might remember my grandparents. Would we want to meet her if she was at home? Heinz suggested we get into his car and he would take us to her home. In this foreign country, we got into a stranger's car and drove to his sister's home.

Elizabeth

We arrived at Elizabeth's home and found her baby-sitting her 5-year-old grandchild. She invited us in and seemed genuinely happy to see us. Immediately, she sent her husband out to the store so that she could serve us coffee and cake. Elizabeth then began to tell me stories about my grandparents as she remembered them from when she was a little girl. When she would knock on the front door, my grandfather would usually answer so that the old people upstairs wouldn't have to navigate the stairs. My grandfather would usually have a piece of candy in his pocket for her and often would take her to the garden (where we met an hour earlier) to see his hen and horses.

Elizabeth gave me pictures of the house and of her uncle, who resided with my grandparents. Curiously, her uncle was dressed in his World War I German Army uniform. I was overcome with joy at hearing about my grandparents and at the thought of finding someone who had actually known them. We continued to talk about the times and our families, both past and present, and then she told us of the day when she heard that "the old people (my grandparents) were gone." She said no one seemed to know where they went or what happened to them. At the time I felt sadness and now I am consumed with rage. Even though we have communicated since then about our families and though I remember the gracious hospitality, I wish that I had been able to know my grandparents as she had. I know I missed a great deal and I feel great resentment. Heinz said that he had heard that my grandfather was buried in a mass grave in a nearby town.

Since that time I have had several letters from them. Heinz sent me another book published by the town showing the life of the Jews in Lippstadt, and several citations about my family and my grandfather were included. Later, I mentioned in a letter that I was sorry that I didn't get to visit the cemeteries in Lippstadt. (Actually, I was so overcome with emotion that I could not entertain the thought of this at the time.)

Heinz then went to the nearby town and found the curator of the cemetery, a survivor of the camps. The curator had erected tombstones for those buried there. Heinz took pictures of my grandfather's tombstone, which also included a mention of my grandmother who had died at Auschwitz and curiously mentioned that my mother had died there as well. Happily, this was incorrect—she had escaped from Germany. I was pleased to know that my grandfather had a proper burial site. It was really special for this man to go out of his way for me and my family. Why do I feel resentment rather than gratitude? After all, he was not personally responsible.

Oral Histories

After my trip, I embarked on a small research study, interviewing seven second-generation survivors. I was touched by their stories and jarred by the commonalties in theirs and mine. Some of the most prevalent themes in the stories are:

- Surviving
- Frightening experiences
- Safety
- Loss
- Denial and minimizing
- Connections
- Passing on heritage
- Identity

Surviving

One of the most common themes was that of survival. Survival stories are amazing. Judy, whose parents came from Germany, is a member of one of a few families who survived primarily intact. Judy is a nurse and a psychotherapist.

I talked with her as we sat cross-legged on her beautiful, new oak bed. Here is a part of her "lucky" families story:

> My mother's family was from Leipzig, Germany. Her mother's family, my grandmother, was born in Leipzig. My grandfather was born in Poland and my grandmother had a big family. They were all able to go to different places during the war. One brother went to Argentina, one sister and a brother lived in France under assumed identities as Christians, and there was one sister who lived in Romania pretending to be Christian. One sister was sent to Poland. Her husband was Polish and that whole family went there. She died, her husband died, and one son died. Two sons were in Auschwitz and were liberated from Auschwitz. My mother's family left Germany in 1939, ostensibly to go to Switzerland to put my mother and her sister in boarding school, but that was just an effort to get out of Germany. They didn't know what they were going to do from that point on, but they were able to get visas for Ecuador. They lived in Ecuador during the war.
>
> My mother was 12 years old when she left. She was always very open and verbal about her experiences up until that time—what it was like living in the Jewish community and having to go to a Jewish school instead of a public school, only being allowed in the Jewish library. She told me only certain park benches were for Jews. So she really remembers a lot of the discrimination against Jews, and as a little girl, I think, it was very, very upsetting for her.
>
> I told you the story about her being in the park and being teased or taunted by some people for being Jewish and going up to a policeman and saying,"Please help me," and the policeman saying, "Little girl, I can't help you." So, the feeling that the policeman who's there to protect couldn't protect her. I feel very upset listening to that. There was, you know, horrible discrimination. Yet, really only now does she say how it felt. Up until now, it's been kind of more descriptive and more what happened. But I think as she's getting older, I'm seeing her feel more of this, she's kind of letting some of the feeling out now, and she's 69 years old. It's many years later. So she was very lucky to get out of Germany in 1939 and go to Ecuador.
>
> And, my father's family also was from Germany and they had a dry-goods business. My father was in the Communist Party. I think he was 23 years old in 1933, and his family said that he should leave because it was dangerous for communists at that point. The stories that I always heard were that he wasn't afraid of the devil and he had false papers and he went all over. He helped his family to hide out in the Pyrenees, on the border between France and Spain. He had a girlfriend who wasn't Jewish and he was able to get his parents and his brother and his family to hide out during the war, to stay there. My grandparents weren't able to talk French so they had to pretend to be deaf-mutes and not talk throughout the war when they were in public. It must have been pretty awful.

> And my father had two sisters. One sister, her family was killed in Poland, and one sister was living in Paris and they had a 4-year-old daughter. I was told that one day the little girl was in the playground and she didn't know any better and told some people that they were Jewish. So after that they were arrested and sent to concentration camps, and they were killed.
>
> All in all, there weren't that many people in my family who were killed. Most of the family did survive, and I always felt that we were very lucky, that there were so many families that did not survive. My mother also left her grandparents behind, and she says that they knew when they left for Switzerland that they would never see her grandparents again. She said that that was really very sad for her, because they had lived next door for most of their lives and they were very close to her grandparents. My father always said that this (the United States) is a wonderful country. He would say that we weren't that appreciative.

Though Judy's father did not talk much about the Holocaust, he shared his feelings about his new country and the fact that his children were not appreciative of the immense differences in how people are treated and respected. Alan, another second-generation survivor, also tells about luck and appreciation in his family.

Alan's parents were married in Poland and lived in a ghetto and were "lucky not to have children" at that time. He has positive feelings about being the child of survivors and felt he has things in common with other survivors' children.

> I had a sense of being very appreciated that I was, that I existed, and I was lucky. You know, a twist of fate and I would have been a statistic. I don't think my parents were always hammering that home, but I think there was a sense of appreciating what you have, because things were a lot different. It could be a lot worse.

Alan talks about his mother and father and how they managed to survive and how they were reunited.

> My mother and father were married while the town was occupied. After about three years the ghetto was liquidated and the Jews were being sent to concentration camps. My mother was sent to Auschwitz and survived. My father and two or three friends from the town were on the train [to a camp], and my father's feeling was that he knew what was going on. So he got one or two guards drunk, knocked 'em out with their own guns, jumped from the train, and scattered. Having done that, my father wound up living with false papers as a gentile for the remainder of the war, about a year and a half. He was the foreman of a labor camp made up mostly of gentile prisoners from Poland who obviously did not know he was Jewish or he would not have had a throat that was unslit.

> And then, after the war was over, neither of them knew whether the other had survived. Finally, word spread and people came to that area and saw him and word spread back to where my mother was. One of my father's brothers who survived and some other friends came to his camp. Upon seeing them, my father had to make it clear that they were not to show any recognition of him or he was, again, dead on the spot. And they just whisked him away, and then reunited, and that was it. My brother was born in Germany and I was born after they came here, early on. And that's just a little bit of our background.

Even though luck is one aspect of survival, there were many more thoughts on how survival impacts the family. Another aspect of survival is that of the recent life of the second-generation survivor. Lilli and Allen B. tell stories that show how the past has affected their lives and survival. Lilli also reflects on who she is and the psychological closure she has realized.

I met with Lilli and her husband Ron in the kitchen of their spacious home in an attractive suburb. They were obviously proud of how far they had come from their childhood walk-up flat. Lilli, a mother and schoolteacher, had set the table with coffee and cake before she spoke with me.

> How did the Holocaust impact our lives? I've thought a lot about it, because I had been in therapy for a while a good couple of years ago and I remember getting very, very angry at my psychiatrist. All he wanted to do was talk about the impact of the Holocaust and growing up in a survivor's home and he thought that was my problem. And I would say to him, "That's not my problem. I have normal, everyday types of problems that I'm trying to work out." My husband was traveling an awful lot at the time. I had three young children. I was teaching. I was back at school to get my certification for teaching. I was president of the PTA. All at this particular time that I was trying to get my life together, and here the psychiatrist talked about the Holocaust, and it had no impact. Looking back and being very objective today, I could say it probably *did* have a very, very strong impact on me because I felt so driven to be supermom and superperson. Being superwife and bringing up three kids and teaching and going to school and being PTA president and showing the world, "Look! I survived it! I can do this." I really think it did have an impact.

Allen B. is a lawyer, recently married, tall, and stocky—the "rabbi of the family," (very religious and keeping a strict kosher home). He is a 30-year-old second-generation survivor whose mother's family survived intact in Vilna, Lithuania, where they were hidden for most of the Holocaust by peasants. His father, who came from Poland in the Galitzia area, stayed alive by hiding in the woods and living with peasants and partisans. His parents sent him away from the ghetto. "He had to sneak in and come back, and he was told by family members that his parents were taken away by train. That was the last time he ever saw them, and it was really hard for him."

Allen B. tells about going to Vilna with his family in 1989.

The Vilna trip, you could tell. I mean, all 40 people went to Moscow and to Leningrad and you could really see a change in the mood of the people how it switched from kind of carefree to very pensive. It was pretty interesting. I took a lot of pictures over there. We saw a lot of things. We did a lot of things. One of our objectives was to find some of the people who helped my mother and grandparents to survive. We were able to find some of these people. It was something. We went to the temple in Vilna. We went to services. We went to the outskirts of the city where the farms are, and that's where my mother, aunt, and grandparents were hidden by some of those peasants.

We found some of those houses. We found some of the people, and it was so backward—water pumps and outhouses. It was really intense. And, you know, these people, the people that helped, these people still had nothing. They had nothing then and they gave of themselves and they still had nothing. And now they were given gifts, they were given money, they were given American dollars, they were given, I guess you could say, some sort of payback. It didn't seem like enough because of what was done and what they did and what they risked. It was very interesting.

My mother and grandparents had come back [to visit Vilna after living in the United States for many years]. Some of them [the population in Vilna] didn't even know that my mother and her family had survived the war. Some of them were in total disbelief. It was something to see. There was one woman in particular who was a single woman at the time of the Holocaust. She was my grandparents' age, now in her eighties. She hid my mother and aunt and grandparents. This was toward the end of the war when it was getting very difficult. At the end she couldn't keep them any longer because people were getting suspicious. Her own life was in jeopardy herself. She got married after the war. Her son was there, so this son was in his forties. He'd heard about my mother and my aunt and my grandparents. He and his mother were crying when we all came together, and her mother was crying. And my grandparents were crying. It was an amazing reunion.

We brought her son over to the United States and he stayed in our house for actually an entire summer and worked over here and made some American dollars and went back. Over there it was really something.

The stories of survival and the gratitude to those who helped truly warm the heart. Often these stories are forgotten. However, the goodness of humanity is also contrasted with the evil, frightening experiences.

Frightening Experiences

Second-generation survivors shared other stories that were heartrending. In these stories people were frequently not so lucky. Often these are their parents' stories.

The second-generation survivors did not learn about these stories all at once. Rather the pieces emerged slowly over the years. Frequently, the second generation did not hear all the details until they were adults. It was not uncommon for silence from their relatives to exist for a period of 10 or 20 years after the Holocaust. Many parents did not talk much about the Holocaust when their children were young.

Marion I met with Marion at a coffee house. We talked while we sipped coffee outdoors, as New York City rushed by. Marion, a slim, attractive, successful writer and mother whose first published works are on the subject of the Holocaust, states that she blocks out the stories that her parents have told her. Others in the group I talked with have done that also. Yet, Marion notes how difficult the time must have been for her parents.

> I guess that I would have to say that the Holocaust—less and less as I get older, but when I was a kid and as a young adult—it was a major part of the relationships I formed. I didn't have gentile friends. I do now, but I didn't then. I think I learned to distrust others until I stepped away from it and formed my own experiences. So I think the effect was very pervasive.
>
> My parents have said something interesting. They said that they would rather have never been born than to have gone through what they went through. And they can say this now as grandparents. So I ask, "Now, 50 years later, you can still feel that after you've made a family, after you have two grandchildren and a nice life?" And that comes to a surprise to me. As much as I know that they suffer pain and saw things that no one should ever have to see or feel, I am surprised.

Others blocked out the stories too. We met Lilli earlier, now we hear from her husband Ron as well. He remembers the stories. Ron is an executive who travels abroad a great deal. When he has traveled to Germany, he notes that he does so with trepidation and thinks of what traveling on a train might have been like for himself as a Jew in the early 1940s. Ron talks about his father. Lilli says "I've heard the story many times and I don't remember it. I sort of block it out."

> He was on many work details that built many of the concentration camps, including the work detail that built Auschwitz. I don't know how long he stayed there, but at the end of the war he was in Buchenwald, which is in East Germany, and I guess as the Russians were advancing, they withdrew from Buchenwald and had the people on a death march, just marching them. And one night on the death march he and one or two friends escaped, and they wandered into the forest, ate some poisoned mushrooms, got sick, and wandered into the American territory near Munich.

Alan recalls his mother's story of his grandfather's death.

> I lost grandparents, uncles, including a younger brother of my father who was in a relatively secure position in Auschwitz, yet his father, my paternal grandfather, had been injured in a fall during a work detail and then was of no use any more. And he was walking to the gas chambers and this youngest son saw his father going and he walked out of his office where he was a clerk of some kind and accompanied his father to the gas chamber. And my mother saw them going and that was the last she ever saw of them.

Judy (the one with the "lucky" family) remembers the story her mother tells of being a very young girl in Germany.

> She told me about a policeman coming up to their home and asking one person from each family to come with him, and she didn't know what they were going to do. But my grandmother had just had a baby and her husband wasn't home and my grandmother wasn't with it. She said that my mother should go with the policeman, and my mother started crying and she didn't want to go with him, and she said that the policeman said to my grandmother, "I'm not an animal, and I'm not going to take her if she's that upset." Later my mother found out that they paraded all these Jewish people through the park and people threw stones and people spit at them and called them horrible names.

These experiences are so frightening that it is little wonder that the survivors often keep silent. Did they try to protect their children or was it simply too painful to remember? Despite this, eventually, the stories were told, and heard by the second generation.

Safety

Remembering the frightening stories, it is little wonder that the parents felt very protective of their children. Almost every second-generation survivor mentioned this. Sometimes it was an unwillingness to let children stray far from the nest; other times it was associated with a sense of being a close-knit family. Marion's comments about distrust and Judy's mother's stories of the police are examples of the precursors. Sara also contributes with her stories about safety.

I first met with Sara on her back porch, enjoying her serene, wooded, flower-filled yard. Sara is an editor, a writer, and the mother of two grown children. She is married to her "soul mate," an artist "filled with the joy of life." He too is the child of survivors. Sara talks and writes about her childhood memories.

> My parents were very concerned about safety. I was 15 years old, but I couldn't take the bus, I couldn't be independent, I couldn't go anywhere. You know, all of my friends could do x, y, and z, but I had to be

very close to home. In our early years in the United States, we lived in a gentile neighborhood, a Polish neighborhood, among those who had been our oppressors in Poland.

We lived in the Polish neighborhood because that's where my parents could work and make a living. My mother worked in a bakery, and my father worked in a grocery store. Later they opened up their own convenience store. It was a Polish neighborhood, so I couldn't have friends. I couldn't have people at my house. I couldn't go to their house because they're goyem, after all, and these same goyem . . . this was America, but in Poland they had beaten them up all the time. It's all true and they lived it. So they didn't trust me to go into the world, and we all had to be like the chickens, always kept very close to the nest.

My sister used to joke that it was like we were cave people huddled around the fire in the kitchen. We always sat in the kitchen, the whole family. Everything was there. We did our homework there. My mother sewed there. She liked it when we were all in the same place. "What do you have to go into another room for?" she would asked. "I want to read in peace," I answered. "There's no such thing," she insisted. "You can sit right here. There's a chair here."

Ron and Lilli also talked together about the protectiveness of their parents:

Lilli: See, they would hold in the tears much more when our kids asked. For us, they tried to shield us a tremendous amount. You were sheltered as a child.

Ron: Protected.

Lilli: Yeah. And I wasn't allowed to breathe without anybody knowing where I was.

Ron: I wasn't allowed to go on overnight Boy Scout trips.

Lilli: I was never allowed to go away to school. My parents were afraid to let me out of their sight.

Ron: But you went to sleep-away camp.

Lilli: I was already 17 when I went.

Ron: I was 18.

Being protective of family is not surprising in view of the losses they suffered. Families were drawn closer and the importance of family was paramount in their lives.

Loss

Sara, the editor, talks about the loss of family and also the feelings of loss related to the inability of her parents to demonstrate affection because of their fear of the "evil eye."

I've written a great deal about my childhood—my childhood memoirs and things about my family—often dealing with the loss. The loss of not having a family apart from my nuclear family. We never had anyone. My friends used to talk about aunts and uncles and cousins. I never had any of those things. So I grew up feeling all this loss inside me. I have made a lot of effort over my life to try to deal with that—that feeling that it can happen again. There's no question in my mind that it *can* happen again. I'm talking about this possibly happening to other people, yes, but definitely to Jews. There is no doubt in my mind that it could again be excused. That people in the world could find ways to look away and not know, the way they did then. I'm sensitive to anti-Semitism. Although I love this country, and there is no question in my mind this is the best place in the world for me to live, I still feel that as a Jew I'm not entirely accepted here. That while it's not a Christian country, I still feel that it's kind of a tolerance.

My parents' approach to life was always to expect the worst in a certain way. They weren't able to get the joy of life back. With their grandchildren, they were more so than with their children. My mother died 10 years ago. She was able to be with her grandchildren what she couldn't be with her children . . . loving and affectionate and doting and all of that, and that was a joy. My son and daughter loved their *bubbi* and *zeddi* and they were doted on by them and it was really a wonderful thing. So they couldn't give it to their children. It was too scary. It was too immediate.

A lot of my personal writing has been dealing with that denial that they practiced in their lives. There were a lot of things I have to conjecture about because they didn't talk a lot about things. It wasn't a family where there was great ongoing communication. As a matter of fact, my father used to have an expression during meals. He would say "*Aza hint est shriet er nisht*"—when a dog eats it doesn't bark. And I would say, "But we are not dogs." So we had this dispute going on for years. But he thought when you eat, you should be quiet, and that's your business. There was a denial of joy, a denial of satisfaction. If something good happened, be careful! Watch out! Because the shit is going to hit the fan soon enough. And my mother in particular was very hardworking. She did everything. She always worked because she had to, and she took care of the family exclusively. No cleaning help, no laundry help, no barbecue chicken from Kings. She raised denial to an art for many, many years.

As she got older, she started indulging herself. She got a mink coat at one point—it was like a baby, the most precious thing in the universe. I wrote a story about it that was published in *Lilith* magazine. And I took some of that into myself, denying myself pleasures or denying myself even, say, the best piece of fruit. If I put out fruit for the family and there were some lousy pieces, I'd eat them.

Ron and Lilli also talk about missing family as they grew up.

Lilli: I felt bad not having grandparents. I had no way of even relating to a grandparent.

Ron: Yeah, I also had no idea of that. I mean, what does a grandparent do?

Lilli: Our parents' friends were generally around the same age as they were. You at least had family in Canada who were much older than your mother, so they had a place to visit.

Ron: On the rare occasion, like once every six or seven years.

Lilli: But I missed that, not having a family. Maybe that's why I'm so strong with the family. I know I would get upset with the kids when they used to fight and say, "You're family. You're family. You have to stick together no matter what." I'm not particularly close with my sister, but we're responsible for each other. Ron's not particularly close with his brother, but we do have a responsibility. We feel a responsibility to him. I think our kids are going to have a tough time with family relationships.

The losses are insurmountable, so it is understandable that some people live with daily thoughts of the Holocaust and must find ways to cope.

Denial and Minimizing

It is little wonder with all the loss and the frightening experiences of their parents that the second generation has daily thoughts about the Holocaust. Sara and Marion both talk about the daily thoughts and the way they deal with them in their lives. Almost all the survivors have videotapes of their loved ones' stories of survival. Curiously, many have said that "for whatever reason" they have not viewed them yet. However, they are grateful that the stories are preserved for posterity.

Sara's husband, a successful artist, has recently changed from painting "beautiful things" that demonstrate the joy of the world to charcoal drawings of the concentration camps as seen from the air. Sara states:

> We are back living with the Holocaust daily. Once again, it's a regular part of my life. My response to that is that I have completely removed myself so that as much as I can I avoid dealing with it. I cannot read any of the books that have come out. I can't watch the specials on TV. I've even withdrawn from what's happening negatively in the world. It's kind of a survival thing in order to keep my equilibrium, because we are breathing that air again. I've had to withdraw from all of those things, and my husband is immersed. So we're zigging and zagging. . . . But to survive I have withdrawn from the constancy.

Marion talks about how, from a very early age, she knew her parents were survivors and she always took care of them.

> I remember being in graduate school and I had a master's degree in counseling, and one of our teachers was talking about Holocaust survivors and she said that they all suffered psychological effects of it. And I stood up and I said, " Well, my parents are survivors and they didn't."
>
> And I was like 25 and I believed that statement. I still believed that. And then I started to think about it. I came to see that they were affected by it, and so was I. I think about it, if not every day, a lot.

Lilli has heard her parents stories, she tells how she copes:

> My mother was the oldest of six children. She survived with two of her sisters. She was in the Brigene ghetto. I've heard the story many, many times and I don't remember it, I sort of block it out. I can remember his parents' when they tell us, but I don't remember too much of my parents'.

Judy recently went to the Holocaust museum in Washington, D.C., and saw things in a different light:

> I saw it more, like, my God! It was really minimized. It really was a lot worse than they ever let on, and I think that was a big realization for me, that they were lucky that they weren't killed, but things were not that rosy. Things were pretty awful. And that was kind of like a more recent revelation to me. I've always thought, oh, nothing that terrible happened, but I see that as my mother gets older, I also hear more from her how this has affected her.

Though they found different ways to cope with the infrequent thoughts of the Holocaust, most second-generation survivors talked about a feeling of connection to the past and to Jewish identity through these connections.

Connections

Although the daily thoughts of the Holocaust and the denial and minimizing were frequently disconcerting, they created important connections. I began this journey with a search for my roots. Others have different connections to the past, to Judaism, and to the Holocaust.

Alan feels comfortable with his upbringing and with his relationship to his parents. He is amazed by his connection to the Holocaust:

> I think it was just an awareness of being a child of Holocaust survivors. It was like, wow! That's amazing that I was that close to someone who was actually in the hell that was going on, and it gives me a little bit of the feeling that there's probably a duty or responsibility or desire on my part to somehow see to it that we just continue, and do whatever needs to be done to not allow that to happen, obviously to anyone but from a selfish standpoint, to us as Jews. You know, it should never have happened, but to think of it ever happening more than once is insanity to me. Yet to think it was only in the 1930s and 1940s. When you think

about how much time history is, it's so scarily close that when I think about it, I'm just amazed, perplexed, frustrated, enraged, you know, that it happened. That it was allowed to happen, that it did happen.

Sara's connection is even closer. She identifies with her mother's experiences, which still impact on her own life:

It's about being good to myself, that I deserve things, that I don't have to continue the deprivation. When I was younger, and I would take a trip or go on vacation, I thought, "Oy vey, my mother never had a vacation. When my mother was my age she was chopping wood in Siberia. I identified so strongly with her loss, with her pain. I struggled mightily and I struggle still with that denial of things, for deserving things that my parents never had or enjoyed."

Allen B. talks about how his father lost faith in religion for a while. But the connection from childhood was strong, and he passed it on to his children.

I think that I felt comfortable in Hebrew school because if your parents were Jewish and survivors from Europe, the people in Hebrew school were also Jewish people and I think they could understand more how your parents were.

Ron talks about the reasons he and Lilli stay involved in the Jewish Community:

Ron: We both are very active in Jewish community issues. I think it is driven by being children of the Holocaust. I know I feel, and Lilli does too, I'm sure, a very strong need to assure the continuity of the Jewish community in order to not give Hitler a latent endowment. And that is an important reason why I'm as active as I am. And, our youngest daughter is now in Israel and when we sent her off it was . . .

Lilli: The first suicide bombings.

Ron: And they went there. People were nervous and some parents wanted to have their kids come home.

Lilli: You didn't even let me put the news on that day.

Ron: A certain amount of people wanted to take off and I said, "No. We're not with them." And that was the response of the Holocaust impact by saying we don't want any more.

The connection to the Holocaust certainly impacts on the family going into the 21st century. Judy has a mission to build a connection for her family with the past:

I was thinking about safety and there was something else that came to mind.

The feeling that I get when I'm at the synagogue is the feeling of really being connected to my past. Feeling like this is what people did thousands of years ago. This is what my family, my families did in Europe. This is what it was all about. I especially feel that with the

> singing. I really am very moved by a lot of the prayers in the synagogue and I feel very, very connected to my past. I feel like it's very important to get that back, to have that connection again. I really feel that it was cut off and I think because of the war what could have been passed down to me was not passed down. My mother, in fact, said she wondered, how could there be a God? They knew they were Jewish but they didn't feel connected to God and they didn't feel like they wanted to really stay connected to their roots in some way. I feel more connected now. I'm going in that direction of trying to build a connection for myself and for my family.
>
> Connections seem to be linked to identity, that is, a Jewish one. This seemed crucial though the format varied from individual to individual, family to family. Will this carry on into the 21st century?

Identity

Thus the connections provided an entree to a Jewish identity. All of the second-generation survivors that I spoke with talked about their idea of a Jewish identity; for some it was religious, for some it was maintaining traditions. Nonetheless, identity was an important component of their lives.

Marion notes that she did not have much religion in her early life and feels the need to do something different for her child:

> For me, it's like, I wasn't brought up with any—with very few—religious rituals, and it wasn't a religious past. My Jewish identity came from the Holocaust. I didn't want Max's to come from that, so he went to Hebrew school and he's having a bar mitzvah and stuff like that 'cause I hoped his Jewish identity would be based on something positive.

Lilli talks about different Jewish identities within her life; she did not always have a strong commitment to this:

> In growing up what I remember is there were two ways that my peers reacted and friends of mine and friends of the family. There was one, like Ron and myself, who became committed to ethical questions. I think I was committed more to the anti-Vietnam movement in the early sixties than I was with Judaism. I think the identity of Judaism came into play when I had my own kids. The second way that I saw my peers and my friends of family and friends of second generation was they wanted no part of their parents. They were embarrassed by their parents.

Lilli relates how she decided to give her children a more Jewish identity.

> I remember there was one time we came back from Brooklyn after Yom Kippur. It was the night of Yom Kippur. I think that's what made me determine that my kids had to go to Jewish day school. In the mailbox was literature about Jews for Jesus. It was the night right after Yom Kippur

and on the bottom of all this literature was a person's name and address and a phone number. They were six houses away from us. I remember how I was livid. I was so upset and Ron was so angry that he decided to call these people up and he went over to talk to them. I remember them trying to talk to him and every time he said something, Ron was able to counter that. Ron went to Yeshiva. It was not religion that I desired, but I wanted my kids to know who they were, not deal from an emotional standpoint, but to deal from fact. You know, so many people went to the gas chamber just because they were Jewish. They didn't know why they were Jewish. They had no Jewish background. They had a mother who was Jewish, or a grandmother who was Jewish. They were gassed the same way as the man with the payis and everything else. I think that made an impact on me, and I think that made an impact on my kids. I remember when my oldest daughter dated, or when she was starting to be very serious about her husband, and I started to put money in these two boxes. In one I put a dollar, and in one I put five dollars. She said, "Mommy, what are you doing?" And I said, "The dollar one, I'm saving for your wedding." She said, "What's the five-dollar one?" I said, "I'm saving for a Jewish day school education for my grandchildren." So, in that respect I think they do have a strong sense of self.

Lillie also talks about her siblings.

I have some wonderful memories. I remember when my sister was born. We are about five years apart. She has a very strong sense of Jewish self. However, she has no commitment to Judaism.

My brother also has a strong sense of Jewish self but really has very little commitment to Judaism. Ron talks about his identity as a son of survivors. When he read a book on the Holocaust, he was touched even more profoundly.

Ron talks about the book.

It is a core element of my identity that I am a son of survivors. There was that famous book by Helen Epstein, *Children of the Holocaust*. And when I read that I couldn't believe, having never met that person, how come she knew so much about me, because all of the many of the idiosyncrasies that she talked about in there I could see in myself, and I could see in my brother. Some of them are crazy things. I went to high school and college in the city. I took the subway back and forth. Subways are crowded. I often imagined I was on a cattle car going to a concentration camp. That's what I was relating to. I go to Europe quite often, and when I go into Germany there's a nervousness in my system.

Judy did not grow up with much religion in her life, but a Jewish identity was very important to her on some level. She went to Israel and met her husband, a Christian Englishman who later converted to Judaism.

> I know that the fact that I was Jewish was a very important part of me, and to me passing on this Jewish identity has a lot of meaning for me. I know that I got all this information about what happened during the war and my parents' experiences, but they were never religious in any sense. They did go to synagogue on the high holidays but that was it, and I really didn't have much of a Jewish education. And we were traditional. We really didn't know anything. There was very little knowledge, I felt, behind what we were doing. So now I feel like I need to give my children more of the feeling of what it is to be Jews. And it's not just the identity, because I think that it's hard to pass on this identity to another generation just based on what my parents gave me. I'm trying very hard to give my children a Jewish education. We're affiliated with a reform temple here, and we're pretty involved with the temple.

The Jewish identity led everyone I talked with to the theme of passing on the information about the Holocaust and Judaism to future generations. For some it is a Jewish education, for others it might be the traditions, and for still others just the stories about the camps and the cattle cars.

Passing on the Heritage

For some reason [could it be a Jewish identity?] the people I spoke with have all been involved with passing on information about the Holocaust and Judaism in some way. Some have written books and articles, others have spoken to groups, others have arranged or participated in Holocaust memorial services and have contributed to the establishment of Holocaust memorials.

Alan wonders about the future:

> Based on those feelings I try to attend and participate in things that are related to keeping the memory of the Holocaust going. And I think as we go into the 21st century, as we get older, I think it's important. I wonder what will happen when there's no second generation, and then with the third and fourth, and so on. We'll be dead and gone, so what will happen? When there are community observances and programs, I try to go. I try to have my children go, but I'm not good at forcing the issue. If they're willing to come with me, I'm very pleased, and they generally go, which is good. I kind of keep a bit involved that way. I don't coordinate or lead efforts in that direction, but if I'm called, I'll usually participate. I'll ask my children to do the same thing as they get older and have children.

Alan shares his experience of passing on the heritage to others in the community.

> They have this society in the metropolitan New York, New Jersey area. The president recently called me and said, "You know, we've been having speakers now from the second generation and we noticed

you've never done it." I knew that I'd never done it, and I'd been conscious of the fact that I haven't done it, and I was always thinking, "Don't call me. Please don't. I hope they don't call me." Even being a lawyer, I'm not that comfortable speaking in front of a group, usually until I've done it or I'm in the middle of it. Then I'm told I get better, more comfortable, and it's good. So when he called me my first reaction was, "Well, let me think about it." And he said, "I'm not going to force you." This was my father's peer, so he couldn't have made me feel guiltier quicker.

But he didn't. I basically said to myself: " 'How could you not do it? Why not? He's right!' You know, don't let my little inhibitions or my schedule stop me. And I prepared something, and I did it, and I felt great about it, and it was well-received." It was a very personalized presentation of my memories of growing up as kids with parents running to meetings of this society, and what it all meant. Then we started to understand what it meant as we got older and what the society meant.

They built a monument to the 6 million Jews that stands right in the center of their area of the cemetery, where members like my father are buried. But there's also a large stone with names of the relatives of the members of the society who died in the Holocaust. So I can relate to, "Not now" or "Why me?" and then do the right thing.

Allen B. sees his parents as his heros. He appreciates their strength in surviving. He relates to the loss of his father's childhood and thus cherishes the time they spend together as a family.

I definitely don't want to be ashamed of it because I am glad they lived through it. I'm not proud of the fact that the Holocaust happened, but I am proud of how they survived and that they *did* survive. It's a great accomplishment. I think that also [children] should learn about it partly because it's their history, it's their heritage. The Jews were oppressed. I think it's important that they learn about Passover, about Egypt, and about Purim. I think the Holocaust has its place in the history. They should really learn about this.

Marion felt that she was living with the ghosts of the Holocaust, and while she was pregnant, she wrote an article for a national parent's magazine on the subject. Later she felt a strong urge to communicate about this to her son.

When Max was just a few years old I had to think about whether I wanted to talk to him about it, and I did. Abe, my husband, thought I was wrong. He would have waited. I just couldn't.

Judy also feels a strong obligation.

I think that there's a really strong feeling in me that this is like a mission, that it's very important that I, as a daughter of survivors that weren't in concentration camps but are survivors of the Holocaust, part

> of European Jewry that was pretty much wiped out—I feel that I have a duty to pass on this religion to my family, that I have an obligation to do that. Maybe I didn't really know how to do it until recently. I think I really didn't. I did know that I had to.

Thus, the heritage, and knowledge about this history, has become important to the second-generation survivors. I can better understand why I had such a strong urge to discover my roots. Though the journey started with a trip to Germany it lead to my Jewish heritage. When I began this research I asked my children if they would tell me about their thoughts on the Holocaust. My youngest daughter, Janice, wrote me the following letter.

> As a child, I was forced to recognize the validity of the Holocaust. My classmates were cruel, as most children are, and taunted me, drew swastikas on my books, told me horrible jokes about the Jewish people, and basically made fun of me for my family and my suffering. As I grew up, I began to realize how much hatred people felt toward myself and my religion. People always make ethnic jokes, then find out my family suffered and perished in the Holocaust, then for some reason they apologize, and are rueful of what they said.
>
> But it makes me wonder—if I wasn't the person whose family was brutally murdered in the concentration camps, would they feel any different? Would they still go on making jokes about the Jews in their slavery, in their untimely and unfair deaths?
>
> I remember back to sixth grade, I had to do a report on my grandparents, which meant surviving the Holocaust. My grandmother, Berta Goldschmidt, was the only remaining elder in my family, on both sides. She was in her eighties, spoke mostly German, and could barely understand me. I proceeded to ask questions for my report with my mother's help. My grandmother became upset and ill at ease, yelling about fires and the terror. I couldn't bear to see it anymore. My grandmother was not able to really talk to me. Leaving me feeling deprived, my mother tried to help her. The effort was futile. My grandmother could no longer talk about it.
>
> When I was 16 years old, my best friend's father, who was 69 at the time, was a Holocaust survivor. He took my friend Susan, myself, and his wife with him to a Holocaust reunion. There we met his brother, who was also a survivor, and his wife.
>
> In the beginning no one could have known more distinctly than I what pain these people have endured. Being in a room with 500 first- and second-generation survivors was very intense, to say the least. So many were crying that it meant nothing to shed a tear in public, though I would have not done it before. People were comforting each other in a way I have never been conscious of. People were joined in remorse, not hate; sadness, not fear; loss, not of integrity, but of those they loved. It opens your eyes, but more than that, it makes you realize how

the wrongdoings of one individual can disturb millions of people, generations to come and generations past.

Janice's painful story was very surprising to me. I did not realize the extent of her suffering. I wonder about the painful heritage I am passing on, yet I know it is a subject that cannot be forgotten. Can we pass on the heritage, eliminate the destruction to human lives, and present a positive viewpoint as our families move into the 21st century?

Perhaps keeping these stories alive may prevent future atrocities. The individual stories make the words "Never again" thunder to life. It is life and the family that we want to preserve, and understanding the effects of the Holocaust impacts the preservation of the family. We can enlist the assistance of our government to act early and forcefully when we see tragedies occurring. This is not just for Jews but for all people in our world. We can no longer tolerate such atrocities.

References

Epstein, H. (1988). *Children of the Holocaust: Conversations with Sons and Daughters of Survivors.* New York: Penguin.

Felsen, I., and Erlich, H. S. (1990). Identification patterns of offspring of Holocaust survivors with their parents. *American Journal of Orthopsychiatry,* 60(4): 506–520.

Harari, E. (1995). The longest shadow: A clinical commentary on Moshe Lang's "Silence." Therapy with Holocaust survivors and their families. *Australian and New Zealand Journal of Family Therapy,* 16(1): 11–13.

Herman, D. (1991). "Ruinboys" or rainbows? Survivors of the Holocaust and their children. *The Jewish Quarterly,* 38(2): 21–26.

Jucovy, M. E. (1991). Psychoanalytic contributions to Holocaust studies. *International Journal of Psychoanalysis,* 73(2): 267–282.

Keller, R. S. (1988). Children of Jewish Holocaust survivors: Relationship of family communication to family cohesion, adaptability and satisfaction. *Family Therapy,* 15(3): 223–237.

Lang, M. (1995). Silence: Therapy with Holocaust survivors and their families. *Australian and New Zealand Journal of Family Therapy,* 16(1):1–10.

Mazor, A., and Tal, I. (1996). Intergenerational transmission: The individuation process and the capacity for intimacy of adult children of Holocaust survivors. *Contemporary Family Therapy,* 18(1): 95–113.

Rose, S. L., and Garske, J. (1987). Family environment, adjustment, and coping among children of Holocaust survivors: A comparative investigation. *American Journal of Orthopsychiatry,* 57(3): 332–344.

Rosenman, S., and Handelsman, I. (1990). The collective past, group psychology and personal narrative: Shaping Jewish identity by memoirs of the Holocaust. *American Journal of Psychoanalysis,* 50(2): 151–170.

Shoshan, T. (1989). Mourning and longing from generation to generation. *American Journal of Psychotherapy,* 43(2): 193–207.

Waldfogel, S. (1991). Physical illness in children of Holocaust survivors. *General Hospital Psychiatry,* 13(2): 267–269.

Wardi, S. (1994). Bonding and separateness, two major factors in the relations between Holocaust survivors and their children. *Clinical Gerontologist,* 14(3): 119–131.

Winik, M. F. (1988). Generation to generation: A discussion with children of Jewish Holocaust survivors. *Family Therapy,* 15(3): 271–284.

VOICES SEVEN

Families Bearing Challenges

CHAPTER 20

THE IMPACT OF AIDS ON THE FAMILY

Sande Garcia Jones and Patricia Ruth Messmer

It was about three o'clock in the morning, and I heard him call softly, "Mama, Mama". I held his hand, and it was still so hot. He said, "I want you to make a party for me. Take me back home and have a party with everyone for me." I told him, yes, of course, I would do that. And I talked on and on about who would be there and what we would have to eat. I just held on to him, because I knew it was the end. His fever had been so high for the past two days, his skin had felt like it was on fire, but now he felt cold. And then I knew it was over, and he was with the angels. This terrible disease had taken my boy, my special boy. . . . And now I had to make arrangements to bring him back home and bury him.

E.'s *mom*, *May* 1996

In June, 1999, Six Blum, the AIDS inpatient unit at Mount Sinai Medical Center, Miami Beach, was permanently closed. The few patients on the unit were transferred to other medical floors at the hospital, and the nurses were floated to other units. Since the early 1990s, the unit had been busy and alive with activity, caring for AIDS patients and their families. Now the beds were empty, the rooms were dark, and the corridors were silent.

The closing of the unit reflected the dramatic change that has taken place in AIDS care throughout the United States. All over the country, the census of AIDS patients has declined so much that special AIDS units were closing in hospitals everywhere (Morrison, 1998; Napper, 1998). The age-adjusted death rate from HIV infection showed an incredible 47 percent decrease from 1996 to 1997. HIV patients had 71,000 fewer hospitalizations in 1997 than 1995, resulting in 878,000 fewer days of hospital care for HIV patients (NCHS, 1999).

Combinations of new HIV medications, known as highly active antiretroviral therapy (HAART), were credited with having a major impact in helping people with HIV live longer and healthier lives. But the promising future of HIV care is clouded. The drugs have not helped everyone, and resistance to the drugs has become a major barrier to effective care. The medication regimes are complex and arduous, and adherence has become an issue. Uncertainty and a variety of questions abound regarding HIV infection and treatment as we begin the new millennium.

This chapter will discuss the impact of AIDS on the family in the 21st century. Findings from nursing research studies are discussed, along with predictions for the future. Woven throughout this chapter are personal stories about patients and families, shared by nurses in AIDS care. Their stories bring to life the voices and perspective of those infected and affected by HIV, and highlight their thoughts, concerns, and conflicts.

THE WORLD OF AIDS

For hundreds of years humans have suffered from diseases. Epidemics like bubonic plague and smallpox have taken heavy tolls. The epidemic called AIDS (acquired immunodeficiency syndrome) has become a household word in our lifetime. To many people, AIDS is still associated with fear of infection, contagion, and death; others still view the illness as punishment for immoral behavior.

Cancer, once the dreaded "Big C," has now become socially acceptable. Obituaries frequently state, "*He died after a long struggle with cancer. Please send donations instead of flowers to the American Cancer Society.*" But AIDS is still unacceptable to many people, and families, racked by grief and anger that death could happen to someone so young, must bear the additional burden of maintaining the secret.

As we enter the third known decade of HIV/AIDS, we are seeing new consequences of this epidemic. Once considered the "4-H Club" (homosexuals, hemophiliacs, Haitians, and heroin-injecting drug users), HIV/AIDS has shown that it does not discriminate. In the last decade it has become clear that the face of the HIV/AIDS infected population is changing.

A significant epidemiological shift has emerged over the last few years. While gay white men accounted for the largest proportion of cases 10 years ago, women and minorities are the new emerging populations. A total of 665,357 persons with AIDS had been reported to the Centers for Disease Control and Prevention (CDCP) as of June 1998. While minorities made up only one-fourth of the total U.S. population in 1997, over one-half of all reported AIDS cases were among racial and ethnic minorities.

Globally, HIV/AIDS is a disease of families, with women and children dramatically impacted by the disease (Sowell, et al., 1999). The hopeful future of HIV/AIDS in the United States is not reflected around the world. A December 1998 report by the World Health Organization (WHO) and the Joint United Nations Programme on HIV/AIDS (UNAIDS) revealed that the epidemic was progressing rapidly. Around the world, 11 men, women, and children are infected every minute—about 6 million people a year. More than 95 percent of all HIV-infected people now live in the developing countries of the world, which have experienced 95 percent of all deaths to date from AIDS.

By December 1999, the estimated number of people living with HIV had grown to 33.6 million. Women now represent 43 percent of all people over the age of 15 living with HIV and AIDS. Since the start of the epidemic, HIV has infected more than 49 million people globally. Although it is a slow-acting virus that can take a decade or more to cause severe illness and death, it has cost the lives of nearly 16 million adults and children around the globe. An estimated 2.6 million of these deaths occurred during 1999, more than ever before in a single year.

The Early Days: Solving the Puzzle

Ruby W., now retired after years of nursing, recalled what AIDS care was like back in 1981. A young Haitian male lay dying in his hospital bed in a large Miami teaching hospital. He was experiencing high fevers and increasing respiratory distress, and he was not responding to an array of powerful antibiotics. The interns and residents were perplexed and frustrated. The man was dying of *Pneumocystis carinii* pneumonia (PCP), a seemingly impossible situation: according to the textbooks, PCP was usually found only in patients who were taking immunosuppressive drugs.

The man died, but soon, several more cases—young men, some Haitian and some not—appeared in the emergency department. Signs were hung over the new patients' beds alerting everyone that this was another case of the life-threatening "Haitian disease."

Fire and rescue personnel were soon warned by the hospital staff to begin wearing gloves, because this disease might possibly be contagious. The doctors tried everything that was available. Experimental drugs were being flown in to Miami from around the world. The same scenes were occurring in San Francisco, Los Angeles, and New York City. As reports came through to the Centers for Disease Control regarding acquired immunodeficiency in previously healthy young adult males, pediatric immunologists in the four cities noted increased numbers of infants with unexplained immunodeficiencies. Doctors from New York called attention to injecting drug users, who were exhibiting a similar picture. Thus, the epidemic associated with HIV infection began almost unnoticed with the suffering and deaths of a few people—gay men, minorities, hemophiliacs and other people who had received blood transfusions, injecting drug users, their sexual partners, and their children (Casey et al., 1996).

In June 1982, Dr. William Darrow, a behavioral scientist at the sexually transmitted diseases unit of the CDC, was finally able to solve the puzzle. The pieces had started to come together after a phone call in March to the Los Angeles Public Health Department. Darrow's evidence showed that HIV in homosexual males was sexually transmitted. "Back then, the issue was fairly simple," says Darrow, who is now a professor at Florida International University in Miami. "We had a problem and we needed to find what caused it. But the riddle is, why is it that 15 years later we haven't seemed to progress? What can we do to stop the spread of AIDS? And, more importantly, why don't people change their behaviors? Do they really think that it's not going to kill them?" p. 10 (Ojito, 1996).

Living with AIDS: The Second Decade

In the early 1980s, being HIV-positive was considered by many to be a death sentence. The introduction in 1986 of the antiretroviral agent Zidovudine (AZT) brought about new hope for treatment, and people started to talk about "living with AIDS." With proper medical treatment and a healthy lifestyle, the HIV-infected person could be asymptomatic for 10 or more years, without progressing to AIDS.

In 1995 the introduction of a new class of HIV drugs, the protease inhibitors, promised new hope for people living with AIDS (PLWA). As of April 1999, the FDA had expedited the approval process for 10 nucleoside and nonnucleoside antiretroviral agents and 5 new protease inhibitors. More drugs are being researched and expected to obtain approval for distribution in 2000 and 2001.

However, the drugs have not helped everyone. Scientific discussions now abound on "salvage therapy," what to do for a person who has "failed" drug therapy. Genotype and phenotype tests are being conducted to determine resistance to HIV medications. Maintaining maximum antiretroviral potency requires exquisite adherence to demanding medication regimes (Williams, 1999). The more complicated regimes that require multiple pills and dosing every 8 hours may not be the protocol of choice for active or disorganized people (Jones & Baggett, 1999). Patients are blamed for noncompliance with the prescribed doses and dietary requirements for the drugs. AIDS activists have decried a biomedical model of care that has failed to consider quality of life (Jones & Brown, 1999). The new medications have not solved the problem of AIDS. A variety of questions and unresolved issues still abound.

HIV in the Third Decade

Practitioners and researchers are now beginning to consider HIV infection as a chronic disease rather than a terminal one, at least for people with finances and access to care. Perhaps someday, with continued advances in technology and pharmaceutical agents, HIV will be like diabetes—not curable, but controllable. Just as blood glucose is checked at home by a fingerstick test to determine the needed dose of insulin, perhaps HIV viral load tests will be done at home, and the medication dosage adjusted daily according to the viral level.

A needs assessment study of caregivers of people with AIDS reveals a desire for more educational programs about the disease process, dealing with grief, dealing with emotional concerns, home versus institutional care, and skills training (Theis et al., 1997). Caregivers need help with and information about coping with loss, coping with responsibilities, readjusting routines and finances.

The impact of AIDS on the infected person and the family unit is tremendous. The new HIV medications do not cure AIDS. However, they do prolong survival and, most importantly, help improve the quality of life for people with the virus. We still face the challenge of meeting the complex health and social needs of HIV-infected people. Much of the enormous burden is shouldered by the family unit (Phillips and Thomas, 1996).

People and families do not exist in a vacuum; they are part of a greater whole, the community. Thus, the impact of AIDS on the community is also an issue of concern. The stigma of AIDS and fear of contagion have made this disease different from other chronic diseases, such as diabetes or asthma. Like the lepers of old, HIV-infected persons complain of being treated as outcasts by the community. Why is this fear present? How can interventions be introduced that will change this community perception and lead to changes in national public policy?

THE FAMILY UNIT: CHANGING THE RULES

Friedman (1992) states that never in recorded history has a society been composed of a greater multiplicity of attitudes, values, behaviors and lifestyles. These social, behavioral, and cultural differences are reflected in a variety of family forms. Nontraditional family forms include the unmarried parent and child family (usually mother and child); the unmarried couple and child family (usually a common-law marriage); cohabitating couple (unmarried couple living together); gay or lesbian family (persons of the same sex living together as "marital partners"); and commune families. Each family form represents a different adaptation to the environmental demands placed on society, and each form has its own particular strengths and vulnerabilities. There is no right or wrong, proper or improper, form of family. Families must be understood within their own context. Labels only serve as a reference to the family's living arrangements and primary group network.

In the 1960s, the communal family became synonymous with the flower children of the hippy generation. In the 1980s the impact of AIDS on certain demographic groups caused a major change in the way health-care providers and facilities thought of and defined family. Since the start of the AIDS era, homosexual males have been hard-hit by this disease. Their chosen family units are often nontraditional, and frequently include gay partners, lovers, or friends. In the 1980s, the addition of *significant other* to the definition of family member forced changes in many institutional policies and protocols. Including these significant others in care planning as part of the family is now recognized as vital to providing social support to the person with HIV/AIDS.

By the 1990s, it was not uncommon for hospital special immunology (SI) units, which were usually the designated AIDS units, to provide cots or sleeping chairs so that the partner or lover could spend the night. This is a far cry from the early 1980s, when hospital visiting hours were strictly enforced and intensive care units had strict regulations governing when and who could visit the ICU patient. Allowing partners to continue in their caregiver role while their lover is hospitalized was also a common scene on SI units. The partner was included and consulted on care-planning decisions. Acknowledging and using the expertise of partners in symptom management is a key feature in being able to negotiate partnerships with family caregivers to deliver high-quality care for people living with HIV infection (Powell-Cope,1994).

Social Support and AIDS Family Caregivers

Research indicates that social support has a direct effect on health, buffers the effects of physical and emotional stress, and mediates immune dysfunction. As summarized by McGough (1990), there can be profound psychosocial consequences for people with AIDS. They often experience social stigma from families and friends, loss of lovers and significant others, loss of occupational and financial resources, denial of shelter and health care, and profound prejudice from society. Abstinence from sexual contact may diminish the person's social contacts. Social abandonment may occur when significant others and friends are lost as they die from AIDS. These people may have been perceived as the patient's "family," particularly if they have been abandoned by their natural parents and siblings.

A study of long-term nonprogressors with HIV disease (Barroso, 1999) revealed human connectedness to be a major part of the experience. This involved support from friends, families, and partners. This theme was also noted in a metasynthesis of qualitative research on the experience of living with HIV (Barroso & Powell-Cope, 2000). Human connectedness involved initiating and sustaining meaningful relationships with friends and family members in the face of increased alienation and separation from others. It included coping with the loss of some relationships; reconstructing old ties; reaffirming positive ties with family, friends, and lovers; and constructing new social networks.

Using grounded theory, Brown and Powell-Cope (in press) described the experiences of AIDS family caregiving. Their study represented AIDS caregiving from 1985 to 1988. Caregiving during this time was linked to several issues: a silent government, a vocal gay community, an unresponsive bureaucracy, inexperienced health-care providers, and a frightened, uninformed, and homophobic populace.

The term *family caregiver* used in the study included family of origin and family of choice. Unique psychosocial stressors for AIDS family caregivers were noted as issues of communicability; stigma; and multiple and premature losses. Findings revealed the basic social-psychological problem of uncertainty, and the core category of AIDs family caregiving to be transitions through uncertainty.

Five caregiving subcategories included: managing and being managed by the illness; living with loss and dying; renegotiating the relationship; going public; and containing the spread of HIV. In a second study, using some of the original study group, Powell-Cope (1994) explored AIDS family caregivers' interactions with professional health-care providers. The basic social process was negotiating partnerships, defined as working out care with one another for the common good of the person with AIDS. Dimensions of this process included: conveying information; knowing; being accessible; and maintaining belief.

From the Parents

To many parents, no matter what the age of their son or daughter, they will always be their child, their baby. Parents expect to be buried by their children. Thus it is a tremendous shock when the parents must make arrangements to bury their child. Learning that one's child is infected with HIV can produce many different emotions. Some parents may also be confronted with the knowledge that their child is homosexual, an IV drug user, or involved with a drug abuser. In this case families experience double grieving: for their relative's behavior or identity and for his or her terminal illness. Parents may feel guilty if they believe that they are responsible for their child's lifestyle. This is especially true of mothers who traditionally have been blamed by society for their children's actions (Flaskerud, 1995). Another social stressor that the family faces is whether to disclose the HIV diagnosis. Having a child with HIV subjects the family to the powerful threat of social stigma and rejection. This stigma is particularly intense in some ethnic groups (Flaskerud, 1995).

A study by Phillips and Thomas (1996) explored extrapunitive and intropunitive anger of HIV caregivers. The study group consisted of four male and four female caregivers of HIV-positive males. Findings revealed that extrapunitive anger involved anger at the disease; the loved one with HIV; other family members; desertion by friends; God and organized religion; society; the health-care system; isolation standards and practices; and discrimination. Intropunitive anger involved self-blame for a loved one's AIDS and treatment choices. Study participants used several strategies for managing anger, including writing poetry and prose; keeping a diary; public speaking; and writing publications. Some parents use anger and denial to deal with the disease and its eventual outcome. The following case study illustrates a difficult situation on the AIDS unit with a family in conflict.

> NK was a 28-year-old African-American female who had been diagnosed 3 years earlier as HIV-positive, in good health, and with a CD4 count of above 500. However, NK did not keep her follow-up appointments. It was a year before NK reappeared in the doctor's office, and she was now 4 months' pregnant. Concerned about the outcome of this pregnancy, NK complied with the doctor's medication regime for Zidovudine [Retrovir, ZDV, AZT], and her child was born HIV-negative.

Delighted, NK named her daughter after the doctor. But it was another 18 months before NK came back for her follow-up appointment. At this time she was extremely dyspneic, and her chest X-ray revealed diffuse bilateral infiltrates. NK was immediately admitted to the AIDS unit with a diagnosis of PCP. Apparently, NK had not complied in the past months with any of her antiretroviral medications or her prophylactic medications to prevent opportunistic infections. NK's CD4 count had dropped to below 100. Her mother was constantly on guard at the bedside. When questioned regarding the need for social service and financial support, NK's mother would firmly state that her daughter had a good job and did not need any assistance. When the mother was in the room, NK would not speak, only nod her head in agreement with her mother. The nurses stated that she was very quiet—polite and cooperative, but reserved and hard to communicate with. When the HIV/AIDS clinical nurse specialist entered the room, NK was polite.

NK's condition deteriorated, and she went into respiratory failure after a spontaneous pneumothorax. Intubated and with a chest tube, she was transferred to ICU. NK's mother angrily insisted that the medicines given in the hospital had caused her daughter's complications and reported the attending physician to the hospital's risk management department, declaring she was going to sue for malpractice. NK survived, was transferred back to the AIDS unit, and appeared to be getting better with medication. In confidence, NK told the social worker that her lover had been taking AZT when he had died earlier that year. NK's mother would still not allow any social service referral for financial assistance with medications, and NK would never speak while the mother was in the room.

NK was discharged but readmitted 5 days later in extreme respiratory distress. Again, it did not appear that she had taken any medicine while at home. NK's condition continued to rapidly deteriorate, and she suffered a sudden cardiac arrest one afternoon after a second spontaneous pneumothorax occurred. NK did not survive the resuscitation attempt. Everyone working the resuscitation code was upset; everyone wanted the young woman to live and return home to take care of her baby.

Upon arriving back at the hospital, the family was extremely upset, angry, and hostile to the staff. The social worker attempted to help them deal with their loss. The mother continued to be as hostile as ever. She got on the phone and stated she was calling her lawyers, because the hospital had killed her daughter with medications. She would not listen to anything that the doctors said, except to agree to an autopsy. She wanted it proved that the doctor's treatment had killed her daughter. She stayed at the bedside with her daughter's body for several hours. Most of the time she was on the phone, calling people and speaking in a loud, angry voice. The father seemed sad, and appeared to want to listen to the doctors, but the hostile mother controlled the situation.

MOTHERS AND SONS: RETURNING TO THE NEST

If there is no significant other or family member living with the HIV-infected person, parents can be faced with the dilemma of how to care for their son or daughter when they live far away. Families who are geographically distant experience severe situational stresses in attempting to visit. They have no place to stay and can't afford the expenses of travel, and they are unable to provide emotional and physical assistance because of distance (Flaskerud, 1995). HIV-infected people may be angry with their family for not staying with them in their newly chosen community. The following case study demonstrates the challenges a mother faces dealing with her son's illness.

GA was a 28-year-old African-American male. He had been diagnosed HIV-positive only 3 months before his first hospital admission. His CD4 count was already low. GA later confided that he had gone to an anonymous testing site several months earlier and found out his status. GA decided not to let anyone except his lover know. GA's lover was tested, and was HIV-negative. During the first days of his hospitalization, this relationship with his lover appeared to be stable. But several days later GA told the nurses on the AIDS unit that he had broken up with his lover, who no longer wanted to be a homosexual; instead, he wanted to marry and have children.

Without a partner, GA now turned more to his mother. By his second hospitalization, he was showing early signs of AIDS dementia. GA had periods of anger followed by calm moments of intelligence and lucidity. GA told the nurses that his mother had many questions about his disease and had asked to speak with a nurse or doctor. However, a different story emerged when the clinical nurse specialist called GA's mother. She was very knowledgeable about AIDS and her son's condition, and had been trying to convince him to move back home to Alabama with her.

"I have told him that I will do all that I can to help him. He doesn't want to move back home with me. He wants to stay here in Miami. He's always been very strong, in his mind and in his body. That's why he's done so well in his business. Also, you know, he's very organized, in both his business life and at home, and can face any challenge. I know he's going to be okay just as long as he takes care of himself. That's why he's upset with me—because I have to fly back home and go back to work. I can't stay here with him, like he wants me to, and he refuses to come back home and live with me. What can I do?"

Mothers' Voices: A Grassroots Movement

In the fall of 1991, five women met to discuss an idea. They had two things in common. They had each come to understand the urgency of AIDS, and they believed that a movement of mothers, working together, could stop the epidemic. From that simple beginning, an organization called Mothers' Voices was born. Based in New York City, Mothers' Voices is now a national, grassroots, nonprofit organization dedicated to mobilizing mothers as educators and advocates to end AIDS. The organization was a vehicle for mothers—and for all those concerned about AIDS—to transform grief and fear into a national movement to change attitudes and public policies.

A premise of the organization is that every child deserves the chance of a lifetime, so volunteers work together to create a world where AIDS is cured and all children are safe. An underlying belief is that mothers have the moral authority to challenge the stigma associated with sexuality and HIV disease. Mothers' Voices provides resources for parents to become informed educators to their children and to other parents about HIV prevention and sexual health. A goal of the organization is to educate and empower mothers, to raise their voices and promote public policies that advance efforts for AIDS education, prevention, research, treatment, and, ultimately, a cure (Mothers' Voices, 1998).

By 1996, the organization had chapters in Los Angeles, Miami, Houston, Georgia, and Atlanta. Ann Kurth, a former president of the Association of Nurses in AIDS Care (ANAC), agreed to serve as national executive director. In 1997, the Mothers' Voices conference was held in Miami Beach as part of the U.S. Conference on AIDS. Through lively and interactive dialogue, mothers and fathers were encouraged to reach out to community allies to build networks of empowered parents as educators. Whether "community" was defined as home, workplace, school, church, or neighborhood, the group addressed how different outreach methods and education tools could maximize their efforts in reaching their targeted populations. An educational video, *Raising Healthy Kids: Families Talk about Sexual Health*, was introduced for community use. Mothers' Voices also put out a new book, *Finding Our Voices: Talking with Our Children about Sexuality and* AIDS. Helping lead the group was Barbara Gaynor. In 1984, Barbara was a middle-class professional with three healthy children. By 1994, she had lost her son, Johnny, to AIDS and watched her other son battle the virus. After Johnny died, Barbara wrote: "*He and I shared the experience together, although my heart was crying and my soul was empty. There was no one to show the way, few to share the secret with. . . . It took many years to realize how depressed I was.*" Barbara realized she had to do something and not just sit around and feel sorry for herself. So she left her Miami job as director of major gifts for the March of Dimes and established the southern Florida chapter of Mothers' Voices.

Barbara tried to get Hispanic and Catholic women involved, but at first the chapter was composed of a small group of Jewish mothers who used all their talents and energies to succeed. Over the next few years the chapter grew and programming increased to include a variety of programs to train parents on sex education for their children. By 1999, the chapter had raised over $123,000 to support their parents training programs. The chapter also began working with communities of faith and addressing the special needs for HIV education and prevention efforts in the African-American and Hispanic communities.

In 1999, Miami had the third highest rate of AIDS in the nation. The chapter pursued local government to address the issue. Finally, in July 1999, as a result of the crisis response team sent by CDC, arrangements were made for the first southern Florida HIV/AIDS town hall meeting. Representatives from the mayor's office, county legislators, and local spiritual leaders and health professionals were scheduled to attend and address the issues facing Miami. Pleased to see community action, Barbara wrote an article that was published in the *Miami Herald*:

> Two weeks ago I received a frantic call from a woman who had attended one of our Mothers' Voices educational workshops. Her daughter was in the end stages of AIDS, and she couldn't get any useful information on her condition from either the doctor or the hospital. I had experienced the same maddening lack of communication during my son's final days. Finally, we turned to a family friend who was a nurse specializing in HIV. She took a look at Johnny, explained the situation, and reassured me that we were doing everything possible.
>
> I shared that experience with the frightened mother who had called, which gave her comfort. I gave her my home number and a couple of other numbers to call whenever she needed to talk. This mother is poor and Black. Yet despite our apparent contrasts, we are more alike than different. Mothers all over the world are very much the same, particularly when it comes to loving their children. Thankfully, our community leaders have gotten the message at last. Now it's time for the rest of us to do the same.

SONS AND LOVERS

In the nontraditional family unit, when one of the partners becomes ill with AIDS (characterized by a CD4 count below 200, frequent bouts of opportunistic infection, and a potential increasing viral load), the other partner must face the burden of becoming a caregiver. If the other partner is also HIV-positive, he or she must deal with the impending death of a loved one, as well as a clear picture of their own probable future. When that happens, who will care for them? Powell-Cope (1996) used grounded theory to study the experiences of nine gay couples in which at least one man was diagnosed with symptomatic

HIV infection or AIDS. "Being a couple affected by HIV infection" in the context of a committed relationship was defined by the concepts of transitions and loss, and the processes of hitting home, mutual protection, and moving on. Results of this study confirm that symptoms of HIV infection among gay men in committed relationships must be understood in the context of a culture that focuses on independence and self-reliance; of a primary relationship defined by commitment, love, and care; and of a disease that is defined by multiple and ongoing losses. The following case study reveals the struggles and stresses of an HIV-positive couple coping with their hospitalizations on the AIDS unit.

> RJ and ND have been together for over 10 years. RJ is Hispanic, and ND is Jewish. Both were HIV-positive, and now they both have AIDS. ND also suffers from a circulatory disease that resulted in a below-the-knee amputation 5 years ago. ND has had increasing hospitalizations over the past 4 years for bouts of opportunistic infections. RJ was always there, by his side. It's tougher now, because at times ND has alterations in mental status; he suddenly becomes extremely angry, upset, and hostile. A few hours later he is back to his normal, quiet, caring self.
>
> Last year RJ was hospitalized because he was "just not feeling well." A routine diagnostic workup found that he had non-Hodgkin's lymphoma. It was a rough time for RJ. The nurses discussed his feelings about cancer. RJ said, "You know, in some ways it's kind of a relief. There's a lot of people that I will not tell that I have AIDS. Now I can tell them that I have cancer, and I know that they will be sympathetic. It's okay to have cancer; it's not okay to have AIDS."
>
> Several months ago, RJ and ND were both admitted to the hospital at the same time. Because they were a well-known couple to the AIDS unit, other patients were moved to other rooms on the unit so that RJ and ND could share a room together. RJ was discharged a few days before ND. RJ admitted that he was going home to get some rest, because caring for ND sometimes was a major strain for him. RJ was concerned because, with his combined AIDS and cancer diagnosis, he had to avoid stress and keep up his own physical and mental health status, to avoid dangerously accelerating both of his disease processes. But he loves ND and will never leave him, even at the risk of decreasing his own life expectancy.

End-of-Life Decisions and Conflicts

Except in Hawaii, gay marriages are not legally recognized. Without formal protection of a marriage contract, the gay partner has no legal rights to either divorce settlements or death benefits. This may often set up a conflict between parents and gay partners.

Paul Crockett is a Miami lawyer known for his work in estate planning for gay couples. Crockett explains to his clients that they must protect their property by making a will. Since there is no common-law marriage in Florida, if a person dies without leaving a will, the property will be inherited by (in the following order): a spouse (does not include a same-sex life partner); children; parents; brothers and sisters; siblings' children. Many gay men do not have children, therefore all property at death will go to the parents if there is no will. This can cause conflict between parents and the lover. Crockett (1996) recounts horror stories of lovers and parents battling at the hospital bedside over the estate, and the conflict and anguish that occurs in the dying AIDS patient. He also advises his clients to check and see how their home is titled, and make sure that rights-of-survivorship language is included.

Crockett advises the gay community on advanced directives and healthcare planning. He states that people need to make sure that a healthcare surrogate is selected who shares the same philosophy and understands what the person wants done if he or she enters a terminal state. This should all be written down and notarized, although that is not required by law. Planning for future healthcare decisions (advanced directives) will make it easier for the designated healthcare surrogate to enact the loved one's wishes at the time that he or she becomes incapacitated (when one or two doctors certify that the person is no longer capable of making his or her own healthcare decisions).

This advice regarding preplanning is extremely important in terms of life support and do-not-resuscitate decisions. Making decisions about when to withhold life support can be difficult for anyone, because it may make us acutely aware of our own mortality. However, legislation regarding advanced directives for health care implies that people want to choose who will carry out their healthcare wishes. The following story demonstrates the many dimensions of end-of-life decisions and conflicts for AIDS patients.

> FD is a 48-year-old Jewish male who had been HIV positive for 15 years. FD was relatively healthy until 2 years ago, when he began having frequent bouts of opportunistic infections that necessitated hospitalization. FD's latest problem was related to multiple small pulmonary emboli that would cause sharp chest pain and difficulty breathing. Although FD had always been sharp, articulate, satirical, and extremely witty, lately he had become much more serious. The nurses talked with FS about how he felt his disease was progressing and about his plans for the future.
>
> This admission had been extremely hard and stressful for FD; he has been in a lot of respiratory distress and pain from a variety of complications that have occurred. At the same time the AIDS unit staff had also been undergoing stress. One of their patients, CN, had gone bad and been sent to ICU, intubated and on a ventilator, with multisystem failure. CN was a 32-year-old Cuban female whom they had taken care of for over 4 years. Just 3 weeks ago CN had been telling the nurses all

about her new boyfriend, and how she was educating him on how not to get infected. Now the doctors were trying to convince her mom to take CN off life support. Her mother would not accept the fact that this was the end. She did not want them to let her daughter die.

FD starting asking the nurses about CN. When the nurses told FD they could not talk about her because of confidentiality, FD told the nurses several of his friends had called him about CN. The nurses were surprised and silent when FD told them that, because of what was going on with CN and her mother fighting not to let them take CN off life support. FD had made some decisions and finally had a talk with his lover about when to let go. FD said it was one of the toughest times he had ever faced, dealing with death and deciding under what conditions he wanted life support stopped. FD decided that he wanted to be "let go" if he suffered over 25 percent loss of his brain functioning, along with over 50 percent of his renal function. FD wanted the nurses to know so that they could help his lover and give him the strength to carry out FD's wishes if it occurred when FD was a patient here in the medical center.

Two days later, CN's mother finally authorized taking her daughter off life support. Several of the nurses from the AIDS unit attended the viewing services at the funeral home. CN's mother rushed over to them, hugged them, and cried. The nurses shared stories of her daughter. Afterward, the nurses realized that the suit the mother was wearing was an exact copy of the one that CN was wearing in her coffin.

When Dad Has AIDS: The Sandwich Generation

In the 1990s families may be faced with caring for an ill parent while still raising their own children. People in the "sandwich generation" may have to deal with their parents' health-care bills while worrying about how to save up money to send their children to college. Further problems arise when there is a chance of the parent's health problem being detrimental to the children. The following situation shows the unique aspects of cultural expectations among family members coping with the diagnosis of HIV/AIDS.

MM lived with her husband and her two small daughters in a small house in the Hispanic community of Hialeah, Florida. MM and her parents had come to the United States from Cuba when MM was a little girl. MM's mom and dad had divorced when she was 12; she lived with her mom but kept up visits with her dad. Twenty years later, her dad was diagnosed with AIDS. Because of his deteriorating health, MM had brought him to her home, where she cared for him.

Now he was in the hospital diagnosed with AIDS dementia along with TB. Because of close contact, MM and her family had gone to the public health department to be checked to make sure that they had not contracted TB from the dad. MM was relieved when the tests were negative. But now MM's dad was in the hospital; today he was screaming uncontrollably in his room, and even MM could not get him quiet. MM had to make decisions; Should she bring her dad back home and care for him or put him in a nursing home? Because of his altered mental status, the doctors were concerned that he would not take either his TB or his AIDS medications.

MM was concerned because of his bizarre behavior at times, which frightened her little girls. What should she do? Should she take her dad home, like a good daughter? In the Hispanic community, you take care of your family. That is what people would expect of her. But suppose he was not careful, and her daughters got infected with TB? Was having a crazy man in the house, ranting and raving and spitting on the floor, a good thing for her little girls to hear and see? If she took him home, would she not be a bad mother?

MM's dad was finally placed in an AIDS long-term care unit because of physician and infection-control/public-health concerns regarding his mental status and his need to be supervised in taking his TB medications. Although MM was relieved that a decision had been made, she also felt guilty that her dad would be in a nursing home instead of being home, cared for by her.

HIV and Women

Throughout history, women have generally been viewed as subordinate to men. Although differences between the sexes are readily acknowledged, the characteristics attributed to women are not always laudable or even biologically correct. Fortunately, in recent years, Americans have experienced an awakening about the importance of women's health. But more research is needed into the causes, treatments, and prevention of conditions, disorders, and diseases that rob women of their health.

Sowell et al. (1999) have conducted an extensive review of the literature on HIV and women, using a biologic-social-psychological framework. They stress that for women, HIV/AIDS is a disease that must be addressed in the framework of women's roles within the family, because an HIV/AIDS diagnosis has significant ramifications for both the structure and functioning of the family unit. It is impossible to consider the impact of HIV disease on women without taking into account factors such as poverty, discrimination, gender-role expectations, and cultural and ethnic considerations.

Although few studies looked at HIV in women in the 1980s, a tremendous body of knowledge has now been developed and continues to evolve (Sowell et al., 1999). Five conditions at diagnosis were found to serve as barriers to self-care for a group of low-income white women (Leenerts, 1998). These included health-care provider failure to mobilize resources; health-care provider devaluing of women; social devaluing; economic problems; and legal problems, including termination of employment, loss of housing, and being victims of rape. A study on self-care burden in HIV-positive women (Anastasio et al., 1995) found that the health-deviation self-care task reported as most burdensome and difficult was obtaining necessary resources to deal with the illness, such as special equipment, pharmacy, and home care. Eating a special diet and administering home treatments (taking medications) were reported as above average on the difficulty and burden scale. Concerns addressed were the expense of nutritional supplements and difficulty with meal preparation related to anorexia and loss of energy.

Rose (1993) also noted problems with nutrition. Women in her study reported a lack of appetite and a need to force themselves to eat, while lack of finances was mentioned as a factor in not eating a balanced diet. The women in her study also reported that prayer, cleaning house, sleeping, eating, and watching television were their coping mechanisms. Implications of the study included the need to identify support systems for women with HIV/AIDS, to identify ways to encourage women to focus on their own health, to assess for depression and suicide risk, and to refer women to appropriate community resources in a timely fashion.

Reproductive Rights

Reproductive decision making by HIV-infected women is a complex process (Bradley-Springer, 1994). While the elimination of new cases of HIV infection among women and infants is an appropriate goal, this goal must be approached without infringing on women's rights to make reproductive decisions and with the realization that some women are willing to accept risks. A survey of HIV-positive women found a relationship between knowledge about AZT and women's indication that they would consider pregnancy based on knowledge of AZT and women's report that they would consider use of AZT if they became pregnant (Vitiello & Smeltzer, 1998). Another survey of HIV-positive women found that when they were informed about the reduced risk of vertical transmission with Zidovudine (AZT), nearly half the women indicated that information regarding AZT would affect their future pregnancy decisions (Duggan et al., 1999).

Nursing attitudes toward mothers who transmit HIV to their children could have significant impact on the quality of care provided (Robillard, 1996). A descriptive study conducted with female pediatric staff nurses at a large Massachusetts teaching hospital found that nurses indicated an empathic response to mothers who transmit HIV to their children. However, younger nurses felt more anger toward mothers that gave birth to HIV-positive children than older nurses. The following case study describes an incident on the AIDS unit regarding nurses' reactions to pregnancy in HIV-positive women.

> RK was a 30-year-old Haitian female who had been admitted to the AIDS unit several times for opportunistic infections. This time she surprised all the nurses and physicians—no PCP, but she was 3 months pregnant! The nurses asked her what had happened with all their talks about safer sex and using condoms so as to prevent the spread of her virus. RK just smiled and said, "I knew that what I wanted most of all in my life was to have another baby. I just need to hold my own baby in my arms. I can't explain why—it was just something that I needed to do, right now, for me."
>
> In most of the nurses' hearts and minds, they understood her yearning. But in patient care rounds, one nurse was vocally hostile and though it was terrible that an HIV-positive woman would deliberately get pregnant, knowing her baby might be born infected. Since RK also had another child, who would take care of her children when she died?

HIV-Infected Mothers: Protecting the Children

HIV-infected women who are mothers have an especially heavy burden—to prepare for the care of their children who will be left motherless or orphaned (Sharts-Hopko et al., 1996). Mothers who are HIV-infected experience the stresses of caring for their children, guilt over eventually abandoning their children, and physical fatigue from the care of children who are also infected (Flaskerud, 1995).

A descriptive study by Rose and Clark-Alexander (1996) on quality of life and coping styles of HIV-positive women with children found three styles of coping. Confrontive was used more frequently than passive or emotive. Significant relationships were found between coping and quality of life, with implications to nursing for the need to enhance decision making and coping skills within the context of the family unit. Another study of caregivers of HIV-positive children found that alternative caregivers, usually grandmothers, scored higher in all areas of quality of life than mother-caregivers (Rose & Clark-Alexander, 1998). The mothers used passive and emotive coping significantly more than the alternative caregivers. The study concluded that nurses need to provide interventions for these caregivers, to improve coping mechanisms, decrease stress, and thereby improve quality of life.

In the 1995 movie *Dead Man Walking*, a mother of a convicted murderer described how the community's hatred and negative feelings toward her son was reflected by insults, whispered gossip, and direct threats toward her children and herself. Mothers with HIV-infected children often exist in a world of secrecy to protect their children from an unsympathetic and frightened community. Children need other children to play with and have fun, and peers and their parents can be extremely cruel if they learn that the child or mother are HIV-positive. If a family fears the stigma often associated with an HIV diagnosis, they may be secretive and may isolate themselves (Boland & Czarniecki, 1995).

> NR was a 42-year-old Hispanic woman with two children who had recently moved to Miami. NR had been diagnosed HIV-positive when her last child was born and found to be HIV-positive. This was NR's first admission to the AIDS unit. During an interview to assess her nursing and psychosocial needs, NR described how, when she first moved to Miami, she carefully went about asking people who was a good pediatrician and then diligently and privately sought out a pediatric immunologist for her HIV-positive child. NR discussed the fact that her main interest was in keeping the child's HIV status a secret, because she was afraid that other children might fear him and not play with him, or that, if their parents found out that he was HIV-positive, they might not allow their children to play with him. NR kept her own HIV status a secret because she feared social reprisals against her children.

CONCLUSION

As we enter the 21st century, issues and questions about HIV and AIDS have come along with us. There are no easy solutions, or cut-and-dried answers. HIV-infected people deal with their problems every day, and each family affected by AIDS must also struggle to find and provide the support that is needed during the up and down periods of this disease. AIDS is also a community issue. Therefore, an agenda for the future must include how to best educate people in a manner that acknowledges the unique differences of lifestyle, age, culture, and ethnicity; how to empower HIV-infected people and their families to live their lives in the best way that they can; how to provide affordable health and wellness care without financial worries; and how to change society's perceptions so that the words HIV and AIDS will no longer be associated with fear, stigma, and shame.

REFERENCES

Anastasio, C., McMahan, T., Daniels, A., Nicholas, P. K., and Paul-Simon, A. (1995). Self-care burden in women with human immunodeficiency virus. *Journal of the Association of Nurses in AIDS Care*, 6(3): 31–41.

Barroso, J. (1999). Long-term nonprogressors with HIV disease. *Nursing Research*, 48(5): 242–249.

———, and Powell-Cope, G. M. (2000). Metasynthesis of qualitative research on living with HIV infection. *Qualitative Health Research.*

Boland, M. G., and Czarniecki, L. (1995). Nursing care of the child. In J. H. Flaskerud and P. J. Ungvarski, eds., HIV/AIDS: A *Guide to Nursing Care*. Philadelphia: W. B. Saunders.

Bradley-Springer, L. (1994). Reproductive decision making in the age of AIDS. *Image*, 26(3): 241–246.

Brown, M. A., and Powell-Cope, G. (1991). AIDS family caregiving: Transitions through uncertainty. *Nursing Research*, 40 (6): 338–345.

Casey, K. M., Cohen, F., and Hughes, A. M. (1996). Preface. In K. M. Casey, F. Cohen, and A. M. Hughes, eds., *The Association of Nurses in AIDS Care's Core Curriculum for HIV/AIDS Nursing*, Philadelphia: Nursecom, Inc.

Crockett, P. (July 1996). AIDS and the law: Taking control and planning for the future. Paper presented at the Miami ANAC chapter meeting, North Shore Hospital, Miami, Florida.

Duggan, J., Walerius, H., Purohit, A., Khuder, S., Bowles, M., Carter, S., Kosy, M., Locher, A., O'Neill, K., Gray, A., and Chakraborty, J. (1999). Reproductive issues in HIV-positive women: A survey regarding counseling, contraception, safer sex and pregnancy choices. *Journal of the Association of Nurses in AIDS Care*, 10(5): 84–92.

Flaskerud, J. H. (1995). Psychosocial and psychiatric aspects. In J. H. Flaskerud and P. J. Ungvarski, eds., HIV/AIDS: A *Guide to Nursing Care*. Philadelphia: W. B. Saunders.

Friedman, M. M. (1992). *Family Nursing: Theory and Practice*, 3rd ed. Norwalk: Appleton & Lange.

Harden, J. T. (June 1996). National Institute of Nursing Research (NINR): Research on women's health. Paper presented at the Sigma Theta Tau 8th International Nursing Research Congress, Ochos Rios, Jamaica.

Jones, S. G., and Baggett, T. H. (1999). Clinical update: New drugs for HIV/AIDS. MED-SURG *Nursing*, 8(2): 108–112

———, and Brown, C. (June 1999). Life in a pill bottle: The lived experience of persons on HIV combination therapy. Paper presented at the Sigma Theta Tau 11th International Nursing Research Conference, London, England.

Leenerts, M. H. (1998). Barriers to self-care in a cohort of low-income white women living with HIV/AIDS. *Journal of the Association of Nurses in AIDS Care*, 9(6): 22–36.

McGough, K. N. (1990). Assessing social support of people with AIDS. *Oncology Nursing Forum* 7(1): 31–35.

Morrison, C. (1998). HIV/AIDS units: Is there still a need? *Journal of the Association of Nurses in AIDS Care*, 9(6): 16–18.

Napper, R. L. Jr. (1998). Census trends in AIDS specialty units. *Journal of the Association of Nurses in AIDS Care*, 9(6): 42–46.

National Center for Health Statistics. (June 9, 1999). New data show AIDS patients less likely to be hospitalized. Centers for Disease Control and Prevention. Retrieved July 16, 1999 from the World Wide Web: htpp://www.cdc.gov/nchswww/releases/99news/97nhds.htm.

Ojito, M. (1996). Detective Zero. *Tropic Magazine*, supplement to the *Miami Herald*, July 7, 1996, pp. 6–11, 18–19.

Phillips, K., and Thomas, S. P. (1996). Extrapunitive and intropunitive anger of HIV caregivers: Nursing implications. *Journal of the Association of Nurses in AIDS Care*, 7(2): 17–27.

Powell-Cope, G. (1994). Family caregivers of people with AIDS: Negotiating partnerships with professional health care providers. *Nursing Research*, 43(6): 324–330.

———. (1996). HIV disease symptom management in the context of committed relationships. *Journal of the Association of Nurses in AIDS Care*, 7(3): 19–28.

Robillard, R. (June 1996). Nurses' attitudes towards mothers who perinatally transmit HIV to their children. Paper presented at the Sigma Theta Tau 8th International Nursing Research Congress, Ochos Rios, Jamaica.

Rose, M. (1993). Health concerns of women with HIV/AIDS. *Journal of the Association of Nurses in AIDS Care*, 4(3): 39–45.

———, and Clark-Alexander, B. (1998). Caregivers of children with HIV/AIDS: Quality of life and coping styles. *Journal of the Association of Nurses in AIDS Care*, 9(1): 58–65.

———. (1996). Quality of life and coping styles of HIV-positive women with children. *Journal of the Association of Nurses in AIDS Care*, 7(2): 28–34.

Sowell, R. L., Moneyham, L., and Aranda-Naranjo, B. (1999). The care of women with AIDS: Special needs and considerations. *Nursing Clinics of North America*, 34(1): 179–199.

Sharts-Hopko, N. C., Regan-Kubinski, M. J., Lincoln, P. S., and Heverly, M. A. (1996). Coping in HIV-infected mothers. *Image*, 28(2): 107–111.

Theis, S. L., Cohen, F. L., Forrest, J., and Zelewsky, M. (1997). Needs assessment of caregivers of people with HIV/AIDS. *Journal of the Association of Nurses in AIDS Care*, 8(3): 76–83.

UNAIDS Joint United Nations Programme on HIV/AIDS. (1998). AIDS epidemic update: December 1998. UNAIDS and WHO.

Vitiello, M. A., and Smeltzer, S. C. (November 1998). HIV, pregnancy and Zidovudine: What do women know? Paper presented at the 11th Annual Conference of the Association of Nurses in AIDS Care, San Antonio, Texas.

Williams, A. B. (1999). Adherence to highly active antiretroviral therapy. *Nursing Clinics of North America*, 34(1): 113–129.

Chapter 21

Shadow Families

Carolyn L. Brown and Patricia M. Siccardi

Each of us has a psychological heritage that is no less real than our biological one. This inheritance includes a shadow legacy which is transmitted to us and absorbed by us in the psychic soup of our family environment. Here we are exposed to our parents' and siblings' values, temperaments, habits, and behaviors. Often, the problems our parents have failed to work out in their own lives reveal themselves to us in the form of dysfunctional coping patterns.

Zweig & Abrams, 1991

Once upon a time, Ozzie and Harriet ruled the land. The limelight was shared by June and Ward Cleaver. The vision of the ideal family was pumped into every American household, through radio, television, and the great American sitcom. Did the comedy reflect or create the image of the ideal American family? Was it an ideal we seek to emulate even today as our presidential candidates of the year 2000 toll "family values?"

The great American dream family acts like a blueprint and it then becomes a standard for us all. For example, the right number of children to fit the blueprint of the great American dream family is two—preferably a boy born first and then a girl. The family has two parents, the man works at a white-collar job, and the woman either works at a lesser job or stays home to care for the family and keep house.

The dream family has a few problems, which can all be solved by the end of the half hour or hour episode. Problems for the great American dream family are simple and easy to deal with if the family adheres to the appropriate family values of hard work, conscientiousness, and honesty and lives in a town called Ideal Town, USA. Our dream family lives happily ever after in a single-family house, with a two-car garage housing neat, staid sedans and station wagons. The house is surrounded by a well-manicured lawn with just the right number of shrubs and trees, on a street where the houses look pretty much the same. Each house contains a replica of the great American dream family, or so it would seem.

Today, many political leaders say, "If we could just get back to the old family values that made this country great," we would come closer to reaching that supposedly utopian ideal of uniformity. Set against this backdrop, we will tell you a story of another side of the great American dream family.

This is the story of two little girls, Polly and Susan. In reality, they lived far apart from one another in different towns in different states on opposite sides of the country. But they also both grew up with their families in Family Values Lane, in Ideal Town, USA—just like you and me. This is also the story of Polly and Susan as adult women. Like characters in *Star Trek*, they live in a time warp that holds the past and future together. Pay close attention. Time warps are very important to this story.

Susan's Story

Let's take a look at 1200 Family Values Lane, where Susan lived. The year is 1955. The father, Joe, is a skilled laborer in the electronics industry. He drives a Chevy sedan, leaves for work at 6:00 A.M., and returns home at 4:30 or 5:00 in the afternoon. The first thing he does when he arrives home is head to the refrigerator to find a cold bottle of beer, pops the top, takes a long swig, and heads to the "big chair" that holds his form for most of the rest of the evening. Joe flips on the television set, or if it is already on because others are watching, he flips the channel to *his* show, without asking, of course, because this is *his* house, *he* is the head of the household, *he* "brings home the bacon", *he* "rules the roost." The rest of the family is there to do his bidding. He turns up the volume on the set, opens the newspaper, lights a cigarette, and begins the nightly ritual.

Mary is the mother and housewife who stays home to tend to the children and the household tasks. There are three children (one more than the ideal number, but the neighbor to the left has only one, so the mean is maintained). Mary works hard all day. She does the laundry, ironing, vacuuming, dusting, sweeping, scrubbing, waxing, shining, cooking, and baking. She gets up at 5:00 A.M. to fix Joe's breakfast before he leaves for work. Mary is intelligent, a former teacher, and avidly pursues the news.

Several years ago, Mary worked outside the home to help boost the family income, but her working made Joe feel inadequate, so he increased his drinking and became even more unpleasant with his family than usual in order to express his displeasure.

Mary quit working to try to bring peace to the family, and to get Joe to quit drinking. She thought that if she were with Joe more of the time, she could stop his drinking, or at least keep it to a low level. However, what really happened is that Mary and Joe started drinking together, both becoming "tipsy" (drunk is more like it, but hardly an acceptable word for Family Values Lane). The more Joe drank, the nastier he became. But we are getting ahead of the story.

You need to know a bit about the three children to understand what life is like at 1200 Family Values Lane. Susan is the firstborn, a responsible child, now about 14. Susan is intelligent, loves to read (spends hours reading to escape from the living hell of life at 1200 Family Values Lane), finds housework *intensely* boring, wants to become a doctor, or a chemist, or something where she can feel good about herself and what she is doing.

Susan has an important role to play in the family. Susan is the caretaker. She takes care of both her younger brothers, feeds the cat, picks up the slack with fixing dinner when Mary is too far gone with martinis to finish up what she had started (oops, I forgot to tell you that Joe and Mary often moved from beer to martinis, a whole pitcher full of ice-cold gasoline with olives and meanness built in), and cleans up after the meal unless she can get her brother, Will, to do it. She also helps with laundry and housecleaning on Saturdays and is a star window washer. All the while she goes about the boring tasks of being a responsible caretaker, her mind and emotions are active with daydreaming and *rage*, with planning for a better future and *rage*, with fantasizing about the perfect life she will have when she escapes *this place*! But when she leaves, her rage will travel with her as she carries her shadow family into the future.

Susan has a terrible case of acne, feels ashamed most of the time, knowing that there is something wrong with her family, and most of all knowing that there is something wrong with her. She desperately fears that none of her dreams will materialize, that no one will want her, and she will grow old alone, with no friends and no lover. Throughout high school, she does not date but starts that phase of her life when she escapes her family to live in a college dormitory. But enough of Susan for now.

Will is the second child, a sweet angelic-looking boy, now about 12. He is bright enough, but daydreams his way through school, achieving little, often late with his homework, and always trying to live up to Sis's performance. You see, Susan is only a year ahead of him in school, since their ages are really only about a year and a half apart. Will tries hard to please but never quite makes it. Joe says, "Hey, Will, go get me a beer!" Will, enthralled with the TV show he is watching, gets up slowly, trying to catch the last of his favorite show. "Hey, Stupid! Didn't I say get me a beer? Who do you think brings home the bacon in this family? I deserve a little respect. Get me that beer *now*! Then go to your room and don't come out until I tell you to!"

The tension in the room is so thick and heavy and paralyzing that no one moves. In fact, no one dares to breathe. Will moves to do as he is told, tears in his eyes, because now he will miss dinner and the rest of the TV programming for the evening. He hates to read, so when he is left alone in his room (shared with little brother, Johnny), he plays fantasy games, alone with his rage, alone with feeling he is not worth much, and yearning for a hug, a loving gesture, something to feed his soul.

Instead, he receives "manly" lessons: Men are dictators, physically violent, heavy drinkers and smokers, and generally "sons of bitches!" But he takes it all in, his shadow family, which will erupt again when he is a young man.

Johnny, the baby, is now about 5 years old, angelic and confused, rejected by his father who is too busy drinking to care about him at all. He is becoming a throw-away child, ignored most of the time, but occasionally receiving Joe's wrath, with comments like, "What's the matter with you? Are you as stupid as you look? Can't you do anything right?" Joe resents Johnny because Mary spends time with him, and Mary's job is to be his party partner and drinking companion.

These dynamics leave Mary in a bind. She is torn between children and home, guilt and keeping up a pretty face for the world. The 1200 Family Values Lane must look just as perfect as the rest of the houses on the block. But enough drinking and lying to yourself, or retreating into helplessness and fear, dulls those feelings.

Susan survives all of the tension and craziness by retreating to the world of books. She loves reading novels, especially romance novels. She transports herself out of the mundane, everyday pain and into a place where there is a prince who rides in and sweeps her away into a life of perfect love and harmony. They live happily every after with a perfect home on Family Values Lane in Ideal Town, USA.

In Susan's fantasy home, there are no dark secrets. In reality, because she has so little real experience with healthy families, she has trouble visualizing a life without dark problems. When she isn't starring in a romantic fantasy world, school is the place where Susan shines, when she lets herself. She is bright and intelligent but afraid to raise her hand for fear the answer will be wrong. When someone else answers, she learns she was right all along. She learns to take the easy path, with guaranteed success, fulfilling someone else's dream for her, rather than pushing forward to realize her own dream. In fact, she tries very hard to keep herself invisible, because if no one sees her, all her dark shadowy family secrets won't show.

She is anxious about a lot of things, but it's normal for her and she doesn't think much about it. The state of high vigilance is the normal state of affairs. The uncertainty comes from not knowing when Joe will get "crazy." He gets angry and lashes out at anyone in his path. It is always unpredictable. She also has trouble sleeping at night. It's normal for her, so she doesn't think too much about it. She worries about a lot of things and gets relief when she can escape.

Her parents move to another street on Family Values Lane in Ideal Town several states away. Susan stays behind to continue her college education. She lives in a dormitory with other young women her age. Now she feels *free* and frightened, *free* and anxious, *free* and sure she cannot make it on her own.

She knows she never wants to live at home again. She cuts a few classes (well, maybe more than a few), dates a little, drinks a little, and tries to find her way in life. She joins the armed services, again not her dream, but certainly her father's dream. Here she meets her future husband, a man who also lived on Family Values Lane in Ideal Town, but in another corner of the USA.

He comes with his own version of looking fine on the surface, coming from a God-fearing, (child abusing in the dark corners of the ideal), perfect family. And later, they marry to begin their own life journey of creating a perfect life. They have not learned too much about each other. They keep their own vulnerable selves safe from scrutiny for a long time into their marriage. Things begin to fall apart.

Susan meets Polly somewhere in the middle of the falling-apart phase of Susan's life. Polly doesn't know Susan's life is falling apart. Ironically, everyone thought Susan was the epitome of perfect family values. In fact, most people she knows still do.

Even Susan herself didn't realize she was in a falling-apart phase. Family chaos and craziness were so normal for her that she didn't think much about how she felt or realize that things really were pretty awful.

Susan and her family looked pretty good on the surface. And isn't that mostly where our lives are lived? She had put into place all of her usual ways of coping. After all, they had always worked pretty well. She had learned very early that she could block out the anxiety, tension, and awfulness around her by throwing herself into a frenzy of activity. When she was a teenager, she read two to four books a day. When she was in college, she wrote long, detailed papers that were masterpieces. They would go far beyond what was expected. People told her how smart and clever she was. And now as an adult, she was smart, clever, and creative. She could avoid the pain and get much praise and recognition. What more could you ask?

So she threw herself into work as a way of numbing and forgetting. It was all repressed and she didn't feel the tears of sadness and rage. But deep in her soul there was a bubbling cauldron, waiting to spew forth like a volcano. She was unaware of the consequences of repression.

Polly's Story

Years ago, on a cold March morning, 2-month-old Polly, and 2-year-old Molly were packed up by their mother, Marcia, and left to live as boarders in another house. It was 3200 Family Values Lane, far, far out in the country.

Marcia had located the address for the boarding house through an advertisement in the big city paper. When Marcia called on the telephone to ask about the house and living arrangements, Mrs. Donaldson told her there was room for the two girls. Marcia was looking for a temporary place because she had decided to leave the girls' father. Marcia and Godfrey were fighting most of the time.

Marcia believed that her children needed to escape the intolerable home situation. Marcia had decided that it would be better for the girls to have one parent who was alive than to have two parents, one dead and the other in jail for murder.

When the three of them arrived at the Donaldson house, Marcia looked around the house and found it to be neat and clean. Marcia did not notice how quiet the house was even though it was the home for eight other children.

Most of the other children were playing outside so Marcia didn't pay much attention to them. Lisa Donaldson was friendly, so Marcia felt secure in leaving the two girls with her, even though they had just met a few minutes ago. Marcia talked with Lisa about returning to visit the girls in about a month. As it turned out, the Donaldson house, a place miles from where they used to live, was home to Polly and Molly for eight long years.

During those years the girls did all the things that children do in their early years. Polly learned to walk and talk and eventually joined the older children on the bus for school. Polly liked going to school and learning how to read and write and count numbers. Even though Polly excelled in schoolwork, she was happiest when she could play outside in the big yard at home. This yard was Polly's favorite place in the whole world; it was the only place she really felt free and safe.

Polly and Molly also learned about another world at the Donaldson house. It was a world of drinking, violence, and sexual abuse. Lisa and her husband, Howard, had a second business that catered to local men who liked to have sexual activities with children. The foster home provided a never-ending supply of children for this business.

This was the dark, secret, shadow side of the foster home. What everyone saw, however, was that every Sunday morning the children were all washed and dressed up and carted off to Sunday school while Lisa went to church services.

People told the children how lucky they were to have such a wonderful foster mother and home. It certainly was a crazy-making experience for the children.

Polly was loyal to the Donaldson family. She learned never to speak of the evil shadow side of the family when she was out in the light of the outside world. As damaging and hurtful as the abuse was for Polly, the terrible pain was deepened because of the dark secret that *must* be kept. She experienced the craziness of being told how lucky she was to have such a good Christian woman care for her. Polly learned not to trust herself or her world; it was far simpler to believe she was wrong and bad than to think Lisa was wrong. Lisa Donaldson was the one who dispensed security. She was "home." She was Polly's family, a buffer from the dangerous world. As with many kids, Polly believed that Lisa was OK, even though she did things that hurt and scared her. Years later, Polly read how kids believe their caretakers are OK, despite overwhelming evidence to the contrary.

Lisa instilled fear in Polly by telling her that God was always watching her and he would see her badness and punish her. Polly tried to be good, but was never sure just what that meant. It seemed like a mystery to her.

Lisa deepened the terror and alienation Polly was experiencing by blaming her for the abuse experiences. Lisa told Polly it was her fault she was hurt. She told Polly she should go along with the men and not fight them. She would lock Polly in a dark closet for hours to try to get her to give up her stubborn resistance.

Eventually Polly stopped fighting. She was too little and alone to figure the whole thing out. So she kept quiet and did as she was told. It was less trouble that way. Besides, it was awfully hard for a little girl to fight the dark shadowy evil all alone and in silence, especially when everyone else thought the Donaldsons were the ideal American family. After all, they provided a home for children who needed it. Wasn't that nice of them? So Polly should be grateful. Polly, Molly, and all the rest of the "Donaldson children" also learned values from their foster family.

The family rules firmly extolled power and control over love and kindness. In fact, rigidity, perfectionism, busyness, secrecy, and creating a good impression were *the* important values in this home. Goodness, generosity, and friendliness were displayed as surface values for all the community to see. Polly learned *all* the values of the family in order to survive, and she eventually brought them forward into her adult world as part of her shadow family.

The shadow family is the family that lives inside each of us. It lives on in our children and children's children. It is the evil, hurtful side of parents, and parent's parents. It is the dark, secret stuff we are not supposed to talk about because it isn't much like Beaver Cleaver's family, all sunshine and light, with parents who have only the best intentions.

And like it or not, the shadow family is a part of us, influencing who we are and how we live every day. Polly's shadow family also included the years she lived with her biological mother, Marcia, who eventually came back to get them. When Polly was 8 years old she left the foster home in the country and moved to an apartment in the city, with her sister and real mother. There was no backyard for playing and feeling safe; only endless yards of pavement. The sexual abuse stopped but physical abuse took its place.

Once again Polly was confronted with the need to figure out the family rules so she could avoid her mother's rage and violence. This new family had similar values to the Donaldsons. Perfectionism, rigid adherence to rules, keeping family secrets, hard work, and self-sacrifice were highly valued.

Polly figured they must be terribly important, so she learned them well. Even though she came to know her family wasn't anything like Beaver Cleaver's, or even like her friends' families, Polly learned to create an image on the outside that looked pretty good so she could fit into the ideal culture of Family Values Lane. If she pretended, and made herself as much like other kids and their families as possible, she would be able to fit in. What she actually lived and what she projected as an image were very different. Poor Polly felt so confused! In the world of Family Values Lane, families were supposed to be lighthearted and good, and always safe. And everyone thought she lived in a house a lot like the Cleavers. In fact, she pretended so hard to make that story real, she became very confused. She wasn't sure about what was really real.

Polly grew up, married twice, and had her own children. She still felt confused and conflicted. She tried to live a happy and productive life. Instead, internal turmoil brought Polly into therapy in an attempt to make sense of her upside-down world. About the time Polly began to explore the conflict she felt and the memories of the terrifying experiences of the past, she met a new friend, Susan.

Insight/In Sight

Have you ever met someone you connect with right away? Someone you know will be a significant part of your life for a long time to come? Susan and Polly experienced that when they met.

They started out by sharing the usual things, but the level of sharing quickly became deeper, to the level of secrets. Sharing about themselves from past, present, and future times. They quickly became "old friends" with a comfort born of trust.

About the time Polly was deep into her therapy, Susan and her husband also started seeing a therapist, and through the therapeutic work they did as a couple, Susan began to have some nagging feelings that something about her wasn't quite right. She began to question why she kept having the same arguments over and over again, and why some things made her feel so anxious. At the same time, she was having horrible nightmares. These nightmares culminated in blood-curdling screams that woke the whole house.

When everyone in the house woke up, they always asked her what the nightmare was about and who was in it, but Susan could never remember. One day she went to a bookstore and saw a book on repressed memories. She stood there and stared at the book, feeling her anxiety climb to the top of the barometer. She walked away and felt a little better.

As an intelligent woman, she thought, "This is really weird, I can't be *this* anxious about a dumb book," and went back to the bookstore. She reached for it. As she picked it up she could feel electric anxiety coursing along her nerves. Quickly, she put the book back on the shelf and walked out of the bookstore. Partway down the block, she stopped short and said, "This is ridiculous! I am a grown woman. This is only a book." She marched back into the bookstore, went to the shelf, and picked up the book. At once, her knees turned to jelly. Anxiety soared to astronomical heights!

Susan stood there a second, put the book back on the shelf, looked away, looked back at the book, and made herself pick it up again. She took a deep breath, held on to it firmly with cold, sweat-slick, fingers, and walked to the cash register, where she forced herself to pay for it. She took *the book* home and let it sit on her bookshelf until she and her husband went in for their next session with the therapist.

Near the end of the session she tentatively said to the therapist, "I am starting to wonder if I was abused as a child? Could this be possible?" Susan answered her own question.

Eventually, when she felt safe enough, she read the book. And over time, Susan came to know that she and Polly shared a history of sexual abuse.

Susan is still struggling to figure it all out, but the nightmares are fewer and farther apart, and now she can remember most of them. Now she knows that the anxiety about the book was the small child living inside her in her shadow family, struggling with all the family rules about *not* telling and keeping family secrets.

Don't tell anyone that Daddy beat on her brothers, that he got drunk, that he crawled into bed with her and did nasty, hurtful things that scared her. Don't even say it out loud in your family because it might destroy the image of a happy, normal family living happily ever after on Family Values Lane.

So far, Susan has had snatches of memory, more in the realm of dreams, all saying she was sexually abused as a young child. Saying all of these things out loud to Polly (and, of course, to the therapist, and also to her husband), and to people who would listen without saying, "How can you even think that, let alone say it?" brought a huge sense of relief to Susan.

It allowed her to move forward, to figure out lots of other problems that had kept her stuck in repetitive patterns and abiding by old family rules about keeping secrets. (For an excellent description of the power of secrets in women's lives, see Munhall, 1995.)

Susan's shadow family was finally being exposed to the light, and this began to diffuse the power of the shadow. As Susan and Polly deepened their friendship, they learned more and more about each other and their lives on Family Values Lane. They became close friends. They never said, "You must be crazy to think or feel that way." They didn't have to pretend that they had grown up in an Ozzie-and-Harriet household.

Polly and Susan learned about how their dark shadow families lived inside them, influencing their lives every day. And they learned they were not alone. Other women and men live with shadowy families inside themselves. These shadows silently control their lives until they choose to crack the door and shed light on the dark secrets.

In fact, many people today are writing about all sorts of shadows that influence people's lives. Shedding light on these shadows makes them less scary and dissipates some of their energy (Hillman, 1989, 1991; Zweig & Abrams, 1991).

There Must Be a Moral to This Story

As children, we learn that fairy tales and fables have a moral, a nugget of truth, a lesson to be learned. So what is the moral in this story of Polly and Susan? Not all of these stories have been told here. The message is clear to us. Hillman (1991) expressed it well:

> Loving oneself is no easy matter just because it means loving all of oneself, including the shadow where one is inferior and socially so unacceptable. The care one gives this humiliating part is also the cure . . . as the cure depends on care, so does caring sometimes mean nothing more than carrying. The first essential in redemption of the shadow is the ability to carry it along with you, as did the old Puritans, or the Jews in endless exile, daily aware of their sins, watching for the Devil, on guard lest they slip, a long existential trek with a pack of rocks on the back, with no one on whom to unload it and no sure goal at the end.

Shadow work goes beyond merely acknowledging and carrying. It extends to loving the shadow, and even playful and joyful acceptance. This poem expresses the moral of Polly's and Susan's stories.

My Shadow Family: A Sinister Playmate

Living with a playmate far back in the dark secret self of a life already half over
A playmate who lives in the dark, dark, darkest corners of the self
A deep, dark shadow of well hidden, hideous evil
A playmate too terrible to be let out but a playmate who cannot be denied
Who sneaks out to play in the dark of a nightmare
Who sneaks out to force me to take on yet one more task to keep the scary monster playmate hidden away
Who sneaks out to keep a marriage to recreate the shadow world of the family with its self-destructive denial
After all, one should never tell a story that doesn't have an ending.

But there is a problem with such an ending. Fairy tales end with "and they lived happily ever after" and then the characters are never heard about again. No one tells you that Cinderella's prince lost the family throne; that they had five children; that Cinderella helped out with the family income by taking in laundry; that the prince tried to regain the family wealth by betting on the horses.

So we will provide you with an afterword to help you know a bit more about how Polly and Susan are today. In fact, there are still lots of unanswered questions; however, both stopped living the myth of Sisyphus. Sisyphus was a man doomed to push a rock up a hill each day, knowing that when it neared the top it would simply roll down again and he would have to start over, repeating the pattern day after day and year after year (Bradshaw, 1992).

Now, when the shadows threaten to sneak out and overpower them, both women are better able to bring them to the light, allowing shadow to fuse with present and future identity. The dark shadows of families who were far from the great American dream family no longer rule by silent and unrecognized coercion.

Now, both women know that their very real shadow families have brought them strengths and skills. They can allow their shadows out to play because neither fears they will lose themselves in their shadows. They recognize that the strengths that helped them to survive, the horrors of the shadows past, fuse with their tender, vulnerable inner selves, creating a healthier whole person. Today Polly and Susan work at very responsible jobs. They still look as though they have it all together, but now are quick to assure people, with a healthy dose of humor, that they too, are human. Both can now say no to a request to add on more emotion-numbing tasks to keep the shadow at bay. This is a skill they are still working to perfect.

Polly's marriage of 20 years ended after much reflection when she realized how her shadow family so strongly influenced her life, keeping her stuck in a relationship that wasn't healthy. She, like Susan, is mother to adult children. Both women have stronger, healthier relationships with their children (notice, we did not say "perfect," but "stronger").

Stronger means more honest, allowing for all (children and parents) to be less than perfect and to grow as they are intended to grow. Susan and her husband still struggle when their shadow families sneak in to wreak havoc with their relationship, but they can now recognize and confront the shadow's attempts to take over.

Both women still struggle with their shadow families. Their shadows do sneak up on them at times, but one brought to the light, shadow power is fused with self giving them greater strength. They learned that only when we let ourselves play with our shadows in the light of the sun can we fuse with their power, harnessing their potentially destructive energy for life-giving purpose. Owning the shadow involves confronting it and assimilating its contents into an enlarged self-concept.

Such healing encounters typically occur in midlife, but meetings with the shadow can happen whenever we feel life stagnate and lose its color and meaning. Healing occurs when we recognize and feel the constricting effects of denial. Or when we doubt the values we live by and watch our illusions about ourselves and the world shatter. We heal when we are overcome by envy, jealousy, sexual drives, or ambition, or feel the hollowness of our convictions. Then shadow work (or play) can begin (Zweig and Abrams, 1991).

We hope Polly's and Susan's stories will allow you to invite the shadow to come out to play with you in the sunshine, where you too can fuse its power with the rest of your being, revisioning your past, living the now, and creating a freer future.

If the journey seems too scary to take alone, ask a friend or a therapist (who is a good friend in need) to join you.

REFERENCES

Here are a number of readings to help you understand the meaning of shadow families and the purpose they serve in our lives.

Bradshaw, J. (1992). *Creating Love: The Next Great Stage of Growth.* New York: Bantam Books.

Hillman, J. (1989). *A Blue Fire.* New York: HarperCollins.

———. (1991). The cure of the shadow. In C. Zweig & J. Abrams (eds.), *Meeting the Shadow: The Hidden Power of the Dark Side of Human Nature.* Los Angeles: Jeremy P. Tarcher.

Johnson, R. S. (1991). *Owning Your Own Shadow: Understanding the Dark Side of the Psyche.* Harper: San Francisco.

Jung, C. G. (1963). *Memories, Dreams, and Reflections.* New York: Pantheon.

Munhall, P. L. (ed.). (1994/1995). *In Women's Experience, vols.* 1–2. New York: NLN Press.

Van der Kolk, B. (1995). *Counting the Cost: The Lasting Impact of Childhood Trauma.* (Film, available from Cavalcade Productions, PO Box 2480, Nevada City, CA 95959.)

———, McFarlane, A. C., and Weisaeth, L. (eds.). (1996). *Traumatic Stress: The Effects of Overwhelming Experience on Mind, Body, and Society.* New York: Guilford Press.

Zweig, C., and Abrams, J. (eds.). (1991). *Meeting the Shadow: The Hidden Power of the Dark Side of Human Nature.* Los Angeles: Jeremy P. Tarcher.

CHAPTER 22

A FAMILY IN DIVORCE, AS TOLD BY SHEILA

Sheila J. Hopkins

Separation and divorce terminate more than the social and legal contract of marriage. They signify the breakup of the family. For me, divorce not only represented the end of a particular, constant emotional suffering, it also meant an opportunity for personal growth. Yet the experience of divorce, initially, was devastating to me. I was angry, fearful, and lonely. I missed the comfort of the known daily routine. I believed I had failed.

I met my first husband in 1953, at a time when the United States had again taken a financial upturn. In my lifetime, we had been through nearly a decade of troubled financial times and four terrible years of the Korean war. Family values were strong, Americans desired stability in their lives, and educational opportunities were available to those who would not have been able to afford them without postwar government benefits.

Widespread alterations in divorce laws reflecting previously prevalent beliefs about matrimony and its essentials were also changing. The strains of war and associated problems that produced more divorces also made the practice more prevalent, conspicuous, and acceptable.

Simultaneously, the growth of women in the workforce resulting from men leaving for war, among other reasons, afforded women an opportunity for economic independence. Marriage was less essential. Life as a single individual was gradually losing its stigma. During the civil rights movement in the sixties, women struggled to shed the subordinate position of a lesser version of their male counterparts. Women resisted becoming a mirror image of men who value power, and these women fought to establish equality, trying to retain the feminine qualities of tenderness and gentleness.

Challenges to institutional authority were commonplace. There were large and vocal movements challenging conventional sexual and marital norms,

---

Reprinted from Munhall, Patricia L. and Fitzsimons, eds. *The Emergence of Women into the 21st Century*. New York: NLN Press 1995.

censorship, the war in Vietnam, and educational policies. The no-fault divorce laws and the increasing numbers of women in the workforce signaled a profound shift in the way divorce was to be handled. By the seventies, decisions about divorce were no longer the prerogative of the state, and church authority was being challenged. Divorce was becoming the privilege of the married couple.

Marriage had been redefined. It was no longer primarily an economic institution, but was now outlined largely by its emotional significance. Love, companionship, and overall compatibility became the essential components. Commitment to the institution of marriage waned, while the relationships between men and women became of paramount importance. But women were still held responsible for the success or failure of their marriages. Meeting such high expectations remains difficult; sustaining them is very near impossible.

My Situation Then

In the mid-1950s, I was a middle-class Jewish 19-year-old from New England. Regardless of what was happening in the world around me, I was imbued with and acted upon the culture and mores of my family and immediate community. For me, early marriage to someone who was Jewish was the major symbol of beginning a successful life. It was anticipated that I would continue my education beyond high school and by graduation from a secondary school would be ready to be married. It was expected that one's life be patterned along a very specific timetable. In fact, a common saying, referring to young women was, "Ring by spring or your (college tuition) money back." Also, we women who came from ethnic enclaves (which didn't begin to disappear until suburbia and civil rights flourished in the sixties) had been impassioned by an image of the prototype we would marry. He would be college-educated, of a similar ethnic background, and would be involved in the rebuilding of a universal Jewish community. The horror of the Holocaust had touched and changed the lives of most American Jews. Whereas assimilation had been the goal in previous generations, Jewish youth who were coming to adulthood after World War II were struggling with the fear of extinction. The feeling was that the only way Jews could survive was through solidarity.

So there I was. It was my first year away from home. I was living in a dorm, studying nursing in Boston, and at 19 (although I was not overtly aware of it), right on track and ready to "fall in love" with a nice Jewish man.

Divorce in Judaism

Marriage is one of the cornerstones of Jewish life. "No man without a wife, neither a woman without a husband, nor both of them without God" (Genesis Rabbah 8:9, Old Testament). Yet divorce is regarded as an alternative when it is "given for the sake of peace . . . and those who divorce when they must, bring good upon themselves, not evil" (Eliyahu Kitov). According to Judaic law, companionship, satisfaction of physical and emotional needs, peace, harmony, kindness, respect, and thoughtfulness are the significant tenets upon which a marriage must be built.

Judaism permits divorce and makes provision for it on grounds no more severe than simple incompatibility, but divorce must never be carried out arbitrarily or with hostility. The law of divorce is given only where every hope of healing the breach is gone and strife and bitterness prevail. Then, for the peace and unity of the family, divorce is granted.

It is acknowledged that the human tragedy inherent in any divorce is especially poignant when there are children. Often it is when there are children that divorce becomes a lifetime burden. Because of Judaic teachings about divorce, I did not feel encumbered by religious beliefs when contemplating my divorce.

SIGNIFICANCE OF DIVORCE

Divorce is of significance on several planes. Sociologically, it is an indicator of the stability of social systems (marriage). It is also an important transition in the life of individuals (a meaningful event in the biography of family members) and it is a microsocial descriptor of associated events such as industrialization, poverty, educational attainment, war, law, religious trends, and historical events. Although the 20th century began with very little divorce, it draws to a close with national surveys predicting that as many as two-thirds of all recent marriages will end in divorce. It is remarkable that similar trends in divorce exist throughout the Western world despite differences in forms of government, national economics, and the role of religion.

The redefinition of marriage in the latter part of the 20th century throughout the West reflects profound changes in relationships between men and women. Marriage is no longer an economic institution; it is defined by its emotional significance. Love, companionship, and equality are essential to its success.

As the meaning of marriage changes, so do the reasons for divorce. Conversely, now that it has become more difficult to sustain a marriage, it has become easier to terminate. Divorce is less costly financially, legally, and reputationally than it was in the past.

There are some documented demographic and personal characteristics that correlate with the probability of divorce. These include early age at the time of marriage, premarital births, divorce from a previous marriage, low educational attainment, and employment. I fit the profile only in terms of early age. In the 1950s, many women married young.

Consequences of divorce on children are difficult to address because longitudinal studies are just now beginning to offer evidence. It does appear that children of divorced parents feel the cumulative effect of the failing marriage and divorce at the time they enter young adulthood. They appear to have difficulty with the developmental task of establishing love and intimacy, making the new families appear vulnerable to the effects of divorce. In many ways, my marital life was reflective of social, community, and family mores prevalent at the time.

Falling in Love

Falling in love at 19 was more like a high tide crashing to shore over rocks rather than the delicate flight of a bird. It was later I learned how tenuous love can be.

I met Milton, my first husband, in 1953. We were both in school, he studying to become a Jewish communal worker, I a nurse. I knew I had met the man who would fulfill my dreams and make my family proud. In those days, our parents' expectations shaped our plans for the future. I was in love. Part of the aura was that he appeared to be in love, too—after a whirlwind courtship (on a very limited budget), upon knowing he would have to serve in the Korean conflict, he insisted we marry before he went into the service. How romantic. I would continue my studies for the next two years while he was away. We could save from his increased allotment as a married man toward our graduate education. I was ready to "merge." In her book *Passages*, Gail Sheehy speaks about, "The urge to merge." I not only felt, as the romantic soundtrack from the film *American Graffiti* shouts,

> *Only you can make this change in me,*
> *for it's true, you are my destiny.*

about him, I was also starry-eyed about my own professional career. I felt that the need for expressing myself in a career of my own would mean growth outside of marriage. Early on I realized that it would not be simple to persue a "destiny" outside the marriage. I was still bound by the myth that happiness, acceptance, and success were, as my mother had found, in being a good wife and mother—in subjugating myself to family needs. This meant being Supermom and wife—consistently making decisions that are best for others. Whereas to persue an occupation was the anticipated commitment for men with the "urge to merge," women were expected to make a commitment not only to husband and children, but to cooking and baking and cleaning and handling the finances and advising. Independence was not one of the anticipated achievements. June, the mom in *Leave It to Beaver*, was still the role model.

Milton and I had both planned to go to graduate school at the same time. I would work full-time and study part-time. He would study full-time. We would live on my salary and take advantage of the many private and public scholarships available.

We married, he went to Korea, and I finished school. We were to begin our married life with all our dreams intact when he returned from the conflict. Graduate school, here we come. But I became pregnant the first week he was home. . . . "You fear it might be silence" . . . and we began our marriage very differently than either one of us had expected.

The Marriage

Milton was furious that I had become pregnant. He was afraid that he would not be able to attend graduate school. After much cajoling and offering up plans, sacrificial to me initially, but ultimately (I thought) good for the family,

Milton agreed upon one. We could live with my cousin to save rent and household expenses, I could work full-time and he could go to school full-time and work, if time permitted. It seemed fair that I take on the burden of solving the problem because I truly believed him when he indicated it was my fault for getting pregnant. What I hadn't expected was his continued anger at me for being pregnant. I listened and I prayed, but never did I think of leaving the marriage. My pregnancy was the first crisis in the marriage. He spoke to me only when absolutely necessary, sex became a chore, and I gained 40 pounds.

Thereafter crises occurred each time a family change or decision was to be made. We did not learn to talk to each other. In fact, whether the issue was limited finances, a new baby, imminent relocation, or as simple as who would baby-sit, handling the situation was agonizing. The problem was usually resolved with my doing what I thought he wanted. There was never a question of my leaving. I believed marriage was forever. I defined myself in terms of my husband and my children. I still believed being a better wife and doing more was the only route to happiness. I felt the failure or success of the marriage was my responsibility. After all, Milton didn't drink, he didn't beat me, he didn't squander money on gambling, nor did he (to my knowledge at that time) have other women. In the 1950s, this was a portrait of a good husband. I was overwhelmed being a "modern woman" working and trying to be a perfect wife, mother, and homemaker. I shall never be able to make up the sleep lost during those years.

As the years went by and my youngest child entered school, I began to, as other women were, look toward what I wanted professionally. In the 1960s, women were striving for their own identity in the work world, in relationships, in published works, and through public demonstration. Not unlike other women of the times, I ached for equality in the marriage, companionship, sexual satisfaction, and professional fulfillment. Although I never entertained the notion of relinquishing my "marital" responsibilities, or leaving the marriage, I was able to go to school part-time and continue supplementing our income while caring for the family.

Milton worked hard and was well-respected in his field of social work. Compared to other pay in occupations, his salary, although adequate, was not competitive with many of his friends' incomes. Although he enjoyed the respect his position afforded, his need for more money and some semblance of fame led us to relocate several times. He was always clear that the moves focused on his career. A community with good resources, schools for the children, and opportunities for my professional advancement were secondary. I flagellated myself for having negative feelings about his self-centeredness. After all, I still believed that the process was correct. It was OK if other family members subjugate their needs to the well-being and occupational success of the husband-father. In turn, the whole family would prosper from his occupational rewards. I believed my future was totally dependent upon him.

As we entered the 1970s, I began to realize that I had a responsibility to myself—I began to grow up. I no longer needed to behave as my mother had . . . I relished the idea of having a life that was part of, yet separate from, the marriage. I continued to try to be supermom and wife, but my focus was shifting. I finally embarked on a path to meet my needs, to fulfill my dreams, to shed the dormant woman I had become. I went back to school. The marriage was a prison and my relationship to Milton was largely one of inane limited conversation about operational necessities and angry exchanges about how to handle every day "crises." I was trapped. I did not want to be divorced. I wanted the family, the "marriage," not the relationship with him. Gradually the marriage became a structure not unlike a movie set, where we used the empty framework to plot and act out our separate lives. My time was spent in school, at work, with the children, and with friends. Supposedly Milton was busy, busy, busy getting ahead at work. He had decided that if he did not receive the directorship of the agency where he currently worked in the next year, we would move again. I had established a life of my own and was very reluctant to go.

Once more I listened and I prayed, but what I had learned was that love can be forever or it can be fleeting, it can be nurturing or destructive, it can be happily bestowed or cruelly withheld, and that a love object can be falsely perceived, distorted by the image of our own fantasies. I did not have a good love.

We did move to Washington, D.C. The older children were to remain in Connecticut. The oldest was in college, already living in an apartment of her own, the middle child would finish his last year of high school living with our friends. Milton would leave in May to become acclimated to his new position. I would remain in Connecticut to sell the house, finish school, complete my work responsibilities, and allow Mike (the child who would be moving with us) to go to horseback riding camp one more time. It was during the summer that Milton met "the love of his life" in Washington. Apparently it was very difficult for him to leave the marriage, although he had become alternately angry and depressed. He did not tell me that he wanted to dissolve the marriage until several weeks after I had arrived in Washington with Mike, who was 11. We had come to closure with all our friends and activities in Connecticut, had begun to be established in Washington, and now Mike and I were to return to Connecticut. I was furious that Milton had not said something earlier, devastated about losing my identity as a wife, frightened about finances, ashamed that I had failed, and most of all, terribly worried about the children. I felt destroyed when he told me that he had never loved me, but had married to have roots.

The Separation

I returned to Connecticut with Mike, a car in poor condition, our clothing, and $500. It was the mid-1970s. Women had made some advances, but were not viewed as being capable of caring for themselves financially. With much humiliation, I had to have Milton sign a lease before a landlord would rent an apartment to me, a female single parent. Of course, my having a job that paid well, which I was fortunate to be able to return to, made no difference. Because of my "marital status," I was also required to pay two months' rent in advance. While my daughter was hounding me to stand up for my civil rights and prosecute the landlords, I was eager to leave my friend's home where Mike and I had been staying. We needed a home of our own, more conveniently located. I wanted to return to the town we had left so the children could reestablish relationships and routines. The town was also midway between school and work for me and I had a cadre of friends waiting to welcome me back. I received no financial support from Milton during the separation. Fear of destroying any possibility of reconciliation kept me from pressuring him.

Becoming

By the 1970s there had been multiple attitudinal changes toward women from previous decades. Society was beginning to entertain a tolerance for diversity in the role of women. Women were beginning to assert their gender in ways other than being wife and mother. We had additional opportunities to find fulfillment and earn respect. Once I was settled into a routine of children-focused activities, work, and school, I was able to spend time introspectively. What a wonderfully exhilarating time! I read about other women, I wrote poetry, I felt free. I viewed my life situation with clarity; the beauty of the world around me was breathtaking. I was exhilarated by cross-country skiing with Mike, awed by the intensity of the beauty in sunsets and sunrises. I felt as though a tremendous burden had been lifted from me . . . and yet there were moments when I was overwhelmed by sadness. I mourned the probable breakup of the family (never the loss of the relationship with Milton). I worried about the effects of divorce on the children. I soared when I felt good. I was immobilized in the pits of despair when I was low, but having been well trained in 22 years of a bad marriage, I was able to carry on with my daily routine and reach a level of fairly consistent contentment.

My life and the lives of the children had stabilized. I wanted a legal and a Jewish divorce. Apparently, Milton was content to be with the "love of his life" and remain married to me. He agreed to the divorce with reticence and went through the process in as small-minded and spiteful a way as one could.

The Divorce and Now

The flight of love may be quick, but some of the pain may last forever. It has been almost 20 years since my divorce. My children are successfully married and have children of their own. Each has established a relationship on their own terms with their father. I have had a wonderful second marriage, yet, whenever I remember my first marriage I'm surprised at the rancor I feel. I relish the excitement of having learned who I had been and who I have become. I remember having cried watching romantic movies because I had not had the romance I expected from my relationship with my first husband. I felt during that marriage that my days were filled with sacrifices and compromises. Everything I experienced during the separation was extraordinarily intense and poignant. I was despondent with grief, exhilarated with pleasure, I sobbed embarrassingly loudly with sadness, I wet my pants with laughter. Sunsets and sunrises were spectacular—the dam had burst. I no longer wrestled with my own private hell. This was the most profound growth period of my life. I am both grateful and proud of the way I changed. I had thought my family knew nothing about my difficulties in the marriage. After the divorce I found that was hardly the case. I am no longer ashamed of that marriage.

Slowly I began to no longer feel incomplete without a husband. I believe I was growing up and I reveled in the process, excited about the potential outcome. It was time to make my separateness complete, to complete school, to be open to romance. Unfortunately, during the divorce proceedings I had slipped into old behaviors. I had spent many hours during the separation working hard to learn about who I had been in the past and reshaping my life so that I could be who I wished to be in the future. Retrospectively, I was appalled to find that during the divorce negotiations I had regressed into the compliant, agreeable, unsure "girl" I had been in the marriage. My need to be what I considered fair, just, and honest, and 20 years of being subordinate, preempted my following my lawyer's advice and I accepted a divorce decree without provisions for alimony, with child support less than aid to dependent children payments, and with very little financial support for the children's college education. Also, in some ways, I thought this to be a show of independence. Foolish me! I am happy to admit that I weathered the financial storms and have a sense of pride that I was able to accomplish my goals and help the children accomplish theirs on my own.

The bereavement I feel about loss of the family recurs with weddings, birthdays, and other family occasions, but I'm largely content, having had a wonderful second marriage, a fulfilling career, and a spirited social life.

Although love is a little white bird that comes to us fleetingly, there need not be disenchantment. There is strength and beauty in the song of past loves. We as women plucked from our innocence of dependence upon men can move forward toward a transformation. The trauma of divorce is a lesson in how to meet adversity. It teaches us that if the intent to bring about our own development is there, we have the ability. We learn that we can stand shoulder to shoulder with men and other women to contribute to a new world. A new world where one's style is respected and both toughness and tenderness add to peace, equality, and development. A new world where diverse logic, values, choices, and prayers are accepted with rectitude.

As we move into the postmodern era, women will remain intact as total beings themselves, not as a lesser version of our male counterparts. We will have equality, married or single, in all walks of life, without forfeiting our womanliness.

CHAPTER 23

Housing for the Single-Parent Family: A Blueprint for Women's Educational Support

Judith Mathews, Maureen Hreha, and Marilyn Burk

Single-Parent Housing: One Formula for Women's Development

Each year qualified applicants to the Muhlenberg Regional Medical Center School of Nursing in Plainfield, New Jersey, include single parents. They inquire about student housing for themselves and their children and then withdraw their applications when they find out that the traditional dormitory residence halls available for the nursing students have no accommodations or facilities for children. The lack of appropriate housing for families creates a barrier that prevents some qualified applicants from pursuing a degree in nursing.

Judith Mathews, Dean of the Schools of Nursing and Allied Health at Muhlenberg, directed a study that would determine the feasibility of providing housing and other services for single parents. The study was a component of Project TLC (Transcultural Leadership Continuum), an ongoing project funded by the Robert Wood Johnson Foundation involving Muhlenberg, Union County College, Kean College, and Elizabeth Regional Medical Center, all New Jersey–based institutions.

Project TLC proposed to increase the retention of minority women in nursing education by supporting the students' academic and economic needs, thereby enabling them to return to their communities as independent professionals. These students would also increase minority representation in the administrative ranks of nursing as they progressed in their profession. The ultimate goal of Project TLC was to increase the representation of minority nurses in leadership roles within the profession. Attaining the nursing degree was the first step in that process.

Project TLC's feasibility study for single-parent nursing students included three goals:

- To determine the requirements for converting existing student residence space into housing for single-parent students and their families
- To determine the need for such housing
- To determine the needs for additional support services for the single-parent students and their children

Accomplishing the first goal required identifying physical space and planning the renovation. Addressing the second and third goals required research into the nature of the single-parent student and the needs of that student.

Basic Peace: A Roof Over Our Heads

The number of young, single mothers in the United States is increasing. The 1990 census counts "other families" as a category of households, defined as households not headed by married couples. Single mothers head about 7 million of these families. The Census Bureau projects that by the year 2010, 8 million households will be headed by single mothers. The number of these families headed by single mothers under the age of 25 will increase by 50 percent by the year 2010.

The 1990 census showed that households headed by single mothers are often low-income households. About 45 percent of single mothers with children under 18 live in poverty. The number of families headed by single mothers is increasing and many of these are families in need.

These families are frequently minority families. In 1992, "67 percent of births to African-American women were out of wedlock, compared to 27 percent for Hispanic women, and 17 percent for white women. . . . it is among Hispanic and white women that the greatest increases have registered" (Patterson, 1993). If Project TLC proposed to address the needs of minority students in nursing education, it had to address the single parent as well.

Does the single mom with her children require support services? Corporate America thinks so. According to the 1994 *Small Business Reports*, 25 percent of today's American families are headed by single parents. Employers who address the issues of diversity in the workforce often find that some of those issues include family demands. Employers are willing to invest in supporting workers affected by various family issues to enable employees' productivity and well being. Demographics indicate that single parenting is now recognized as one of those family issues (Dow, 1993).

Single parents' needs are often addressed by employers who provide assistance, such as child-care programs or flextime scheduling arrangements. Dow Chemical provides day-care programs, school-age child care, flextime, and even lactation support programs at a number of its plants to assist single parents and dual career families (*Occupational*, 1992). Sony is another company that provides day-care facilities at some of its sites (Jorgensen, 1993). American companies are taking advantage of the diversity of the workforce and addressing employees' lifestyle concerns to enable increased success on the job. Companies want to "harness the diversity of the U.S. workforce to increase productivity and profit share" (Dow, 1993).

Single-parent students have needs as students, as parents, and as individuals. Colleges that have begun on-campus residential programs already know this and address these needs.

Single-parent housing, child care, and other support services for nursing and other postsecondary students are already provided at schools such as Trinity College, Goddard College, Texas Women's University, and St. Catherine's in Minnesota. Douglas North of Goddard College wrote:

> Everyone who works with single parents recognizes that among their primary needs are relevant education, skilled counseling, quality child care, and a job that pays enough to make it financially advantageous to work. (North, 1987)

Texas Woman's University program for single-parent students in need is a quality program in increasing demand. Nancy Murphy-Chadwick of Texas Woman's University describes her school's services, which support not only the adult single woman student but the child of that student.

> The on-campus family population has grown yearly with a 363 percent increase since 1983. . . . Single parents have a secure environment to make a home while attending classes. . . . The accessibility of quality child care and convenient, secure housing can relieve two of the major pressures students with young families face. . . . (Murphy-Chadwick, 1989)

The College of Saint Catherine recognized a need for special housing and additional services for its population of students, several of whom were single mothers. St. Catherine's programs include several health-related degrees, including an associate's degree in nursing. St. Catherine's recognized the need for:

> . . . odd-hour day care . . . necessary for students who must take early morning clinicals in hospitals in support of their school work. . . . Living . . . with other single parents and having access to regular and odd-hour child care would reduce scheduling hassles and enable a community of support to occur. . . . the support and people connections that provide a 'safety net' for . . . students. (Wroblewski, 1990)

A 1989 doctoral study from Ball State University compares the impeding and enabling factors for the traditional fresh-out-of-high-school student to reentry students in Ball State's nursing program. The older, reentry students list the cost of college and arranging for child care as impeding factors, or barriers, to their enrollment in the nursing program. Two potential enabling factors listed by reentry students are encouragement from college personnel and change in responsibilities at home (Scott, 1989).

All of these programs recognize that housing and child care are basic requirements for the single parent in need who wants to enroll in postsecondary college and nursing programs. Additional support services allow that student to succeed, increasing not only enrollment, but retention and successful completion of the programs.

As Muhlenberg Regional Medical Center addressed the issues of housing for its single-parent students, it also addressed the issues of programs to support those students. Based on information from these colleges, Muhlenberg Regional Medical Center's Feasibility Study Team developed plans for three counseling approaches that would address the single parent as student, person, and parent.

A Blueprint: The Muhlenberg Plan

Once Muhlenberg decided that the physical change was feasible, it developed its support services plan. Students admitted to the nursing program are fully qualified applicants as well as single parents in need. Support services also include housing, child care, counseling, and academic support. The program addresses the well-being of the children living at Muhlenberg. The program was called Project Hope (Housing Opportunities for Parents in Education).

This program targets the enabling factors cited in the Ball State Study—child care and support from college personnel—as well as housing as the basic needs of these students and their families. In many cases, however, these single-parent students have extraordinary needs.

Local New Jersey shelters that also provide housing for single parents were surveyed. They all affirm the necessity of providing support services, such as counseling. Several of their residents are from a world of poverty, abuse, or other crisis situations. Identifying the potentially successful student is not enough. The single-parent student may have a history of complex problems to overcome.

Project Hope respects the single parent as a person. A personal counselor is available for scheduled individual and group counseling sessions. The sessions focus on improvement in self-esteem, problem solving, interpersonal relations, and conflict resolution within the group. This counselor helps students adjust to dormitory living and enables each to function as an individual, student parent in a communal public setting.

The program also supports the single parents as parents, and that begins with safe, dependable child care. The women have the services of the Muhlenberg Child Care Center, which provides care from 6:30 A.M. to 6 P.M. for children from the ages of 3 weeks to 5 years of age Monday through Friday. Evening child care is included and scheduled for two weekday evenings twice a week within the dormitory setting. A cooperative program of baby-sitting was organized for weekend, odd-hour, and sick child care, gradually assuming more of the child care responsibilities.

Project Hope facilitates additional parenting support by providing a family mentor. The family mentor is available formally and informally for the purpose of fostering the family unit and supporting the student as a parent. Formal sessions are presented in parenting, safety, child growth and development, decision making, goal setting, health and wellness, socialization, team building, and peer interaction. The family mentor also assists in an initial orientation period for the incoming families.

Finally, this project supports the single-parent nursing student in academic and clinical training matters with an academic counselor. This counselor focuses on the student as a student, identifying and addressing any learning problems or disabilities. The academic counselor also builds study skills, test-taking strategies, and time- and project-management skills.

CONTRACT FOR DEVELOPMENT: FAMILIES TOGETHER

Project TLC has family residential and academic policies in contract form that ask the women and their children to commit to academic performance and housing responsibilities.

Accepted women enter the program screened for motivation, sense of responsibility, and aptitude for college academic work. This screening process is in addition to a preparatory six-week period before classes begin. It is essential that both the women as single parents and their children are familiar with their new living conditions and expectations. This orientation period gives the families time to get to know one another before the entire class meets as a whole.

Careful screening of single-parent applicants combined with a full network of professional support for the women and their children enable these women to achieve their educational goals.

The program is not simply a gift. It demands from the student the ability to study and achieve academically as she copes with communal living and parenting.

The program asks that the woman return to her community as an educated nurse ready to serve as a role model of achievement and independence.

References

Dow programs address child care, dual-career couples, and other work-family issues. (October 23, 1993). *Chemical & Engineering News*, p. 47.

Healing's bedside revolution: Health care reform could further expand role of nursing. (December 31, 1993). *Washington Post*, p. A1.

Health-care reform should bode well for nurses. (January 11, 1994). *Wall Street Journal*, p. A1.

Hennenberger, M. (August 21, 1994). For nurses, new uncertainties: Managed care means fewer openings, specialized needs. *New York Times*, p. 45.

Jahn, B. J. (1990). An investigation of changes in perception of career mobility with advanced formal education by registered and vocational nurses. Doctoral dissertation, East Texas State University.

Johnson, S. (August 28, 1991). Helping single parents find success in college. *Wall Street Journal*, p. B8.

Jorgensen, B. (September 1993). Diversity: Managing a multicultural work force. *Electronic Business Buyer*, pp. 70–76.

Murphy-Chadwick, N., et al. (1989). *Family housing and services*. Washington, DC: American Association of State Colleges and Universities. ERIC ED316148.

North, D. (1987). AFDC goes to college. *Public Welfare*, 45(4):4–12. *Occupational Outlook Handbook, 1992–1993 Edition*. (1992). Chicago: VGM Career Horizons.

Patterson, M. (July 14, 1993). Single motherhood on the rise. *Star Ledger*, pp. 1, 15.

Scott, J. (1989). Traditional and reentry nursing majors: Motivational factors, vocational personalities, barriers and enablers to participation. Muncie, Ind.: Ball State Indiana.

Single parents. (July 1992). *American Demographic Desk Reference*, pp. 14–15.

Single parents. (December 1993). *American Demographics*, pp. 36–37.

Single parent support. (September 1994). *Small Business Reports*, p. 20.

VOICES EIGHT

FAMILIES LIVING WITH VIOLENCE

Thinking about violence, whether in a country, a family, or a workplace, Patricia Munhall wrote this verse.

Killing Spirits

Ambulatory schizophrenics walk the earth,
We pull levers to vote, marry with trust, or work with them
And the pain begins, some say torture

Is there not a screen to sieve potential of aggression "to come"
And more important the impulsiveness of the release

Of the inner ledger of retribution
The sins trespassed against them
Where they seek vengeance
At some ungodly hour

And we at their untender mercy
Are in the process of annihilation through evil
Where suddenly to a skip heart beat, we wonder,
Could this be it?

CHAPTER

24

DOMESTIC VIOLENCE: A LOSS OF SELFHOOD

Evelyn Ortner

I am Evelyn Ortner, founder and executive director of the Unity Group, Inc., advocates for battered women and their children. Prior to founding Unity, I had been an adviser and speechwriter for then-secretary of Health and Human Services, Margaret Heckler. My area of concentration was women's issues and domestic violence, in particular. Even then, through the Reagan period of the 1980s, Surgeon General Koop referred to domestic violence as the number one health problem and leading cause of death and injury for women in the United States.

When I returned to my home in suburban New Jersey, I founded Unity, a nonprofit all-volunteer group (no one is on salary) that provides a multitude of services, all without charge, to meet the daily needs of our clients. We offer support group services, other monthly public service programs, and referrals to pro bono legal and medical services.

I first learned of the nightmare of abuse and its pervasive nature while in Washington. These statistics provide some idea of just *how* pervasive it is.

- Every 15 seconds a woman is battered in the United States.
- Between 1959 and 1975, 58,000 American soldiers were killed in Vietnam. During that same period, 51,000 American women were murdered by their male partners.
- Each year, approximately 1,400 women die as a result of domestic violence.
- 95 percent of domestic violence victims are women.
- Industry loses $3 billion to $5 billion per year through absenteeism because of injuries caused by domestic violence.
- Each year, 2 to 4 million women are beaten by their partners.
- Domestic violence is not limited to any geographic area, income level, or religious affiliation.

Adapted from Munhall, Patricia L. and Fitzsimons, Virginia. *The Emergence of Women into the 21st Century*. New York: NLN Press 1995.

- Each year more than 1 million women seek medical assistance for injuries caused by battering.
- 15 to 25 percent of pregnant women are battered.
- Approximately 35 percent of women with injuries who use emergency room services are abused women.
- Battering is the cause of one of every four suicide attempts by women.
- There are three times more animal shelters in the United States than shelters for women.
- 87 percent of children witness the abuse of their mothers.
- Children in homes where domestic violence occurs are physically abused at a rate 1500 percent higher than the national average.
- Boys who witness the violence are more likely to batter their female partners as adults than others raised in nonviolent homes.

During the period I served in the federal government, I read countless books and articles on the subject of domestic violence, including Dr. E. Shein's *Coercive Persuasion and Brainwashing*; *Conditioning and DDD (Debility, Dependency and Dread)* by I. E. Farber, Harry F. Harlow, and Louis Jolyon West; and Biderman's "Chart of Coercion." Having digested these materials, I understood that battered women are hostages and that there are literally *thousands* of women who are being held hostage in their own homes. Though there may not be bars on the windows and doors to keep them in, there are invisible bars that control the minds of these victims, and they are stronger than any iron bars could be.

Let me describe the function of the three D's.

- *Debility*: This first D is induced by semi-starvation, fatigue, disease, isolation, chronic physical pain, loss of energy, all of which leads to an inability to resist minor abuse, which then leads to inaction and a sense of total exhaustion.
- *Dependency*: This second D is produced by the prolonged deprivation of sleep, food, fresh air, social contact, factors necessary to maintain sanity and life itself. Occasional respites from the abuse teach the victim that, should he want to, the abuser can stop the abuse. This leads the victim to harbor false hopes of change and keeps her there eternally, hoping for release from her agony.
- *Dread*: This final, ultimate D is the fear of death or of permanent disability or deformity.

The three D's keep a victim in her place in a constant state of panic, hoping to please, never knowing what will incur the wrath of her abuser. Dr. Saul Shengold has termed this condition "soul murder"—a victim's soul in bondage to someone else. Jefferson said, "I have sworn upon the altar of God eternal hostility against every form of tyranny over the mind of man." And what, if anything, has society done to practice what that great patriot preached so very long ago? Precious little.

TABLE 24–1 BIDERMAN'S CHART OF COERCION

General Method	*Effects and Purposes*
Isolation	Deprives victim of social support (for the) ability to resist
	Develops an intense concern with self
	Makes victim dependent upon interrogator
Monopolization of perception	Fixes attention upon immediate predicament; fosters introspection
	Eliminates stimuli competing with those controlled by captor
	Frustrates all actions not consistent with compliance
Induced debility and exhaustion	Weakens mental and physical ability to resist
Threats	Cultivates anxiety and despair
Occasional indulgences	Provides positive motivation for compliance
Demonstrating "omnipotence"	Suggests futility of resistance
Degradation	Makes cost of resistance appear more damaging to self-esteem than capitulation
	Reduces prisoner to "animal level" concerns
Enforcing trivial demands	Develops habit of compliance

A victim is told that she has provoked him and therefore must be punished, that if she did not provoke him, he would not be forced to hurt her, but she persisted, and therefore she must be punished. She, in fact, made him do it. One abuser actually told me that his victim now hits herself, also; he has trained her to do that. Dr. Biderman's "Chart of Coercion" encompasses DDD and depicts the descent into hell of emotional imprisonment (Table 24–1).

These methods can reduce anyone to a slavelike condition. I have often drawn the comparison between Holocaust victims and domestic violence victims—the macro as opposed to the micro, but is it really the micro? After all, the Holocaust had a beginning and an end, while the victimization of women, like a mobius strip, seems unending. Anyone undergoing DDD is a dehumanized being who is unable to distinguish herself as a separate person and often is unable to distinguish right from wrong. These women are survivors in the same way that Holocaust survivors are. They do what they need to do in order to survive. One of my clients has referred to herself as a sacrificial lamb. Unfortunately, there are those among us who insist and persist in calling the battered woman a masochist—a shocking lie that the public must be disabused of.

I would like to introduce to you a few of my clients. The very first call I received was from a woman who had two daughters, one about 3 years old and the other about 18 months. Her husband, unbeknown to her, was having sexual relations with their 3-year-old daughter. One night the husband took his two sleepy daughters out of the house, locked his wife in her room after beating her unconscious, and set the room afire. Fortunately, she regained consciousness, jumped out the window, and fled to a hospital. Those horrible events took place over six years ago. To this day, the older daughter has severe emotional problems. Her mother suffers from the physical aftereffects of the fire and innumerable emotional problems. She is a strikingly beautiful woman and is still struggling to keep legal custody of her daughters.

Another equally beautiful young woman from a cultured upscale family met her abuser in 1982. He is an uneducated, perennially filthy drug user and dealer, unemployed, and from a dysfunctional family. Being the con man that all abusers are, he convinced her of his loneliness and his needs. Within a month or so she was reduced to abject servitude. He said, "Call me Mr. Jones of Jonestown. I can do all this by drugs, starvation, and beatings." Currently she lives in poverty, has had major surgery, is losing her teeth, and is not permitted any connection with her family or friends. She is free only to work and support her abuser.

One client in her mid-fifties has been brutalized for years. Her story is unique in that her husband first told her she was too thin and insisted upon her gaining weight and forcing her to eat only high-calorie foods. Once she was truly obese, he took her to the hospital and had her undergo intestinal bypass surgery to help her reduce her weight. As a result of that surgery, she suffers innumerable disabilities and currently weighs 180 pounds and is 5 feet tall.

Another client, beaten while pregnant, aborted at home and carried the fetus about, crying for help. Her husband, who had caused the tragedy, called her names and refused to take her to the hospital.

These behaviors are not without repercussions. When victims do not receive the appropriate support and intervention, they suffer secondary injuries—what I call *revictimization by the system*. The victim feels numb, a kind of paralysis sets in, she is unable to make rational decisions, she feels vulnerable, lonely, and confused. Her selfhood is gone. To question a victim's response or lack thereof is to inflict a secondary injury. Even those who escape suffer from post-traumatic stress disorder (PTSD). Some symptoms of PTSD involve sleeping and eating disorders, nightmares, flashbacks, extreme tension and anxiety, nonresponsiveness, and memory trouble.

Support from the medical professionals, the court system, law enforcement, and lawyers, to say nothing of friends and family, is essential. To blame the victim is a crime in itself. Failure to recognize the importance of the crime is to invalidate the victim, who requires that very validation to recover.

The AMA has admitted that they are delinquent in recognizing and providing the necessary help that victims require. Doctors do not even ask how the injuries that they are treating have been inflicted. I think we can safely say that it is indeed a rare occasion when someone runs into a door or does a somersault in the tub. The reluctance to address the real issue increases the sense of isolation of the victim and discourages her efforts to leave the abuse. This refusal to recognize and validate the victim is a significant factor in the development of subsequent psychopathology.

Research shows that in 96 percent of the cases, there is no psychosocial history taken and no psychiatrist is consulted. In 92 percent of the cases, no social worker was consulted and in 98 percent of the cases, no referral was given. Dr. Malcolm G. Freeman of Emory University said, "Probably the greatest thing physicians can do to help victims of domestic violence is to be emotionally supportive." Prescribing tranquilizers and pain medicine is not a remedy. It is a Band-aid solution and a poor one at that. Triage nurses often are aware of the abuse, but refuse to get involved and instead refer the patient to police.

Anne Flitcraft, M.D., states that 45 percent of the women in alcohol treatment started out as battered women who drink or succumb to the drugs that doctors prescribe to make them feel better. The previously mentioned client who referred to herself as a sacrificial lamb had called doctors constantly, none of whom recognized her problem. A prominent specialist to whom she went for ultrasound for three consecutive months decided she was in need of therapy. He claimed that she is suffering from Munchausen's syndrome, a feigning of ailments. Doctor, can you not decipher her clues, her silent call for help? By concluding that she is unstable, he is colluding with her abuser. The doctor is simply not listening.

Who are these women who become victims? They are all about us and can be anyone and everyone. Customarily, these are women who want to please and have low self-esteem. They define themselves in terms of others. But none of these factors are essential. All women are potential victims. By the time the victim is aware that conditions are abnormal, it is usually too late. Wooed by the silky tones of adoration, lulled by champagne and flowers, she descends step by hideous step down the path to hell.

Who are these abusers? They can be anyone and everyone, the mayor, the teacher, yes, even the clergyman. A major characteristic of assailants in domestic violence cases is their capacity for deception. They are masters in the art of finding ways to blame other people and external events for their inappropriate behavior. A lifelong pattern of avoiding consequences for their own behavior effectively limits a sense of personal responsibility for their actions as well as limiting their motivation to change. An abuser has an intense desire to control an individual. This individual becomes the repository of all of the abuser's inner conflict. In a kind of symbiotic dance, the abuser and his victim feed off each other. The victim often thinks that by being "good" she can eliminate the next beating. But as long as the abuser blames the victim for his own problems, the beatings will continue.

The assaults are a product of the abuser's personality and bear little relationship to the victim's behavior. Unless the abuser takes responsibility for his own behavior, the violence will continue.

It is a misconception to believe that the abuser "loves." The attachment to the victim has nothing to do with love. It represents a pathological dependency on the victim. This factor is so extreme as to result in murder if the victim should leave or even speak of leaving. Often she is persuaded to stay by his pleadings of his absolute need of her. This bolsters her shattered sense of self. Often she is moved to remain as he fills her need to be needed. A "honeymoon" phase may ensue when no assaults take place, but that is short-lived and the tension and assaults are renewed. Society tends to blame the victim and fix the responsibility on her to leave. We fail to hold the abuser responsible for criminal behavior. Claiming alcohol or drug addiction as an excuse for their behavior is outrageous. There is no excuse for abuse. Abusers abuse because they want to abuse.

Here is a list of the abuser's common characteristics:

- Jealousy of their partner
- Control and isolation of their partner
- Jekyll and Hyde personalities
- Explosive tempers
- Have legal problems, served time in jail
- Projection (blame others for own behavior)
- Verbal and physical abuse
- History of family violence
- More violent when partner is pregnant
- Denial (he never did anything wrong)
- Cycle of violence

There are some early warning signs to be aware of and to run away from as fast as possible should you see them:

- Physical abuse during courtship
- Violent family environments
- Cruelty to animals
- Inability to handle frustration
- Poor self-image
- Extreme possessiveness and jealousy
- Police record for a violent crime
- Overt and excessive concern (a cover for control)
- Chronically unemployed
- Use of force in sex
- Past relationships in which there were indications of abuse
- Sees women as inferior to men

Though society constantly berates the battered woman for not leaving, and all manner of reasons are given for her staying in the abusive situation, the basic reason for her remaining is mind control and the aforementioned methods employed by all abusers, young and old, rich and poor, ignorant and educated. They are one and the same—hideous. Women are not born with this ailment, domestic violence, nor do they contract it like TB. It is visited upon them by vicious men.

And what can we do as a society to hold back this tide? We must train all of our professionals—including medical, legal, judicial, educators, the clergy, and so on—in the dynamics of domestic violence. We must do as they have done in some parts of the United States, and that is to practice vertical prosecution. What that does, in essence, is to employ personnel who are trained in domestic violence dynamics, from the district attorneys, prosecutors, and judges to the police officers. That unique group works only on domestic violence cases, and their success rates are outstanding. It is understood that domestic violence is a crime against the state and not a private matter. It will therefore be prosecuted to the full extent of the law. Victims need not press charges, nor appear in court, and charges are never dropped. In jurisdictions where vertical prosecution is practiced, battered women have a better chance of survival than in other parts of the country. Since that is the case, it must be implemented throughout the country.

Crisis intervention teams are another tool to save the lives of women and children. Here, trained volunteers from each municipality are on call on a rotating basis. Once they are notified by the police that a victim is waiting at the station, a volunteer goes there to offer practical information as well as solace to the victim. Such help and validation is essential.

One of the easiest methods to avoid future violence in our lives is to raise our children as equals, to let our daughters know that they do not have to marry into status, that they can and should be able to achieve on their own. And when Johnny destroys Mary's castle in the sandbox, he must be chastised publicly for that infraction. Mary needs to know that she need never accept that kind of abuse and Johnny needs to know that he was wrong and that everyone believes him to be wrong.

If that kind of misbehavior is not stopped in the sandbox, Johnny may grow up to be an abuser in some Mary's bedroom, and Mary, if not validated, will grow up thinking that abuse is okay. We might as well hang a placard around her neck that says, "Here I am. I'm a victim." Dr. Carol Gilligan, an expert on female adolescents, says that young girls sacrifice truth on the altar of niceness. Being nice is one thing, being subservient is quite something else.

We cannot allow our young people to grow up with the possibility of violence as a virtual fait accompli. We cannot sacrifice even a single female to this horror. We cannot afford it because our children are our future. Remember the teaching of the Talmud: "He who destroys a child destroys the world, but he who saves a child saves the world."

CHAPTER

25

THROUGH THE DISTANCE: LIVING AS AN OBJECT OF ANGER

Julie M. Evertz

ENDBEGINNINGS

As a soon-to-be-divorced mother of four loving little boys, I would like my story to be about living through some of the darkest of family secrets. Even so, it begins with death, my twin daughters', Nicole and Emily, nine years ago. Nicole and Emily died in a second-trimester miscarriage. They were beautiful and special girls-to-be yet were not entitled to the dignity of being called human beings. They deserved and had the right to be visible; a right not granted to them nine years ago. Nicole and Emily died at 18 weeks gestation. Two weeks stood in the way of their visibility and legitimacy as human beings as society defines it. Two weeks stood in the way of my right to mourn their loss, have a funeral, burial, or birth and death certificates, tangible reminders of their existence. It is a harshness, a distance to which I remain sensitive. Our dehumanization was pervasive. Finally, perhaps inevitably, my girls decided that they would not remain silent, and in 1997 they cried out for my attention and love.

On one beautiful January day, I stood on a balcony 11 stories high and chose to be alive in every sense of the word. I was with 18 other people for the entire day. No one knew of my struggle or the pain that had been released and was now torturing me. No one knew how much I suffered that day. I kept it a secret and swallowed the flood of emotions that overwhelmed me. I hid in the bathroom to cry. I changed the subject to avoid my pain, anything to protect myself. That secret almost killed me. Years of practice at keeping quiet and being silenced in one way or another kept me functional that day. Yet, now my secret was out and there was no turning back. It followed me every moment of every day. The more that I tried to bury it, the more my secret took on a life of its own and demanded more of my energy.

What I now know is that it wasn't only one secret but my response to years of secrecy, my anger at being distanced, punished, abused, and betrayed by my family as a child and adult. It was also the culmination of self-anger unleashed combined with my own perceived shame, guilt, and humiliation.

Three days before my miscarriage, during an argument at home, I slipped and fell in a puddle of water on the floor, water that had been impulsively thrown at me. I remember being told, "You should have watched where you were going." I remember being mocked for my clumsiness. Instead of my husband's concern and remorse, I was made to feel responsible. He told me that I was blaming him so that I didn't have to feel guilty or accept responsibility for the loss. From that moment on, it was my fault. Having been raised to always take responsibility for my actions, I assumed responsibility for the loss of my twins. My unnecessary fall at the hands of another who vowed to love and protect me still haunts me.

It was supposed to be a simple assignment. I was to describe a painful experience as an exercise in phenomenological writing. Little did I know the power of that assignment. My anger at others, and, perhaps more significant, my anger at myself was brought to awareness.

There is much work in grieving. It is tiring. However, it is more tiring not to grieve. So many times I went through the day functioning as expected and appearing superficially fine to the world when the reality was that I was not fine all the time. There was a battle inside of me for months. It was a battle between hanging on and letting go. It was what I called my purgatory on earth. There was no resolution, just pure suffering. I hurt a lot inside. I cried a lot but mostly alone. I just pushed my grief down, put it out of my mind daily to keep functioning. The anxiety from this tug of war seeped out of me daily in one way or another. My tolerance for its presence varied too. There were times when I felt like screaming as loud as I could but nothing came out of my mouth. There were times when all I wanted to do was to sit on the floor and cry without interruption. There was never any time for the luxury of my grief. The supermarket comes before grief. Laundry comes before grief. Everyone was always telling me that I needed to take care of myself. They had no idea what they asked of me. Everything I did was tightly scheduled around what others first needed from me. There was always someone who needed me to take care of them, and it seemed natural for me to do it. I liked the feeling of taking care of others too. Emotionally, though, I lived alone for a long time. That feeling of alienation was horrible. I was everything to everyone in my house and nothing to myself.

Then there was fear. I was afraid of my feelings, my grief, and my anger. My thinking went something like this: If I grieved the loss of my girls, I had to eventually accept their loss. I didn't want to accept their loss. Even though I can't have them physically with me, I miss them so much. I miss what they could have been. I miss what we could have done together. If I accepted their loss, then I had to accept my loss too. Letting my girls in again, to be "alive" with me, was frightening. I wanted to feel closer to them. I kept trying to get closer too, but they never felt close enough. There was always distance. I felt myself being cautious in getting closer to them. For years, I avoided the pain of losing my girls and of any memories of violence surrounding their loss. I was afraid that the emotional pain would consume me. It is a horrible nightmare that no woman should have to endure.

Live or Let Die

My most horrifying memory was the feeling of carrying my dead baby inside of me for four days, the time it took to schedule my surgery. I spent those four days wishing for just one little movement, some sign of life, a kick, something to prove them all wrong. I stared at my stomach constantly and waited. I begged and bargained with God, but nothing worked. She just remained still inside of me no matter what I did. I had seen and felt a living baby growing inside of me, yet now there was nothing but stillness and death. There was nothing as a mother that I could do to save my baby, so I just held her, not physically, but emotionally. I haven't let go since.

I always feel angry when I hear or read distinctions made between perinatal loss and what I guess the professionals call "miscarriage." I don't see them as separate. Loss is the experience. Why is one loss more privileged than another? It seems to me that society has much power when it comes to grief and mourning. It is all right to grieve if there is a physical baby for everyone to see and know. I didn't have that, so I was expected to move on and forget about it all. I was expected to cope, so I did. In the course of one week, I was the mother of one son, an expectant mother, lost twin girls, and returned to work. I went on to have three more sons. Several years later, a colleague of mine lost her newborn baby girl. It was her first baby. The baby had suffered terrible anoxia and died several days after birth. I went to the funeral. I just wanted to be present. It was so difficult to be there, but I felt compelled by something that I couldn't explain. I genuinely hurt for her and I knew that I could only offer my presence. I thought that is what I would have wanted. I was in awe of her strength and faith. I didn't have the right to a funeral or family support when my babies died. I didn't have the right to comfort, to be able to grieve and receive all that goes with that. I didn't have the right to be visible. Everyone around me tried to get me to forget about it. I think that I did so more for them than for myself. I often wonder if perhaps I went to that funeral for me too. As I sat there during the funeral staring at the picture of my colleague's baby, I felt so incredibly sad. My entire body hurt and felt heavy. It was so cruel. The baby was perfect and beautiful but just not alive. Maybe the reason that no one cared for my babies is that they didn't acknowledge them as the beautiful, perfect babies they were to me. I didn't need to see them to love them.

Sometimes I think that my girls and I are on a mission together, a mission of love and acceptance. I embrace my twins and love them openly. I acknowledge their existence at every opportunity. It is the only way out of the loneliness. Closeness has given me comfort. I like talking about them now and realize that I refer to them by names or as "my twins" or "my girls." Sharing them with another who also embraced them with love literally saved me. I know we are not alone anymore. It is unconditional love that humanized them. It is the most precious gift one can offer another. The closer I became to Nicole and Emily, the less empty I felt. I don't think that I will ever be close enough, but I do know that my girls are always present with me and no one will ever separate us again.

When I was growing up, I was always told to try to solve my own problems. It was drilled into my head to avoid being a burden, to avoid intrusion. The message was simple: silence and invisibility will be rewarded. Expression of emotions was not encouraged. To expect or receive any emotional support was out of the question. I also didn't feel worthy of it. I often wondered why I was spared and Nicole and Emily were not allowed life. I try every day to be worthy of my girls. They are with me all the time in one way or another. Some days the reminders are gentler to me than others.

Innocence Lost

Our understanding of children's perceptions of violence within the context of family is limited. Their responses to family violence are constantly developing as mechanisms of hope and survival. "Experts" and parents make assumptions about children's responses to family violence. Children's feelings and possible suffering can be rendered invisible by these assumptions.

Family violence produces suffering. While much has been written *about* domestic violence, child abuse, social responsibility, and the effects of battering and rape of women on the family context (Barnett & La Violette, 1993; Bergen, 1996; Gelles, 1997; Hampton et al, 1993; Lieblich & Josselson, 1994), the actual experience, the meaning of violence as seen through the eyes of its most innocent victims—children—has received little analysis and remains obscure. One possible reason for this lack of analysis lies in the persistence of the socially constructed roles of children as "property" of their parents. This perpetuates invisibility and silence of their experiences.

So how is it possible that families have been violent for centuries, all over the world, yet we have only recently discovered and attended to family violence as a serious social problem? Gelles (1997:12) describes the myths and controversies that have hindered our understanding of family violence and subsequent sufferings as a result of such violence.

- Family and intimate violence is a significant social and public health problem but not an inevitable aspect of family relations.
- Family violence is confined to mentally disturbed or sick people.
- Family violence is confined to the lower class.
- Family violence occurs in all groups—social factors are not relevant.
- Children who are abused will grow up to be abusers.
- Battered wives "like" being hit and/or are responsible for the violence; otherwise they would leave.

- Alcohol and drug abuse are the real causes of violence in the home.
- Violence and love do not coexist in families.
- Violence is usually visible.

Perhaps one of the most enduring problems in the study of family violence has been the difficulty in developing useful, clear, and acceptable definitions of violence and abuse. Ultimately, this difficulty is due to varying cultural views on whether behavior is or is not acceptable. In any culture, children should not have to live in fear or as objects of anger.

In order for family violence to be prevented, fundamental changes in values and beliefs must be reflected upon and critiqued. Gelles (1997:166) proposes some policy steps that could help prevent intimate family violence.

- Eliminate the norms that legitimize and glorify violence in the society and in the family.
- Reduce violence-producing stress caused by society.
- Integrate families into a network of kin and community.
- Change the sexist character of society.
- Break the cycle of violence in the family.

Such steps require long-term changes in the makeup of our society. Such fundamental changes in family life and families are often resisted. Ironically, the alternative is that in not making such changes, the harmful and deadly tradition of family violence continues.

When the Bough Breaks, the Cradle Does Fall

That violence is visible is perhaps the most dangerous assumption. I am a living example that not all violence is visible. It is the invisible violence that worries me. Of course, obviously abused and neglected children deserve and need a voice, immediate protection, comfort, and love. However, the label itself, "abused children," is biasing. It presumes a universal knowing of abuse.

Distance from oneself, others, and experiences can kill. Distance almost killed me emotionally, spiritually, physically—in every way that a human being can be killed. Thankfully, my faith in God and the sustained, unconditional loving presence of another who recognized my pain—my therapist and friend—saved me from being lost in that distance.

Creating life and loving my boys is my passion. They are the core of my strength. Although I was abused as well as a child, I did what I was told to do and kept quiet. I was a good girl and swallowed my feelings so as not to make anyone else uncomfortable. I sacrificed my visibility for my family and to keep peace in the family. When I did that, I stopped being a person and became an object to my family. The person, however, was there all along. I screamed to be seen and fought to stay alive, all alone for many years. Deep down, I wished that I was dead at times. Forcing me to silence damaged my spirit, my innocence, my unconditional trust, and I hated my parents for that. Equally and unconsciously, I hated myself. I remember wishing that someone would save me. Meanwhile, I learned to survive, but at tremendous cost. I kept my secret buried, but over the years it slowly eroded my spirit.

Left unattended, secrets can kill (Munhall, 1995). Individuals in great pain often experience their own bodies as the agents of this anguish. This acknowledgment or awareness can produce self-hatred, self-alienation, and self-betrayal. These emotions are often projected onto others. The world is one distortion. There is a distancing of self that can grow from experiences of separation, shame, and stigma. This distancing is unhealthy and unsafe. Secrets lose their power when they are revealed in a safe therapeutic environment where unconditional and nonjudgmental love can be found. My experience of child abuse changed me forever. It was my initiation into the existence of evil in the world. No child should have to face evil. Every child deserves unconditional love and protection. I remind myself of this each time I think of my four boys.

Through the Cracked Looking Glass

There is nothing positive about enduring violence. Surviving violence, however, is positive and shows strength, insight, and the willingness not to give up. There is nothing positive about feeling invisible. There is no reward or sense of pride for having lived through violence. Further, the quality of that existence is a form of suffering. It is often distance. Suffering people do cope, live, and go on in life. I did. I just didn't know to what extent the violence that I experienced as a child had affected my life as an adult. That is also suffering. It takes strength to endure suffering; therefore, I believe that all individuals enduring violence are strong. Any form of violence, however defined, is a form of suffering, though the responses remain precious subjective interpretations of those who suffer. I have spent much time attending to suffering. Much of this suffering is related to what I perceive as violence and violation, betrayal, the objectification of one as an object of another's or one's own anger, and the subsequent invisibility and alienation of self. If there is anything positive from suffering violence, it is my desire to reach out and help others. I have acquired understanding in a most difficult way, but that understanding cannot, I believe, be learned in textbooks, or through a medical model or behavioral approach. I want to help others heal. In doing so, I will also continue to heal.

Experiencing violence can be compared to a partial dying. It is painful to experience a dying human being. It is painful for a human being to die. It is a distant and lasting suffering without the presence of another. Violence is a loss that can be made bearable when we are not alone in the experience. There is less distance. Throughout my life, I have been very aware and sensitive to distance and the need for authentic presence. Both are important in offering comfort to those who suffer and in impacting family violence. Although our understandings of family violence are unique and contextually interpreted, the connection created within the experience of another's authentic presence is everlasting. Its effects are even more powerful. I am living proof of it. I keep that in mind with my four boys, remembering that they are unique human beings whose interpretations of suffering through their perceived sense of violence in whatever context that may arise, at the very least, deserves and receives my acknowledgment and love.

WASTING AWAY IN MARGARITAVILLE

For the past 11 years I have been told that I am loved by someone who has hurt me, who continues to hurt me. I married a recovering alcoholic, sober for 13 years now, who had also been a victim of child abuse. Unfortunately for both of us, he remains in denial about his own abuse and the abuse he has inflicted on me. My husband found me at a time when I was vulnerable and in need of comfort. In the beginning, he was comforting and charming, but we married too soon. If I had seen any sign of violence at all, I would have run in the other direction, but that was not the case. As the result of feeling unworthy of love as an abused child, I ended up in an abusive marital relationship as an adult and encountered several abusive people in my various work environments. There were times when I felt like a magnet for abuse. However, it is important to understand that none of this was conscious at the time. It has only been through intense and continual self-reflection that much of these connections became a part of my awareness.

One way or another, my husband always beat me down and won. He beat me for years, but mostly they were silent beatings. I understand now that it is absolutely possible to beat someone to the point where they are broken and barely alive, yet leave them with seemingly no visible signs of the beatings. Nevertheless, I believe that all beatings are visible if one looks deep enough beneath the surface. I was mostly beaten inside, and there were times when I felt barely alive because of it, but I have also been beaten outside. I am just good at ducking and hiding.

Since I was an adolescent at least, I always believed that my intuition was strong. I trust it. I also questioned everything, so I suppose that habit of mine annoyed my parents. It was easier for them if I just did what I was told to do without any analysis of the request. Now I can see how I did the same with my husband. One might think it cowardly. I considered it survival. Feeling invisible, being unheard as a child made me afraid and kept me quiet. Being quiet became a reflex, like breathing. No one around me, family or colleagues at work, had any idea what I lived with at home. I had been well trained in the art of secrecy. Over the years, I was brainwashed into feeling like I was someone's property. I think that falls into the category of slavery. The mental control he had over me was powerful to fight and wore me out. He made me doubt myself often. I hated that feeling.

He has often told me that he "doesn't want to hurt me." Maybe he really means what he says. I just wish he could say that he *won't* hurt me. I would feel much more secure, but not relaxed. Words can be empty. I was always kept in suspense with his allusions to revenge when he was hurt by someone. My husband's control over me was pervasive, yet he saw none of it. He always perceived events or others as trying to control him. Virtually everything I did had to be corrected, edited, or negated. Nothing I did was ever good enough or "right" (does any of this sound familiar?). He had to change everything I did. He would have liked to change me. None of this is what the public sees. Most of the people with whom he works believe him to be a nice guy, caring and even funny. In those contexts, he is. But he is not nice to me. How can I fight that illusion? Public persona is powerful and frightening. It is another form of silencing. That ability to silence can be deadly.

For most of my marriage I lived in fear of my husband. When I allow myself the luxury, I often dream of what it will be like to live without fear, to come home relaxed and free. For now, I come home knowing that I will be criticized, scrutinized, interrogated, ignored, or pursued relentlessly about where I have been, where I am going, why I need to go, or how much I am spending. I am questioned about how long I have been gone and why I needed to be gone so long. I live with someone who takes paper towels out of the garbage and lays them out on the counter to dry and reuse, then gives me a lecture on how wasteful I am. I live with someone who rearranges the dishwasher after I load it because I don't know how to do it the right way. I live with someone who tells me I am only good for doing laundry, ridicules my love for books and reading, yells at me for being "stupid" when I forget to save the water in which the potatoes were boiled or the vegetables cooked. If I sit down for a minute, I am accused of being lazy.

My husband mostly speaks about what he doesn't have, what he could have had, or what he can't do. He is a negative and regretful person who also suffers. He suffers from unawareness. He is an all-or-nothing thinker who views compromise as "giving up." When he gets angry I cannot predict his response. Usually he twists everything around so that it is my fault. He rarely admits responsibility for any of his actions. Nothing is ever his fault. It is always because of me or something or someone else that he comes to feel or act a certain way. I don't have that kind of power and I don't want it either.

I can't reconcile my feelings of fear, intimidation, and anger at his presence. My husband always denies being angry. How can he never be angry? I know that I get angry and I don't deny it. I may excuse my anger, but being angry isn't easy. It can be scary. For me, I have to get the thought out of my head that if I am angry, something bad will happen to me. That has been reinforced through years of abuse. Whenever I was angry, something bad *did* happen to me. My husband lives in a world of extremes. There is anger, peace, and nothing in between. So if I disagree with him or protest a decision he made, he perceives it as me trying to control him, and he gets angry. Results of his anger have varied over the years. I remember once I had the nerve to raise my voice to him, and I was hit for it. During an argument, I was trapped in a bathroom and slapped across the face repeatedly. My head vibrated from the contact. What I remember most is how much my head hurt. I had a terrible headache for most of the night and my face was swollen the next morning. He had looked like a wild animal to me. I had never seen anyone so angry. I had never been so frightened in my life. I thought that he was going to kill me. Of course, he tried to downplay the whole incident. He told me that he didn't hit me that hard, even though my lip was bleeding, I felt dizzy, and my face was numb. I remember feeling grateful for the numbness.

What worries me is that I believe that he felt he had the right to hit me, that it was justified. As sick as it sounds, I also believe that, unconsciously, he enjoyed having the power over me at the time. I felt and was helpless. I was very pregnant at the time and my mobility was not very good. He told me to shut up as he hit me and I did. Sometimes, when I close my eyes I can see the expression on his face at the time. I can't forget that experience. I can't forgive it either. I don't want to anymore.

I have tried to impress upon my husband how much terror he has caused me over the years. He always responds by saying that he never wanted to hurt me, that I made him angry and caused the situations in the first place, and he wishes that he hadn't been forced to hit me. He says that he was just trying to get my attention, that he never meant to hurt me, and didn't believe that he had hurt me that much anyway. I guess losing two daughters is not hurt enough for him. I told him that fear and intimidation are not appropriate ways to get someone's attention, but that he had my attention now. Never once has he admitted responsibility or remorse for hurting me. Never has he told the children, who witnessed the violence, that he was wrong to hit me and that hitting is wrong in any context. How can a person live without remorse? I guess the better question is, how could I live with a person who didn't have any remorse? Lessons that I had learned as a child, that silence and distance were rewarded, kept me a prisoner of my own abuse. Fear has been an effective form of discipline. I also kept hanging on because I was raised in a strict Catholic home that espoused marriage until death. I never realized how much power there is in such social constructions. They are hard to change. Guilt was also an effective form of discipline and regulation with me. My husband insists that he has very logical reasons for his actions. The new phone on the wall is a constant reminder. The old one was destroyed by his throwing it across the room in a fit of rage. To me, he just defends and justifies his violence toward me. He is the one person with whom distance feels comfortable.

I believe that our marriage was over the first time he hit me, the first time he humiliated me in public, the first time he chose work over me when he didn't have to make that choice. Our marriage has been over since I lost Nicole and Emily. I know that technically he did not kill them, but in my mind he had a hand in their fate. Whenever I bring up the subject, my husband tells me that I was selfish, that I should forget about what I don't have and appreciate what I do have, my four healthy sons. I love my boys—they are my life—but I miss my twins too. I tried to forget about them once, but they won't have it anymore. They will not be ignored and I don't want to ignore them either. What my husband and others cannot understand is my experience of emptiness, of one minute being full of life and the next having that life ripped from me.

There are times when I think that I am living with two husbands. One is perfectly unassuming, pleasant, even charming in public. The other is obsessive-compulsive, rigid, judgmental, a perfectionist, intolerant, volatile, intimidating, and a chronic victim in his own eyes. No one sees that person except me. He questions and watches everything I do and how I do it. I am always corrected, criticized, or taught the "right" way, which is his way of doing anything. I cannot relax in my own home. I am on constant guard for the next attack. Sometimes it is difficult for me, let alone anyone else, to believe what I have endured. Abuse is a private hell.

I would have to say that my emotional abuse has been greater than the physical abuse. It slowly chipped away my self-esteem, which has required much rebuilding. I never thought that I would let anyone treat me in such a way or do the things that my husband has done to me, but I did. His words and actions mixed with my mother's and reinforced the effects of their abuse of me. On the feeling level, it hurts to the very core of my being. I have begun to replace the experiences of abuse with experiences of care and love. At the same time, I remember to always show my boys love and compassion for those who suffer and provide them with a safe place.

Fumbling Toward Freedom

I was once told that there would be a time when I would scream. In truth, I was screaming for years and in all that time, among all the people I have come to know as friends, colleagues, acquaintances, only one person heard me. Maybe it is my fault for not screaming loud enough. It is hard to speak loud and clear when you are choking on fear and are beaten and wounded inside and out. Over time, my voice became almost inaudible. I was disappearing in every way possible. I felt lost and unheard. I don't feel either anymore. There is much comfort for me in knowing that I have been heard. I have been heard by a therapist I consider as a friend more than as a therapist. It has made my suffering endurable. What kept my screams silent for so long was the fear that no one would believe me—no one would believe in me. How could someone so formally educated be in this situation? How many others are screaming while no one hears a thing? It is a horrifying feeling to be calling out for help, hanging on to hope for dear life, and continue to feel yourself disappearing. To the extent humanly possible, I try very hard to listen for those silent screams. I know them well. I will continue to find ways to make the invisible visible. Most important, I won't give up on those women and children who suffer family violence. I know that they expect to remain unseen, unheard, and untouched. They expect that others will give up on them. Many have already given up on themselves. I almost did. In that expectation is despair and tremendous suffering. I have experienced it as a nurse and I have felt it in my own life. I have come to understand that making the invisible visible requires a complete commitment of self, a closeness and a willingness to be vulnerable shrouded in unconditional love and care that, although always ethically respectful, cannot be edited at will. In the closing of distance, trust builds and healing begins.

Sometimes we can best help others by remembering that what we believe about them may be reflected back to them in our own presence and affect them in ways we do not fully understand. Similarly, the places where we are genuinely seen and heard are sacred and important places to us. They remind us of our value as human beings. They give us the strength to go on. Eventually, they may even help us to transform suffering into wisdom.

Closeness is what heals and allows for the possibility of greater understanding, empathy, and humanness. In order to truly understand, I believe that we must immerse ourselves in the world of those who suffer family violence and let them teach its realities. It is only through realness and the capacity to endure the intensity of a prolonged empathetic connection, with all its inherent ordeals, that those who suffer find comfort and those who comfort begin to understand their experience. We must engage in experiential knowing.

The greatest gift we bring to anyone who is suffering is our wholeness. Listening is a powerful tool of healing. It is often in the quality of our listening, not in the wisdom of our words, that we are able to effect the most profound changes in the people around us. When we listen, we offer an opportunity for wholeness with our attention. Our listening creates a sanctuary for the homeless parts within the suffering individual. That which has been denied, unloved, devalued by themselves and by others, that which has been hidden, can find comfort in our silence and simple presence.

Healing suffering begins with our being real with ourselves and others and having the courage to communicate our realness without preconditions or assumptions; it is giving ourselves without boundaries. It is only through closeness and greater awareness that we can hope to create with those who suffer strategies that impact the effects of family violence and to alleviate suffering in a sensitive, ethically reverent, and effective manner. For it is in our communication with others that suffering surrenders its abstract anonymity and acquires a human face. Abstractions of a universal phenomenon, no matter how artfully described, cannot equal its existential reality in a human life. Theoretical concepts can only be theoretically correct. They cannot capture the richness and uniqueness of the individual experience. Assigning sterile labels to the struggles of those who suffer seems, at best, distance; at worst, it is a betrayal of our humanity.

References

Barnett, O. W., and La Violette, A. D. (1993). *It Could Happen to Anyone: Why Battered Women Stay.* Newbury Park, Calif.: Sage Publications.

Bergen, R. K. (1996). *Wife Rape.* Thousand Oaks, Calif.: Sage Publications.

Gelles, R. J. (1997). *Intimate Violence in Families,* 3rd ed. Thousand Oaks, Calif.: Sage Publications.

Hampton, R. L., Gullotta, T. P., Potter, E. H., and Weissberg, R. P. (eds.). (1993). *Family Violence: Prevention and Treatment.* Newbury Park, Calif.: Sage Publications.

Lieblich, A., and Josselson, R. (eds.). (1994). *Exploring Identity and Gender: The Narrative Study of Lives.* Thousand Oaks, Calif.: Sage Publications.

Munhall, P. L. (ed.). (1995). *In Women's Experience,* vol. 2. New York: National League for Nursing Press.

CHAPTER 26

CANCER OF VIOLENCE: POWER DIFFERENTIALS AND FAMILY VALUES

Patricia L. Munhall

We've just celebrated the 30th anniversary of Earth Day, even though we continue to exploit our land, waters, and air. We continue to deplete limited natural resources. However, progress on the condition of the environment was noted and accolades given to those who are working diligently on these conditions in the natural environment.

I can worry about just so many things at any given time. As far as the environment is concerned, I believe we need to expand our conceptualization of it and prioritize what is most important.

My worry is not so much the trees, soil, water, and air as what it is that keeps people out of this natural environment, behind locked doors, off public transportation, out of parks, and living in a state of fear. My worry is about a "cancer of violence." Like cancer, violence comes when we are least aware, when we thought we took proper precautions, when we are trying to convince ourselves that "it" could not be happening to us. The suddenness, the unpredictable event, or the predictable event we were denying could happen—like cancer, violence, dark, scary, lurks in the micro and the macro environments.

This paper is on the cancer of violence as it affects women in particular. This cancer is pervasive in the world and calls on us to respond swiftly. We cannot bury our heads in the sand. Some may be survivors of violence, but many women have not survived. The survivors bear scars, have nightmares, and carry a lack of trust.

This is not meant to scare you; most women and men are already scared. I hope to raise your consciousness of a critical women's health problem and an environmental, social, and cultural bloodbath—in Burundi, in Rwanda, in Mozambique, in Nigeria, in Bangladesh, Cambodia, Afghanistan, and most

---

Adapted from Munhall, Patricia L. and Fitzsimons, Virginia M. *The Emergence of Women into the 21st Century*. New York: NLN Press. 1995.

recently in Kosovo. Since World War II, 23 million people have died in 150 wars. *One* unnecessary death or act of violence is a tragedy and a travesty.

Today I am writing of other war zones, the "cancer of violence" and women. Women were killed and raped in those 150 wars. The hellish accounts of women's rapes in Bosnia and Kosovo still haunt me. Some were then killed or their children and families were taken from them. And the same phenomenon happens to women in a silent war zone—often their own home, often their office, often their own neighborhood.

Every day, every hour, every minute, a woman in this country is violently assaulted. Every 6 minutes a woman is raped. Spouse abuse is more common than automobile accidents, muggings, and cancer deaths combined (U.S. Senate Judiciary Committee, 1992). When we recast this problem into a women's health problem, we now see a disease that affects 3 to 4 million women. Not only do we have a major *health* problem, but a major *crime* problem that receives little attention, unless it involves a celebrity. Those who keep statistics on these kinds of crimes often discount them as trivial domestic squabbles. Yet, one third of all female homicide victims are killed by their husbands or boyfriends (FBI, 1990).

I would like to share a story about a friend of mine. I'll call her Nancy. You may have a similar friend or you may share some of her story. None of this is fictitious except her name. Nancy was severely physically and psychologically abused as a child, though not sexually that she can remember. She grew up with little self-worth or feeling of safety. Though paradoxical, because her father never protected her, she married to feel safe. Her husband brutalized her, forcibly raped her (just recently declared a crime), hit her, and verbally demoralized her at every turn. *Battered woman* was not a term known at that time, though I do remember her calling the police when she feared for her life. She was told they could not do anything until something actually happened.

Eventually she left him. She left him because she believed it was harming the children. Living at this time with a shattered ego, she could not leave to protect herself. Around this time, the term *dysfunctional family* came into vogue and divorce was commonplace. Nancy had a mental health problem from her childhood and was still pretty much doomed, which is part of the tragedy of domestic violence.

Nancy had lived in a fortress, feeling trapped, sensing suffocation and impending doom, but not entirely a victim. Still attempting to survive, she was caught up in the huge power differential that is the earmark of violence against women.

Nancy was able to leave, but she was scarred. It was not long before she found herself in another abusive relationship. This is all too common; it is part of a cycle of demoralization and dehumanization that continues until someone helps the woman help herself. This situation does not respond to rational explanations. The perceptions of an abused child or woman are so distorted that they become part of the damage. Once again abused, depressed, feeling worthless, she lived in a dungeon of debasement and powerlessness. Nancy had one night that I want to tell you about because she is fairly normal in every other aspect. But it tells you about violence and the powerful and unbelievable collusion of men to maintain power. Nancy eventually left this man. One night she was sitting at an outdoor café in Greenwich Village and he came up out of nowhere and hit her hard across the face, while shouting obscenities at her. A man came to her rescue. The old boyfriend went to her place, broke into it, and rampaged through it, while the hero sat and consoled the visibly shaken Nancy, whose eye was beginning to swell. Her hero took her back to her place and she said goodnight, but he said he would feel better if he saw her into her apartment. He then proceeded to rape her. He did not see this as rape, although she said no. He thought in his powerful way that it would actually be good for her.

In these instances, the women are often blamed. People ask what is wrong with her? Few ask *what is wrong with these men*? A 1992 report by the Senate Judiciary Committee revealed that women aren't just shoved and slapped. "They are beaten with fists, burned with cigarettes, scalded, slammed against walls, dragged by the hair, hit with hammers, broomsticks and gun butts, pushed out of moving cars, run down by cars, sexually assaulted, strangled, stabbed and shot—*by men they know best*."

What women are contending with is the recognized or unrecognized, conscious or unconscious, use of violence as the maintenance of power—the power differential. It's old, but it's still with us and it seems to be coming back in insidious ways that we all must be on guard against. Men's superior strength and control over economic resources still hold women hostage. Throughout the world, women who refuse their husbands sexual intercourse are raped or, worse, killed. And we talk of women's sexual autonomy and reproductive freedom. According to the World Health Organization, more than 84 million women alive today have undergone sexual surgery in Africa alone (Rushwan, 1990).

What about this power differential? In the legislature of this country a bill called the Violence Against Women Act went into committee in 1990 and came out of committee in May 1993. What does that tell us? Anita Hill relates her story and the all-white male Senate Judiciary Committee sits stonefaced, quietly reinforcing our understanding about who controls the rules for social discourse. How precarious is the future for the woman who dares to speak aloud? Anita Hill gave public language to repeated experiences of sexual harassment in the workplace. For this she is called self-serving, a destructive, vindictive woman.

Power has always been an intricate part of women's oppression. This we know. Collusion among men has reinforced the power of power. The use of words spoken by women to the holders of power are conveniently suppressed or marginalized. But that is the power men possess and use—and they know it and they are not going to give it up until there are enough resources to resocialize them and develop a male consensus against the suppression or marginalization of women. A major consciousness raising is essential here as well as severe prosecution for these crimes.

We are walking on land mines. They are on the streets of our cities and the floors of our homes. They are most often planted by men . . . in our minds. Some men are outraged by violence toward women. They would never, and this is said as though it is a virtue, "raise a hand against a woman." Is this not still part of their context, of their power? Paradoxically, women also need the power to protect them. Women need men in order to feel safe. Each time a woman is assaulted this becomes reinforced for the unassaulted woman. The land mines: do not go out at night; do not go out without me to protect you; ask my permission and I will ascertain if you will be safe. And on it goes. The powerful then protects the weaker, at least the one perceived to be physically weaker. Men actually believe this at home, certainly in the office and in society.

That is the *power differential*. Now I must refer to something very closely related to that—something that we as women and good men want to watch very closely and analyze—*the return to family values*.

Let me tell you about a patient I have who today still suffers greatly. Lisa was sexually abused as a child by her father. She was also physically abused, and, of course, her perceptions of the world are so altered that the sequences of her adult life have brought her close to death on several occasions. This is not uncommon for adults with this history. Lisa believes she deserved this. She was the oldest of four children and in a way took her mother's place. Her mother was an alcoholic and Lisa had to assume responsibility for her siblings. She cooked, cleaned, and took care of the household. The role reversal that we now know about is very apparent in these kinds of homes. By outside appearances this was an "intact" family. Lisa had nowhere to go and her survival depended on this. After all, she really was a child.

In my clinical practice and in my personal life, I have encountered enough fallout from the so-called traditional family that the thought of returning to this condition (family values) that existed before the 1960s is frightening. The most frightening aspect of such a return is its hypocrisy—the secrets that were the most intricate part of the maintenance of the appearance of the family. Of all the myriad secrets to keep, the most important were incest and child abuse. The abuse, because of the threat of power differentials and lies, had to be kept secret. Because of a no-way-out scenario, the secrecy makes it possible for the abuse to continue. Other family secrets are parental alcoholism and the battered women.

Returning to family values is to return to keeping secrets and allowing abuse to continue. Also, I suspect that a return to family values is a return to the patriarchal family, and loyalty is the penvitimate family value.

Society has not become violent because of a loss of family values. We now know more about family violence because we opened the Pandora's box of family secrets. This is incredibly important. We abandoned the idea of loyalty in exchange for mental health. What a step backward into mental illness and women's oppression and other scary possibilities under this rubric of family values. This is not political posturing or an ideological statement. When professionals began to look beneath the appearance to what was concealed, healthy action could be taken. Today a child is encouraged to come forth if someone is doing something that does not feel right. Women are encouraged to seek help and, when they are ready, go to a shelter and save their lives and do better for their family in the long run. If a parent has a drug problem, a child is encouraged to seek help for herself in this situation. Where does a child learn violence, prejudice, or hate? These are not family values and neither is patriarchy. Incest is not a family value. Drunkenness is not a family value. *Father Knows Best* is a work of fiction—so might be family values. If there is love and respect, no one will argue. But we must be ever vigilant about loyalty and the toll it takes on women and children. We opened up the family. Let us keep it open for the protection of the least powerful.

All I have shared with you is aimed toward empowering women and understanding the meaning of violence in our lives. War zones are where the powerful demoralize and dehumanize the less powerful. Women have enormous strength, but they must have places to say the unsaid, and women must feel safe. We cannot go backward. We must continue to move forward. Our consciousness is sometimes raised through tragic experience. Women must raise the consciousness of men. We are all—men and women alike—affected by the rape of women and girls. Men need to know that they are intimately related by blood to women. Power is power. Do they want someone to use that power on the women of their blood, on the women whom they care about? Let us keep the family of humans open to values that are about survival and the quality of existence.

Dialogues have started. Bills have been passed. It will take a lot more—I hope not with more bloodshed in the home, in our cities, in the country, in the world, but I am not naive. The power differential must shift. We must be very vigilant to its various appearances and attempts to maintain itself. We must critically analyze this concept of family values. And we must allocate greater funding for a war against violence: the growth of this deadly cancer. In fact, a war against violence is an oxymoron. We must allocate greater funding to find ways to channel violent energy toward working for peace. How many times must it be said? How many women must be degraded? How many women and children must die? To answer this question we must continue our work. We must be heard around the world.

VOICES NINE

Reflecting on Family in the 21st Century

Kimberly Jones wrote this to her mother along her journey toward independence. Or did she write it to herself?

Apples and Oranges (Conversation with Mom, #2)

Some days the idea of packing an overnight bag and hopping a plane to New York seems like a viable option for rejuvenating life. Other days it doesn't. That's when I want to drive. On those odd Tuesdays, I shy away from racking up frequent-flyer miles. I think about how it's only a five-day car trip from the Sunshine State to the Big Apple.

My mother doesn't understand my fascination with New York. She sees used condoms, sullied syringes, and overpriced hamburgers. I tell her to "go down to South Beach and you'll see the same thing, only the majority of the residents will be out-of-the-closet homosexuals rather than rude, fast-talking New Yorkers."

Lately we've been discussing college. I see NYU, in my future, in all the bright lights of naïve Broadway starlets. Nowhere else can better prepare me for the cutting of bureaucratic red tape, power trips, rush hour, and spilled coffee that the rest of adulthood is. I see fantastic English programs, top-of-the-line journalism, and theater so exquisite even Patrick Stewart is awed. I see the chance to be a *wonderfully unique* individual so that I blend into a crowd of people who don't care that I'm *wonderfully unique* 'cause they have a subway train to get in five minutes.

"Why NYU? Why so far away? You have a $24,000 scholarship to the University of Florida. It's a good school, ya know." Why anything if not New York? This is my future. And what sort of future lies in *Gainesville*?

I need bohemia, independence, a chance to actually cultivate my artistic talent, maybe discover that I have no writing talent and my high school attempts at being a poet were only catered to because everybody decided I *was* a poet.

I need to test my talent in a place where if you suck, they have no qualms about spitting on your soul and kicking you out the back door.

I need forced reality, the chance to learn that everything isn't handed to you on a silver platter and being spoiled isn't a perk I'll get anymore when allowances don't flow in and the electricity gets turned off, 'cause my waitressing job will only bring in enough money to pay for the walls of my apartment and my college tuition.

They say that people don't use exterminators in New York 'cause if you killed all the bugs, there'd be nothing left to hold the roof up.

In my opinion, if I make the five-and-a-half-hour trek to Gainesville, I will end up longing for a guy I've been mooning over for three years already, clutching the same group of dorky, reliable friends, making deadlines and writing crappy poetry about unrequited love till I end up a spinster in Montana with six cats and a dog named Hood, after my English teacher in 11th grade.

I told her this, one day in the midst of the 769th argument regarding my undecided COLLEGE PLANS. Her response was a blank expression, then "Get real," she said, brevity being the soul of wit and all, ending the conversation once more.

I've already packed up my room for what to take with me when I leave in six months. Pinky, the stuffed rabbit, is staying home, but my books, knee-high boots, and signed copy of *little earthquakes* are mentally boxed up for the 3 hour plane trip (or car ride, depending on who you talk to).

I don't want to spend the next four years recreating my high school experience in a small town filled with people whose faces I've already cataloged—people who have a predisposed image of *who* I *am, what* I *am, and what* I'*m meant to be*.

I want to be thrust, gloriously naked (figuratively, of course), into a 30-degree winter street, facing the cold with a wary smile and a blank book prepared to catch the shavings of my craft as I whittle away at my old style and discover my womanhood amidst cab fares and 24-hour coffeehouses.

Besides, the University of Florida is number three in hard liquor consumption. Does my mom really want the nearest quickie-stop package store to be the first number on my speed-dial?

I think the homeless bums and reckless creativity of NYC are safer in comparison to drunken frat boys and lost virginity.

And in New York, in the place where all the movies are set and songs are sung—where they're proud of the crime rate and rudeness—I'll be able to look out my dorm window and scream, "I'm a woman and I don't know what I want." The neighbors will scream a reply: "Shut up. It's four in the morning." And I will close my window smiling at the loneliness of it all.

—*kimberly jones*

CHAPTER 27

THE AMERICAN WAY THROUGH HAZEL EYES: A LOOK AT THE CARIBBEAN BLACK FAMILY

Sandra E. Gibson

I am going to take you on a journey through our family experience. An experience filled with sight, sounds, colors, customs, rituals, and language that brings personal meaning to the rich blend of Black Caribbean life that is my heritage.

MY STORY IS HISTORY

I am challenged in this chapter to explore the similarities of African-American and Caribbean family traditions. As I carry you on this journey, I ask myself, Where do the two meet? Some of my African ancestors entered the United States as slaves. They had been transported to the New World from West Africa during the 18th century to work on cotton plantations (Dow, 1995). Their bondage, which lasted through the Civil War, prompted the creation of many African-American families in the New World. In order to survive, these families were forced to integrate African and New World customs and values. Some of my[1] ancestors were brought to the Bahamas as slaves at the end of the 1700s when their Loyalist masters were expelled from the American colonies. This influx increased the number of slaves in the Bahamas to approximately 6,000, double the white population at that time.

With the decline in the cotton trade and the emancipation of slaves in the Bahamas in 1838, a few departing plantation owners gave land to their former slaves. They worked hard to bring agricultural vitality and prosperity back to the islands. However, it wasn't until after World War II that the grandchildren of the emancipated slaves began to experience economic stability through alliances with military, industrial, and tourist groups.

[1]The Caribbean ancestry is from the Bahamas. My African ancestry brought me to the Bahamas which is termed Afro-Caribbean.

In the United States

By contrast, the emancipation of the slaves in the United States in 1863 did not bring economic, political, and social stability to African Americans. Bahamians and African Americans both experienced varying periods of migration throughout their countries in an attempt to find work and prosperity, but African American, seemed to experience more obstacles to economic and educational freedom (Bigelow 1995).

Over a million Afro-Caribbeans have moved to the United States since the 1800s. Throughout this transition they were able to hold onto much of the cultural and ethnic customs of their homelands while pursuing the "good life" in the United States. I think this is where I experience much of the confusion—when I look at the African-American experience through the Caribbean experience—through hazel eyes.

Looking at Black Bahamian families is like looking at a melting pot of cultures. The hazel eyes of my Caribbean brothers and sisters represent a blending of race, color, customs, and traditions. I believe that it is wonderful to blend the beauty of diversity and expand our growth from the similarities and differences we find.

Specifically, the two groups (Bahamian Caribbean & Afro-American) probably both had a sense of excitement about coming to a new land that had a reputation for freedom and prosperity, but the entry and recovery process was so different for each group. As we all know, first impressions are extremely important, and these two groups certainly had initial impressions of the "American Way" that clouded their perception and adjustment.

Me

I am of Afro-Caribbean descent and a member of the baby-boomer generation. I grew up in the civil rights period, a time of racial unrest and the birth of affirmative action.

My parents and their friends have many stories about the Bahamian community. Many Bahamians settled in the area between Key West and Miami, especially in Overtown (the Black section of downtown Miami), Coconut Grove, Dana, Del Ray, and West Palm Beach. All of these areas became, and continue to be, havens for the Bahamian community. The first generation of Bahamian immigrants felt that the United States would be a gateway to increased prosperity, education, and independence, in other words, to the good life.

Although they came for the good life, many left a land that provided comfortable homes and family and friends who were a continual source of social support, beautiful surroundings, and emotional stability. It is amazing that such a close-knit group would risk the loss of family and friends for the unknown. However, from talking to a number of Bal-Bahamians, including my grandparents, I have formed these impressions. As a group, they tend to be fairly assertive and determined. The glamour of coming to someplace larger and filled with choices too numerous to count seemed to outweigh the relationships left behind. Also, trips back and forth to the Bahamas were frequent. As they strengthened their roots in the United States, they slowly brought back little bits and pieces with them and left souvenirs of Americanism in their homeland.

How We Are

What evolved in the United States were distinct communities that typified the familiar treasures of home. Today there are restaurants and small businesses from Key West to Miami that attract Bahamian descendants like a magnet, soothe the lonely, and fascinate the tourist.

Food and social gatherings are of particular significance. I cannot tell you how many pleasant gatherings have formed around a bowl of boiled fish and grits, with a piece of hot Johnny cake and sour (lime) on the side. A harvest from the sea prepared for friends is the champagne of life to the Bahamian. Conch, snapper, kingfish, crab, and lobster, accompanied by the proper side dishes, peas and rice, okra soup, homemade potato salad, couch fritters, with soursop ice cream and guava duff for dessert-these are more than enough to bring a smile to any self-respecting homie from Nassau.

Some Stories

I'd like to share a few stories with you about a group of Bahamian-Americans who immigrated to the United States in the 1940s and 1950s. They're a small group, but they are all friends, and a couple of them are relatives. All of them currently live in the United States after many years of commuting back and forth to the Bahamas. Most of them were born in the Bahamas, and all but four of their children spent their elementary school years in the Bahamas. The entire group are American citizens, including their children, and they meet regularly to socialize and sing the praises of "home." I admire all of them for their spirit, strength, and sense of humor. All of them have such enthusiasm for the Bahamas but equally as much pride in their American citizenship.

This special group meets after church every Sunday morning at Rose's house. They really are a family who know each other so well and seem to work for the comfort and each other's understanding. They take brief vacations apart in the form of church holidays, trips home, or weekend excursions around the country. They often travel together, and it's absolutely delightful to see these 50-, 60-, and 70-year-olds laughing with the kind of abandon that comes from sincere trust and love for each other.

I call them the "fish people." Rose fixes boiled fish and grits every Sunday just for this special group. They've been meeting for about three years now, and I suspect they will continue to meet, laugh, and eat together until they can no longer get around.

Tales of the Fish People

It all started when the church stopped having breakfast directly after service. The breakfasts were originally rotated by several women's groups within the church, but the details of shopping and cleaning up gradually became tedious. Rose was encouraged by her son and her husband to fix breakfast at home for her church friends, all of whom have ties to the Bahamas. The group offers a great deal of pleasure to its members, who laugh, and tell the old stories that they heard from their parents. Some of these stories are embellished, just for laughs.

Elliot's Way

Elliot formed a club from the members who regularly came to Rose's place. He wanted to form a club that was different from the Bahamian Federation and built on the American-Bahamian component of history. He called the club the Bahamian-American Culture Club (BACC). Elliot was the first president.

The BACC has a strong social purpose. It has Joke Night, entertainment for the college students from the Bahamas, a Boxing Day dance the day after Christmas, and numerous social get-togethers. Lately, the group has started to give donations to students to advance their education. The club was a dream for Elliot because he loved his heritage so much. He talked of how he was not accepted as a child by his peers because he was different, that is, from another country. He was teased for receiving a lot of praise from teachers, for knowing the answers to math and science questions. Elliot is retired now, but during his working years he was quite the education leader.

About a Name

Initially, there was resistance to the club's name because some in the group thought it would turn off those who were born and raised in the United States. The turning point came when one of the members noted that many of them were married to Americans who really did not know much about the Bahamas.

Several of the Bahamian men had American wives who were born and raised in the United States although several were of Bahamian descent. Historically, more Caribbean men than women came to the United States. This accounted for many mixed marriages between 1920 and 1930. Approximately 29,000 to 40,000 Black couples consisted of a foreign-born husband and an American wife (Ueda 1980).

Sara's World

Sara was a charter member of the BACC. Her cousin Alice invited her to join. It seemed like a cool idea because there were so many people who shared memories about the traditions and cultural habits of their parents and the difficulties of adjusting to groups that had no idea of the experiences you brought with you. All this meant a lot to Sara because it served as a link to her parents and her childhood. Sara did not grow up in the Bahamas, but she had many memories from Coconut Grove, the mecca of the Bahamian community.

The Grove was like a home away from home for Bahamians. Even today, if you walk down Grand Avenue, you can feel the Bahamas in the coconut trees that line the streets and the flamingo pink frame houses with conch shells in the front yards. If I close my eyes I can envision the excitement my forebears must have felt when they saw the beautiful coconut trees and the clear blue water around the marinas. I am sure they looked around and said, "This is the place!"

GOOMBAY

Every year there is a tremendous festival held in the Grove called Goombay. Goombay is the ultimate Bahamian-American celebration. It lasts for several days and includes dancing, music, and, of course, food, food, and more food.

Sara had memories of good times, and also of sad events that always turned into good times. She especially enjoyed the "rake-and-scrape" and the Junkanoos. The rake-and-scrape is an affair where everybody brings something to make noise with from home—spoons, washboards, cow bells, whistles, sticks. The whole idea is to scrape up something from home that you can easily make noise with, so you can join in with the Junkanoos.

The Junkanoos were directly from Nassau and dressed in very elaborate and beautiful costumes. Sara used to dance in the street with the Junkanoos when she was a little girl. The peak time for the Junkanoos is Christmas and New Year's Day. When the Junkanoos came to town, it was truly an event and continues to be so today. Nobody in the group could remember exactly when the Junkanoos started; they just said that they had always been around. They always brought such excitement to the town—music, competition, and beautiful elaborate costumes. Every member in the BACC had a special story about the Junkanoos and attended the annual dance in memory of the good times. Sara always had a good time with a cow bell and whistle in hand.

ALICE'S GRANDMOTHER

There are certain people in this life who live to be in charge. Bahamian women are known to be somewhat assertive. Alice got her attitude from her grandmother. She grew up listening to her grandmother, and learned to take charge just as her grandmother taught her. Her father was a Bahamian who married an American woman back in the 1920s. Her paternal grandmother was very influential in the family and would often say, "One ounce of blood and that's your cousin."

Alice's grandmother was involved in everything social, religious, and family. She was a generous and highly moral woman who ruled the house and was well respected in the neighborhood. She was a jack-of-all-trades, a good businesswoman, and devoted to sharing the finer things in life with her family.

Alice came from a large family and was the leader in the big house. She was considered a socialite. She knew everybody in town, attended all the important affairs, and coined the term *cousin* as an affectionate term to identify all her friends and associates. Alice frequently says how grateful she is for all her grandmother taught her and for having grown up in such a household. Alice has made the most of the American way. She knows that she has a lot of her grandmother in her.

Families

The families who came to the United States in the 1970s were middle and upper middle class—literate and well educated. Many of them were prominent in publishing, real estate, advertising, banking, insurance, and retail clothing. Families had high educational aspirations and emphasized hard work, saving, and investments (Garcia, 1986).

Several of the families noted that it was very important to help other family members and countrymen. One woman stated that "family was everything." Of course, Alice's grandmother, fondly called "Tika," ingrained in her family the belief that we were all cousins somehow. My friends sing the praises of their extended families. Many of the families lived with and took care of their parents, grandparents, and aunts. They were raised to feel that the elderly, especially their parents, should be well taken care of by their children. The parents were frequently referred to with great affection and commonly took care of the small children. The terms of affection or endearment used by Afro-American children and those of Carribean origin to address their family members, especially their parents, tend to ring with closeness and humor. Grandmothers, aunts, and guardians are called Nana, Madear, Mama, Goddie, and other terms of endearment.

The Culture of the Islands

Weddings, funerals, and church gatherings are among the most wonderful events one can attend in the Bahamian community. Weddings are fairly traditional events, filled with food, dancing, kisses, hugs, and the special rhythmic sounds of steel drums, horns, and guitars. Bahamians believe in very large weddings, even if they can't afford them. It is important to have the most elaborate affair possible. "Showing off" is expected, with as many of your friends attending as possible. It is traditionally the bride's day and it is expected that the bride's parents will bear most of the expense. However, today the bride and groom often share the expense.

The tradition of marriage holds many similarities for Black Americans striving to start a family. The wedding is thought of as a very sacred, usually flamboyant event with all the attention and accessories that time and personal budget will allow. Black-American marriages have taken on a more European flair with time and increasing economic and employment status.

Ellwood and Crane (1990) have found that significantly fewer African-American men and women were choosing to be married, but certainly not to be childless. Younger Afro-American women are choosing to become mothers outside of wedlock. One reason for this is the lack of available Black men. Statistically, there are approximately 81 Black men to every 100 Black women. This makes mating with the same race almost impossible. In addition, when the variables of homosexuality, lack of education, and unemployment are added to the mix, one can see that marriage is very problematic in this period.

Organized Religion

Religion, defined as a higher spiritual power, has always been at the center of African-American and Caribbean family life. Faith in God is typically seen as an extremely powerful tool. Spiritual status is thought to directly affect one's own plight in life, prosperity, happiness, peace, and health. A large majority of Black Americans are Baptist, Episcopalian, Pentecostal, and Presbyterian. However, religious affiliations certainly run the gamut. Generally, it is considered imperative to attend worship service on Sunday and participate in the associated activities that enhance the service, such as choir and scripture readings.

Most African-American services are filled with joyful singing led by youth and adult choirs, ushers, praise teams, well-rehearsed soloists, and a call-and-response style of prayer and singing that invites active participation from the congregation.

The hierarchy within the church is usually very structured, with the minister in a revered place of honor. The minister is frequently given monetary gifts and recognition by the church members. It is not unusual for the minister to be very active in the community as a political leader, and to freely share his views in the pulpit. The family of the minister is also held in high esteem, and the son or daughter who decides to pursue the ministry as a career brings a great deal of pride to the family.

It is preferred that a minister be married. The church members generally pay the minister's salary, maintain a home or rectory, make weekly donations toward the maintenance of church utilities, and make special offerings for the minister and his wife and for various groups throughout the year.

Bahamian Americans are also Christian and have a similar allegiance to their ministers and to the ongoing financial and educational activities of the ministry. Dow (1995) explains that three realms of the supernatural can be identified when exploring Bahamian religious beliefs: God helps the faithful and punishes the wicked; the spirit of the person who dies "in Christ" can go to rest and help the living; if an ungodly person dies, the spirit wanders about, frightening and hurting people.

Church services in the Bahamas are especially festive and dramatic on holidays. On Palm Sunday, Easter, and Christmas the mood is joyful. You have not lived until you have walked through the streets with palm in hand, the pastor and band leading the way. The sounds of cultural and spiritual pride can be heard for blocks.

Of Hats and Funerals

Easter Sunday is a big hat event! A great deal of time and money are spent on hats. Your hat must match your outfit perfectly. In Nassau, the tradition of wearing a hat is still quite prevalent. However, it is a tradition that has not stood the test of time in the United States.

Funerals are a mixture of sadness at the loss and happiness for the new life of the friend or loved one. This philosophy is similar in both African-American and Caribbean cultures. This is an area where variations are often indistinguishable, with more specified details for those born and raised in the Bahamas. Generally, for the Bahamian born and raised in the Bahamas, the grieving lasts from the wake to the funeral reception.

The wake is the central event of the funeral. The purpose of the wake is to celebrate the passing of the loved one into a new life, a life that was meant to be. The wake is usually very well attended by family and friends, and the guests are expected to bring food for the family. Food is seldom catered unless the family is not well known or well liked by the immediate community.

Traditionally, the family is to be served and protected by those around them so that they will not need to spend energy making guests comfortable. Their time should be spent reminiscing about the lost loved one and finding comfort in the "good times." The wake is often thought of as the best part of the death experience because of the stories that are exchanged. The stories that are told are truly amazing, sometimes unbelievable, but always, always, interesting.

There are certain things that have a special place within Bahamian society: hats, bands, singing, and proper behavior at funerals. The church and funeral congregation love to sing and it would not be unusual to sing seven or eight verses of a song. The band, which includes drums and horns, usually leads the march to the funeral site.

Once the family is at the funeral site, there is another service with lengthy hymns and music. The actual funeral service is a little more formal and somber. The focus is on demonstrating how much the loved one will be missed. It is important to cry and scream. A "good" funeral is one where people cry and holler and scream, demonstrating how much the person would be missed.

One woman told a story about the funeral of her best friend's neighbor. She felt obligated to holler and scream throughout most of the funeral service so that everyone would know that a good person had died. And then there was

Tika, who lived in Key West many, many years ago. Tika was apparently very fond of attending funerals. She attended all the funerals in her community, even those of people she did not know.

After the funeral service, the body is taken to the burial ground. A few blocks from the site, the casket is taken out and rolled to the site so that friends and family can walk along. After the burial, the funeral party dances in the streets. My relatives have described this phenomenon as a side-splitting experience.

Shared Issues

There are a number of issues that African Americans and Caribbean Americans have in common. The first is communication and perception of acceptance by whites. Bahamians have a distinctive English accent that is often a source of pride and humor for friends and family but that clearly identifies them as "different." Language was often a point of concern in the past because Caribbeans were not always clearly understood. In southern Florida today, this is not considered an issue. However, I have found that there were some language and accent issues for the children, who say that they are often teased and called names—homie, homeboy, cockney, monkey chaser, and yardy. They were also ostracized by their peer group. One 20-year-old explained that he was routinely criticized once his peers discovered he was from another country. He felt that his speech and phrasing were not acceptable here, whereas in his native country he excelled. This young man was so grateful that he could always go home to his family. His mother was proud of him and always praised him lavishly. He was the oldest, and a boy, and that gave him status in the family. When he was with his family, he was in charge. He did not need to worry about being teased, and his siblings would never question him out loud.

When I shared this young man's story to several members of the BACC, a few of them said that this was a problem years ago but they were genuinely surprised that the children of today were experiencing some of the things they experienced in the 1960s and 1970s.

Initially, when large numbers of Caribbean immigrants came to the country 30 and 40 years ago, adults associated the British accent with allegiance to the British crown. Ueda (1980) explains that economic competition, cultural differences, political disagreements, and separate associational life resulted in mutual suspicion and communication problems between Caribbeans and African Americans.

It is unfortunate that several decades later we still seem to be dealing with the same problems. Rumbaut (1994) explains that the children's psychological adaption is affected by the family context. Specifically, the strength of children's ethnic self-identity tends to mirror the perceptions of their parents, especially the mother.

Perceptions of Acceptance by Americans

I have heard Caribbean families' stories from a variety of members ranging in age from 18 to 70. As a whole, the group is enthusiastic about discussing their adaption to the United States. However, they each had specific areas where adjustment was difficult.

The under-30 group focused on how their American peers did not accept them because they were different. Several of them reported that they got into fights because of teasing and taunts regarding their speech and dress. One man stated that his accent was used as an excuse to eliminate him from a work group.

Children and young adults reported that Americans frequently stated that the immigrant group had an air of superiority. A couple of them mentioned that they were told by their parents that they should ignore the teasing and harsh words, but the majority of them said that the experience definitely colored how they approached relationships with their American peers.

Most of the interviewees stated that they preferred to stay within their own cultural group because they felt understood and safe. It seemed to be very important to the teens to remain with a group of people who had similar problems and understood how they felt. They explained that the communication style of most Americans was not very clear to them. Their peers often didn't say what they actually meant and couldn't be trusted. Although there was a definite air of suspicion, they noted some categories of flexibility. For example, Caribbean women felt a high acceptance by American men.

The teens who had been in the United States for less than five years were distressed by the educational system. They stated that they had come from a setting where educators were respected and revered, and they found it difficult to adjust to an atmosphere where the limits were always being tested. However, they did admit that the United States offered them a wide variety of educational and social choices. Nevertheless, they missed the familiar surroundings of home, and most of them stated they felt that they would return home after they obtained an education and financial security.

The Adults' Perceptions

The middle and older adults stated that they felt that they had done a lot of compromising throughout their adjustment to the United States. They frequently emphasized that they had worked very hard to get the peace and comfort they had for their families, and that the United States had been a blessing to them.

The middle adults focused on their acceptance in the work world and how hard they and their children had to work to be accepted, treated equally, and to get ahead. The adults seemed to be very disappointed that they had to fight for acceptance and equality, especially in the work world. They emphasized that they were laid back and peaceful and found the aggression in the work setting quite an adjustment.

Both the middle and older adults have attempted to withstand the unfair and unequal treatments. Their hard work was always intended to smooth the way for their children. They believed that their sacrifices would make their children's lives less stressful than their own.

It is fairly typical for American Blacks and Caribbean families to be very vocal when it comes to the needs of their children. The mother tends to take a dominant role in the education of the children and solicits the help of the father or male partner when she is not successful alone.

Assimilation

In general, there was great concern regarding their children's exposure to the American way. Older adults stated that they were starting to see their children change in so many ways as they adopted American customs. The parents stated that they could easily deal with the changes in dress, in food, and music, but the change in attitude toward adult authority figures was troubling. They described how their children seemed so rebellious, beyond the point of being outspoken, especially the boys. Gewirtz (1970) stated that minority families have paid a high price for rapid acculturation into the United States.

Is it possible that the children have assimilated in a way that they feel provides them with more protection through aggressive, violent means? Or is this simply a developmental adjustment that has been exacerbated by the move from one country to another? The family unit certainly has a challenge, since it has not only moved from one place to another but from one culture to another.

A few of the parents noted that their children had withdrawn from the mainstream through disassociation with other cultural groups. Others noted that they gave their children a great deal of encouragement to excel academically, stating that this strategy had been successful for others.

Personal Family Insights

Families found that adjustment to the new culture was greatly helped by persistence, faith, friends, support, and family circles. This is demonstrated by the people at Rose's place. A majority also revealed how much the church community had come to mean to them. The families were predominately Roman Catholic and Episcopalian and heralded their strong faith as key to their adjustment and survival in the United States.

Although the adults stated that they found safety and comfort in groups who had cultural experiences similar to their own, their attitude was far more positive than that of the youth. The adults felt that the freedom and opportunities they had been able to obtain in the United States outweighed the hardships they had endured. Caribbean Americans felt they were making significant headway in integrating their customs and traditions as they educate the different cultural groups around them.

FAMILY: THE BOTTOM LINE

How does the concept of family fit into this journey? The family is the engine, the driving force that keeps the members energized to move toward success. Historically, from slavery times to the 1990s. Black families and their Caribbean counterparts have relied on the faith and generosity of their families.

It is well known that you can always come home. Home is a place for solace no matter what your past mistakes have been. You can always bring home to the family whatever or whoever you have gathered along the way. The gift of family closeness is worn like a badge and frequently thought of as a blessing.

REFERENCES

Baptiste, D. (1993). Immigrant families, adolescents and acculturation: Insights for therapist. *Marriage and Family Review*, 19, 341–363.

Bigelow, B. C. (1995). African Americans. In J. Galens, A. Sheets, and R. Young (eds.), *Gale Encyclopedia of Multicultural America* (pp. 16–41). Detroit, Mich.: Gale Research, Inc.

Cohen, C. (1994). What culturally diverse students say about emotion: An exploratory study. *Journal of Multicultural Social Work*. 3:113–124.

Ellwood, D. T., and Crane, J. (1990). Family change among Black Americans: What do we know? *Journal of Economic Perspectives*. 28: 65–84.

Garcia, J. (1986). Caribbean migration to the mainland: A review of adaptive experiences. *Annals of the American Academy of Political and Social Science*, 487: 114–125.

Gewirtz, A. (1970). The price minority groups pay for rapid acculturation in the USA. *International Journal of Offender Therapy and Comparative Criminology*, 14: 86–90.

Hirschman, C. (1994). Problems and prospects of studying immigrant adaption from the 1990 population census: From generational comparisons to the process of "Becoming American." *International Migration Review*, 28: 690–713.

Jones-Wilson, F. (1994). The family. In K. Estell (ed.). *The African American Almanac* (pp. 693–719). Detroit Mich.: Gale Research, Inc.

Otterbein, K. F., and Otterbein, C. (1995). Bahamians. In J. Dow and R. Van Kemper (eds.), *Encyclopedia of World Cultures: Vol. 3: Middle America and the Caribbean*. Boston: G. K. Hall.

Portes, A., and Grosfoguel, R. (1994). Caribbean diaspora: Migration and ethnic communities. *Annals of the American Academy of Political and Social Science*, 533: 48–69.

Rumbaut, R. (1994). The crucible within: Ethnic identity, self-esteem, and segmented assimilation among children of immigrants. *International Migration Review*, 28: 748–794.

Ueda, R. (1980). West Indians. In S. Themstrom, A. Orlow, and E. O'Handlin (eds.), *Harvard Encyclopedia of American Ethnic Groups* (pp. 1020–1027). Cambridge: Harvard University Press.

CHAPTER 28

THE AGING SOCIETY: FULCRUM FOR THE NEW CENTURY

Virginia Macken Fitzsimons

Every five minutes, a baby boomer turns 50. By 2015, when those baby boomers are turning 65, one person in four will be over 50. For the first time in human history, the five-generation family will be commonplace. The parents will be 90, the children 70, the grandchildren 50, the great-grandchildren 30, and the great-great grandchildren will be under 30 years old.

Characteristically, the new-century family will be middle-aged and above. The older family will have to accept the shift in generational roles. The individuals must maintain couple (or single) functioning with interest in face of physiological changes. The older family must be prepared to face critical losses of a spouse, siblings, and peers.

Older couples will have to renegotiate the marital system as a dyad, develop adult-to-adult relationships with their grown children, realign relationships to include in-laws, grown children, and new members subsequent to divorces and new marriages, and maintain their own identity as an older couple.

THE LONGEVITY REVOLUTION

In the 20th century life expectancy increased by 25 years, as a result of scientific discoveries, improved public health, and more stable economic conditions. The 21st century will focus on middle age, the stabilization and prevention of chronic diseases, and an increase in the quality of life—new ways to prevent osteoporosis, cardiovascular deterioration, and Alzheimer's disease. We can also expect gains in genetic research and concommitant applications to clinical practice.

With increased understanding of the complex psychological and physiological conditions of an aging population, focus on the coping and adaptation mechanisms of our society is warranted. Science has moved from the narrow view of aging as a disease to a broad view of healthy aging, with health seen as a matrix of nutritional, physical, social, and behavioral needs.

Common life events for older families include retirement, bereavement, sexuality, and cultural norms. Research offers ways for individuals to continue as active, productive members of their families and communities and as full partners in society.

Family roles supporting the quality of life for the older member address stabilization of self-care in health issues, socialization within the family and the community, economic stability, and other lifestyle and personality characteristics (ability to cope and change and attitudes toward aging). Goals are to retain independence and vigor. Historically, the role of the family is to provide health care directly as needed and to establish a social and physical environment to promote physical and social activity, transmit cultural norms, begin educational processes, and foster psychosocial growth.

There is a wide range of health and functioning among older people. The family unit determines the environmental and social variables that modify the impact of acute and chronic diseases and their outcomes. The individual's self-care supports social status, independence, and empowerment. The family modifies stress by offering social support, expressions of love, connectiveness, stability, and feelings of well-being.

Family stressors in the 21st century will range from changes in current family roles to the implementation of contemporary science findings.

Understanding that family units will be older and knowing what stressors and adaptations are needed for a healthy family life will benefit the entire society looking for reality-based planning and living. Some of the topics widely discussed in the literature of family development follow.

Grandparents as Parents

Today, 3 million children are being raised by their grandparents. This represents a 50 percent increase in the last decade. In most of the homes, no parent is present. In the past, multigenerational households were not uncommon in ethnic and working-class communities, but the phenomenon now includes all social and economic groups. Middle-class grandparents who planned to have freedom and independence in their retirement years are providing an ever greater share of child rearing as a result of their own children's drug addictions, divorces, financial troubles, and two-career marriages. For most of these grandparents, assuming parenting responsibilities again is not a first choice but a last resort.

Social scientists once predicted that grandparents would have more alternatives. Retired persons would be able to take up new areas of work, travel, hobbies, and sports. Their families would have grown and they would be free of responsibilities.

Instead, these grandparents are parents to young children and experience much stress and resentment. The emotional, financial, and legal pressures of their unplanned-for status as caregivers can be overwhelming. While middle-class grandparents feel the added expenses are a burden, those on fixed incomes are particularly distressed. Many of the caregivers are widows and serve as both parents and grandparents.

Some grandparents find the experience frustrating and exhausting. Like all new parents, they experience isolation. These new parent/grandparents are forming support groups and express their anger toward their own children for having forfeited their parental responsibilities. These support groups provide a network for child-care information such as medical care and educational opportunities.

While some grandparents refuse to take on the additional burden, most grandparents set aside their retirement plans and do what they are asked to do: 10 to 20 additional years of childrearing. However, they express considerable anger toward the son or daughter who failed to parent.

Centenarians for the New Century

People over 90 years old represent the fastest growing segment of our population. More than 1.7 million Americans will be 100 at the turn of the century. These hearty people attribute their long lives to the right occupation, the right diet, the right genes, and faith in God. Ninety-five percent of centenarians are nonsmokers. The new-century family will contain many older members. A number of longitudinal studies are focused on understanding this population. Data is being collected in the following areas:

- Demographic information
- Family longevity histories
- Need for social and environmental support
- Personality, stress, and coping
- Life satisfaction and morale
- Physical and mental health
- Nutrition and dietary patterns
- Intelligence and cognition
- Memories
- Religious beliefs and practices

How We Understand Aging

A substantial amount of understanding regarding aging has been gained since the 1800s. However, it is nowhere near the amount of knowledge needed. Our research base is built on the "average man," who is white and 65 years old. In order to understand the laws of human development and aging, we need to extend our research beyond age 65 and include women and people of all ethnic and national groups.

Men of a Certain Age

Hormone replacement therapy for older people is an important field of research with significant health and lifestyle implications for the new century. Estrogen replacement therapy has received wide acceptance. Research is continuing on human growth recombinant hormone for men. Such outcomes as increased lean muscle mass and thickened skin in elderly men are being monitored. Improved weight gain and general improvement in fitness will be the best short-term treatment for the frail elderly, those who are malnourished, and those with poor wound healing who are prone to falls.

Research also continues on testosterone replacement in elderly men. Hypogonadal males are more than six times more likely to break a hip during a fall than those with normal testosterone levels. The men particularly like the feeling of well-being the testosterone replacement provides.

Exercise plays an important part in the hormone replacement question. It is likely that exercise increases the natural production of the growth hormone or the synthesis of the receptors. There are two immediate questions regarding male hormone replacement therapy: What effect will long-term replacement have on the nests of slow-growing prostate cancer cells found in almost all elderly men? What is the appropriate age for hormone therapy intervention? Should men begin at 40 or 50 years of age to prevent problems later in life?

You Are What You Eat

Nutritional surveys indicate that up to one in four elderly persons has clinical malnutrition. Even older family members who are well-educated and financially comfortable may be seriously malnourished.

Good nutrition is the essential ingredient of good health. Poor nutrition aggravates chronic ailments such as heart disease and hypertension. For the older person, it becomes a vicious circle. Strokes and chronic illnesses such as arthritis, diabetes, and depression can greatly diminish appetite and both the ability and desire of the individual to eat. Poor dental health and broken, decayed, or missing teeth also make it difficult to chew. Each problem in turn adds to the malnutrition syndrome.

Poor nutrition may include alcohol abuse (increasingly identified as a major chronic problem in older families); inadequate intake of meat, fruits, and vegetables; or skipping meals altogether. Other contributing factors include poverty, leading to an insufficient food budget, social isolation, and drug interactions, with resulting diminished appetite.

Vitamins particularly formulated for the elderly may help prevent disease through micro nutrition. A multivitamin and multimineral regimen significantly increases immune function and decreases the frequency of infections in the elderly, by as much as 50 percent in people over 70 years of age.

Aging is generally associated with impaired immune responses and an increase in infections, particularly respiratory diseases such as bronchitis and pneumonia. Pneumonia remains the fourth most common cause of death in the elderly. Deficiency in protein leads to muscle wasting and impaired immune responses.

Blood samples taken before beginning the vitamin therapy show many deficient levels of vitamins in the bodies of the elderly. After a year of vitamin supplementation, blood samples demonstrate a uniform improvement in all areas of nutrition. Even in apparently healthy elderly people, levels of essential nutrients are improved by basic doses—not megadoses—of vitamin and mineral supplements.

Many older people find it impossible to alter the food habits of a lifetime. Teaching nutrition and better eating patterns is the key to better health for all family members in the new century. Diabetes, cancer, and heart disease are diet-related and respond to alterations in diet.

Fitness Counts

A less active lifestyle places the older adult at particular risk for depression and physical dependency. Body building with weight training and aerobic exercise is recommended even into the late nineties; exercise will reduce the risk of hypertension, diabetes, osteoporosis, osteoarthritis, heart disease, and the fatigue of muscle atrophy.

Even centenarians can improve with exercise. Weight-bearing exercises hold calcium in the bone and increase the fluid in intervertebral disks, diminishing the loss of height. Increased blood supply to the muscles improves tissue elasticity and muscle mass and strength. Within two weeks of moderate exercise, benefits can be measured in every age group, including centenarians.

Vaccination for the Young and Old

Pneumonia and influenza vaccines are important for the elderly, especially older disabled men. Influenza vaccinations prevent viral infection, and can sufficiently enhance the immune system so that it is as functional as that of a younger person. The vaccine works by energizing the helper T cells. T cells circulate in the blood and retain a trace memory of past viruses. The vaccination helps the immune system remember the virus, enabling the T-cells to respond more quickly, with more robust energy, if the virus enters the body again. Any subsequent illness, either pneumonia or flu, will be of shorter duration, with far less serious symptoms.

Attitude

The new-century family will be counseled to monitor its attitude toward itself and approach to living. When faced with problems in activities of daily living, middle-aged and older adults who identified only aging as the cause of their problems have a far greater risk of dying (up to 78 percent) than those adults who give specific, non-aging-related reasons for limitations. When a problem is attributed to old age, the individual becomes resigned to believing that it is not treatable or preventable and delays or omits getting care. The individual gives up and becomes less self-directed and powerful.

llness prevention will include not only good nutrition, fitness, or rest but also mental attitude. Optimism actually increases the potential for a full life span. An optimistic outlook on life is an essential component of a healthy life.

Making Whoopee

It is a myth, and only a myth, that older people are not sexual. Older people have active sexual lives, although researchers have not frequently studied this age group. Until recently, it was assumed that not much sex was going on, so it was not studied carefully. The classic Kinsey Report on male sexuality devoted only a few passing comments to sex after 60, but there is mounting evidence that older family members are not at all celibate.

Studies show that older adults in good health are sexually active. Among women age 60 to 70 years, 80 percent report that they are sexually active; 65 percent are still active after age 70. Figures for men in the same age groups are 91 percent and 79 percent, respectively. With the introduction of Viagra, these figures for the male may indicate the use of the drug, yet a clear study has yet to account for the extent of increased sexual activity. Drug companies are anticipating a Viagra type drug to be available for women within the next two years. Poor health and widowhood diminish sexual desire and potential. However, more than half of all seniors desire sex well into their nineties if a partner is available. In general, those older persons who reported that sex and sexual satisfaction were important in earlier years still found the same degree of satisfaction—or even more than in younger years. Older men and women masturbate regularly. Male homosexuals remain sexually active after 60. Presently there have been no studies of older lesbians.

Normal aging changes sexual responses for both men and women. Reduced testosterone levels in men result in decreased sexual desire and sensitivity and diminished peripheral neuron sensory fibers. Longer and more direct stimulation of the penis is needed, however some men report that they could keep an erection longer and that an orgasm is possible even in the absence of ejaculation.

Reduced estrogen levels in women allow the action of the natural testosterone in the female body to influence sexual desire. As a result, many women experience an increase in libido. Hormone replacement therapy overrides this effect of the testosterone and the status quo is maintained. Many use estrogen creams to avoid discomfort during intercourse and to improve vaginal lubrication and elasticity. Women can remain multiorgasmic well into their nineties. When a partner is not available, older women masturbate for the release of sexual tension.

It is important that the sexual needs and potentials of the family's older members be respected. Outward displays of affection, such as hugging, kissing, and cuddling, should be possible for older couples, and not negatively sanctioned by younger generations in the family.

In many ways, partners over 60 have an opportunity to enjoy biological and emotional synchrony unparalleled at any other age. The male's tendency to reach orgasm more slowly is well suited to the longer time a woman needs to become aroused. Birth control hassles are over, children no longer need immediate attention, and both partners have the leisure time to enjoy physical intimacy.

However, and it is a big however, sexual function is dependent on good health. After a heart attack, the fear of death is associated with sexual activity. Will it cause too much of a strain on the heart? Will it raise the blood pressure? Physicians recommend that patients resume sex when they can achieve an exercise stress test level heart rate of 120. In patients with angina, nitroglycerin shortly before making love eases the potential for chest pain.

As we enter the new century, surgical advances such as laser and microscope instruments will spare tissue and decrease the damage to neurons, thus protecting the pelvic structures. Fewer colostomies and mastectomies will be needed and insults in body image will be reduced.

Prescription and over-the-counter drugs for hypertension, anxiety, digestive and infectious conditions frequently dampen libido and cause impotence. Pharmaceutical companies, aware of the impact of these drugs, are developing second- and third-generation drugs to reduce these side effects.

Money Matters

Up to 97 percent of older families, whether they live in their own homes or in service agencies, will have some federal assistance such as Social Security, a major source of income. Medicare will account for 18 percent of the federal budget by 2020.

The financial aspects of caring for older family members are as important as the emotional aspects. When parents age, their role in the family unit is altered. It is predicted that all generations of the family will be expected to contribute financially to the care of the elders. With far fewer younger persons to participate in the workforce, older members of the family will work longer and will need financial planning in order to maintain themselves.

Successful multigenerational family communication stresses the need to review options for living 10 to 20 years before decisions must be made.

Experts recommend that discussions be held openly and that each generation be a part of the decision-making process. For example, on par of importance with availability of health care is the decision regarding retirement living.

This new century will offer many more alternatives to retirement housing. One such innovation is the reverse-mortgage loan, which converts equity in the family home into a monthly income. The older people will be able to maintain their standard of living and not be plunged into house-rich but cash-poor poverty. Thousands of reverse mortgages (unknown 10 years ago) are given each year. A reverse mortgage will provide a steady income to elderly homeowners and does not have to be repaid until the property is sold. Additional equity, above the amount loaned, belongs to the homeowner.

As the baby-boomer generation prepares to retire, it is estimated that $50 trillion will change hands from one generation to the next over the next 15 years. Never before in human history has so much capital been moved across so many families. This transfer of capital is in the form of the stocks, bonds, and mutual funds in retirement accounts and in the equity of the homes bought and paid for by the American working and middle classes. This is one cause of the enormous rise in the New York Stock Exchange in recent years.

Intergenerational planning, which includes decisions regarding lifestyle, place of residence, sources of income, health care, and financial planning, facilitate the proper protection of the family's monetary base and ensure that the family remains flexible in the face of market changes.

WORK AND LONGEVITY

It is entirely possible that many family members can anticipate at least four different careers over his or her life! The average age of the workforce is now 39 years old. In 2020, the mean age will have risen to 47 years old.

The new century will have no specific retirement age. Career paths will be determined by the interests, needs, and stamina of the worker. For the older person, continued work will mean a new partnership with a company and mutual planning.

Strategies will incorporate such variables as broader career options, with continuous on-the-job education; attention to self-presentation; maintenance of workplace safety; continued professional and personal development to maintain current work skills and friendship networks; and appropriate workload management for the older worker.

Overall, the aging U.S. population will mean more older workers. Their skills and expertise will be critical to businesses aiming to meet higher production targets. The challenge to older workers will be to learn new skills and keep up with technological developments.

Continued job satisfaction and organizational commitment are the variables inherent in worker longevity. Older workers are more committed to their employers than younger workers. Workforce downsizing, therefore, has dramatic emotional implications for the older worker. Studies are predicting that older workers will consider employment in smaller companies. Small business owners encounter difficulties in staffing, that is, finding, directing, and retaining competent employees.

Small business owners also face increasing pressure to improve productivity and company commitment. Given the high correlation of older workers' organizational commitment and the needs of small companies, it is predicted that older workers will be more likely to hold positions in smaller companies.

The Small Business Administration is projecting some new-century trends. Changing demographics (the aging of the population) will make the senior worker quite desirable. The older worker's expertise, more favorable attitude toward work, and high level of commitment make the employment of older persons a viable option.

Marketing Trends

Many popular perceptions of older adults are stereotypes that are not based on reality. These misperceptions are perpetuated in the attitudes of both the young and the old. Increasingly, advertisers are portraying older consumers in a positive way. Multigenerational families will become a common part of both television and print ads. New-century trends in advertising will include far more families interacting in a intergenerational manner, demonstrating the family roles each generation plays in the development of the other.

The 20th century was the century of the young. The new century will see the older family as the fulcrum of society.

References

Butler, R. N. (1998). Historical Perspective on Aging and the Quality of Life. New York: Springer.

Curry, M. (1996). Vitamins for the elderly: Disease prevention through the use of micro nutrient. *Medical World News*, 33(12): 32.

Gutfeld, G. and Rao, L. (1992). Healthy aging. *Prevention* 44(12):10.

Poon, L. W. (ed). (1998). *The Georgian Centenarian Study*. Amityville, N.Y.: Barnwood.

Smith, P., and Hoy, F. (1992). Job satisfaction and commitment of older workers in small businesses. *Management*, 30(4):106

Stewart, A., and King, A. (1994). Conceptualizing and measuring quality of life in older populations. In R. Abeles, H. Gift, and M. Ory, eds., *Aging and the Quality of Life*. New York: Springer.

Wold, G. (1993). *Basic Geriatric Nursing*. St. Louis, Miss.: Mosby Year Book.

CHAPTER 29

WWW.SEX.FAMILY

Shelley Green

SEX

Sex. The word throws us. We want to talk about it. We're embarrassed to talk about it. We know we should tell our kids about it, especially the parts our parents didn't tell us. And we don't want the kids to learn the wrong thing, the wrong way, from the wrong people. But we don't talk to them. We say, "Next year, when they're a little older." Why? We can't imagine our kids as sexual creatures. We still can't quite imagine our parents as sexual creatures. We don't even talk out loud about ourselves as sexual creatures. Even within the context of the sexuality courses that I have taught for 10 years now, students are reluctant to speak openly.

There is instant, rapt, although somewhat anxious, attention in such classes, and tensions run high. This speaks to me each semester of our culture's ongoing love-hate relationship with sex and all its implications. No other topic (with the possible exception of death, which doesn't count because it's not about now, it's about later) puts us more in touch with our own morality, mortality, vulnerability, and humanness than sex. Sex touches our hopes, our fears, our fantasies, and now, with the reality of AIDS, our mandate to choose between life and death.

PUBLIC VS. PRIVATE

It's an intimately private topic that, in our current culture, has become a vastly public industry. It is used to sell cars, cigarettes, lingerie, and alcohol. It is sold itself in bars, on street corners, over the telephone, and in the mail. As we move into the 21st century, our relationship with sex moves with us. And, as one of my students commented, "There's no such thing as 'just sex'." Our conflicted relationship with our own and others' sexuality influences our daily interactions. Our choice of intimate (and not so intimate) relationships even determines the children we will bring into our world.

How will we find our sexual attitudes, beliefs, and behaviors changing in this new century? What will we choose to retain from our historical values? What will become last week's news? What will constitute our sexual tragedies and triumphs? How will these be defined in a technology-dominated world?

Our cultural relationship with sex covers a multitude of issues. I will touch on a few that seem to me to be most pressing. I will take a look at how we have managed these issues in the past, how we currently address them, and how we may find ourselves relating to them in a future influenced heavily by technology, including the powerful scope of the information superhighway. Each of the issues addressed below has an impact on the definition of family in significant ways.

We cannot speak of sex without implicitly calling into question our connections (chosen and ordained by birth) with other people. As we continue to redefine our sexuality, our sexual relationships will influence our new descriptions of the term *family*. A 7-year-old who lives with her two moms defined it in the following way: "A family is a bunch of people, or not so many, who love each other." Perhaps this child's wisdom can provide the flexibility we need to create new and more encompassing definitions of family.

That Was Then, This Is Now

Forty years ago, the following scenario was a common one: Ozzie and Harriet, or June and Ward Cleaver, hoped the kids got the "film in third grade" but otherwise didn't mention "the topic." Instead they stayed up until midnight Friday nights wondering what was happening in the back seat out on lover's lane. The kids' version of this scenario, of course, was the dilemma of having absolutely no accurate information, which led to furtive searches in the *Encyclopedia Britannica* or the parents' secret bookshelf when they were away, along with the desperate groping on various movie dates. Censored information about sex only increased the curiosity, but left few adolescents with the ability to make wise choices.

The World Wide Web Comes of Age

Today the lack of information is not the problem. Rather, by the age of 10, most kids know much more than their parents about how to "surf the Net," and thus have easy access to graphic materials that provide much more than juicy images of the Playmate of the Month.

The proliferation of sites about sex on the World Wide Web may be the single most dramatic influence on our relationship with sex during the next 20 years, including how we live it, learn about it, and do it. For adults, the distance and anonymity of sex on the Internet provides a safe haven for sexual exploration. The computer allows individuals, in the privacy of their homes, to explore thousands of Web sites that offer information on every kind of sexual practice.

This is not sex education as we once knew it, and the ease of accessibility offers unprecedented freedom to take advantage of such information. Through chat rooms, where people log on from their home computers and engage in sexually explicit conversation, previously forbidden activities, partners, and identities may be explored with little or no risk. If things get too hot, you can always log off. No need to leave a phone number.

Such physical distance may provide welcome relief, not only for those afraid of exposure to the AIDS virus but for those who fear face-to-face sexual encounters as well. Such Internet travels offer an enormous variety of opportunities for sexual experimentation, and as one man told me, these are the only sexual relationships he is willing to risk. No one knows if he "doesn't get it up," no one knows "how big it is," and no one knows if he really has an orgasm. His sexual prowess is as incredible as his linguistic ability, and no one will pose a challenge to his manhood. If they do, he just signs off.

Back to the Future: It's a Man's World

But while sex on the Internet may seem like a dramatic restructuring of our sexual world, in some ways such exposure to sex differs little from the experience of young boys in the 1950s finding their fathers' *Playboy* under the bed. In each case, the sexual images are remote, somewhat surreal, and forbidden. And in each case, the business of sex has been owned by and created mostly for men.

Sex on the Web targets a male clientele willing to pay for graphic sexual images of women. Celebrity faces may be transposed over the nude images of other women' bodies for further titillation and exploitation.

Historically we have assumed that technological advances spell progress, but have we really progressed as we move into the new century? This male sexual world harkens back to the overt sexual mores of the 1950s, when fathers openly (although often not in the presence of their wives) encouraged their sons to experiment sexually, even providing them with prostitutes in some cases, but threatened the life of any male who dared approach their daughters.

A father whose son "got his girlfriend pregnant" could be secretly relieved that his son was a "real man," while the pregnant girl's father could choose to threaten her, abuse her, or disown her. Perhaps these seemingly archaic sexual attitudes have not changed too much. Consider the Spur Posse, a group of southern California adolescent males in the mid-1990s whose initiation rite involved the rape of preadolescent and adolescent girls. When the boys were caught, some of their fathers defended them publicly, excusing their violent behavior with the old "boys will be boys" adage. Perhaps they were secretly pleased their sons were not gay. Perhaps things haven't changed so much after all.

The Quest for Safer Sex

Adolescents and adults in the AIDS era are attempting to find some form of safer sex (as opposed to safe sex, which may exist only on the Internet—your computer may get a virus, but you won't). Computer sex is one way, but there are others as well. A friend told me the following story.

As she was lying on her towel at the beach, soaking up the sun, she noticed a man nearby watching her. He was also lying on a towel, but face down, and she soon realized that he was masturbating as he kept his eyes on her. Being an adventurous sort, she chose to play along, and began slowly rubbing lotion on her thighs and her chest, moving her hand languorously along her bikini line. This went on for some time. The man gradually moved his towel closer and closer to hers and, continually watching her, eventually reached orgasm on his towel. He lay there for several moments, then rose, walked over, and thanked her for the "safe sex."

What makes this story even more interesting is that this woman is a lesbian. In this isolated instance that was irrelevant. Her "partner" had no knowledge of her sexual orientation, and perhaps he wasn't even interested. Many women, both lesbian and heterosexual, would be violently offended at the thought of a man finding sexual gratification by observing them from a distance. However, for this man at least, and perhaps for others, the safety of the anonymous act outweighs the accompanying alienation.

This is a powerful message. When sex equals death, sexual opportunities necessarily come in new packages. Computer sex and masturbation in the presence of strangers are two rather disturbing, but perhaps common, examples. In these encounters, identities, histories, other ongoing relationships, and previous commitments can become irrelevant in the minds of the participants, at least in the moment. There are some advantages to this. It's easy to walk away from a stranger on the beach. An Internet affair presents no threat of disease, no awkward moments of being caught in bed, no dealing with other people's children, spouses, and exes. Nevertheless, read Ann Landers or Dear Abby for a week and you'll see more than one letter dealing with a devastated and desperate spouse, frantic to rescue his or her partner from the clutches of Internet sex.

And the effects of these computer explorations go far beyond Dear Abby. As a therapist, I meet clients whose spouses have become involved with lovers they met on the Net. These relationships are being described as the newest addiction; self-help books and support groups are sure to follow shortly. Already, sex addiction groups tell us that sex is a dangerous substance, and that once addicted, abstinence is the only safe course of action. These stories offer yet another view of our conflicted passions about sex. In a world filled with fear of death by sex with a stranger, the only sane options seem to be abstinence, monogamy, or sex as noncontact sport.

Whence Intimacy?

Of the three options mentioned above, perhaps only the second offers a safe context in which to experience sexual intimacy. When asked why sex is important, women frequently respond with this word, intimacy. Men may use other words—and our culture may not support them in responding with this one even if they want to.

But the intense personal connection that is possible through sharing one's body in the most intimate way with another is perhaps the part of sex we both fear and desire the most. What if you're passionately in love with her, but sex is lousy? What if you dislike him, but have overwhelming orgasms with him? In each case, we tend to assume something is wrong with *us*—either our ability to develop close, intimate relationships or our ability to please the ones we love sexually.

The media tell us that love and sex should be synonymous, and those in love should have multiple, simultaneous orgasms. Right! It's no wonder Internet sex has come of age! Sex experts are more than ready to take our time and our money to educate us about our own particular sexual dysfunction, be it desire disorder, orgasmic disorder, retarded or premature ejaculation, erectile dysfunction, or any number of other possibilities. These "disorders" are all about mechanics: how the equipment works and how to get it to work "right" all the time.

One major sex therapy textbook includes 400 pages on physiological disorders and one paragraph on intimacy. It is not difficult to understand how performance can become the all-encompassing goal, while intimacy takes a back seat. Our cultural and sexual alienation only enhance that likelihood.

AIDS and the Birth of a Sexual Revolution?

By the year 2000, we will have been living in the age of AIDS for almost 30 years. Today's children have no concept of life before AIDS—it is simply the norm until a cure is found.

Currently, the fastest-growing segment of the HIV population is women, and minority women are disproportionately represented in this group (CDC, 1994, 1995; Schoofs, 1997). These women are the partners of IV drug users and gay or bisexual men, or they are prostitutes or IV drug users themselves. Their children are often born with the virus.

However, as medical advances make it possible to live with AIDS rather than simply die with it, fear may indeed diminish (see Chapter 20). Safer sex may be only for wimps. Cool people may be willing to live on the edge, take the risk, and find themselves among the millions affected by the virus. If the medical advances announced at the 1999 World AIDS Conference in

Vancouver are realized, scientists and physicians may eventually find a way to eliminate the virus from the body. If this does occur, will this signal another sexual revolution? As fear gives way to liberation, we may see a replay of the 1960s and 1970s.

The advent of the pill in the 1960s and the legalization of abortion in 1973 offered unprecedented opportunities for nonmarital, nonprocreative sex. Millions took advantage of this freedom, and it took perhaps 20 years for us to recognize the accompanying costs. Pregnancy was, unbelievably, our biggest fear about unprotected sex at the time. Of course, prior to the development of penicillin, we feared disease, but in the 1960s and 1970s that fear became minimal. Gonorrhea? Syphilis? Just make a quick trip to the clinic. The responsibility for contraception was placed entirely in the hands of women. Women ingested the chemicals. Women had the abortions. Yes, we were liberated. And yes, there were costs. We may see similar liberations, and similar costs, as the face of the AIDS epidemic changes in the 21st century.

The research on reproductive technology in this country has not kept pace with almost any of our other research initiatives. And why would it? There is no great desire among men to assume responsibility for contraception. Women still bear the children, and the major responsibility of any sexual encounter.

In an election year, when the politicians use the abortion issue as a battleground for votes, women fear the loss of choice. Perhaps we need to fear the indifference (and covert resistance) to developing reproductive methods that would involve men in the process. This reluctance tells us even more about our culture's consistent position on sex, and about the ongoing tradition of men making decisions that determine women's sexuality. Such decisions have overwhelming implications for our understanding and experience of family, sex, relationship, and intimacy.

THE NEW FAMILY

Twenty years ago, we all knew what family meant: one father, one mother, 2.2 kids, and a house in the suburbs. Regardless of how accurate this view was, it was widely accepted as the norm and universally proclaimed as the only socially desirable option.

Thousands of articles and books were published analyzing and describing the nuclear family and the family of origin, and exploring such concepts as dyadic adjustment, marital communication styles, relationship development, and sexual dysfunction.

The vast majority of such research focused on, and indeed assumed, a heterosexual, monogamous union. While we still clearly live in a heteronormative society, that norm is now becoming much less clear, much less accurate, and in some cases, much less desired. In part, this has to do with our changing relationship with sex.

Currently, there is no universally accepted definition of family, and the term *traditional family* has become most closely associated with the religious right and its family values coalition. This coalition urges us to elect politicians who take an openly antigay stance so that we can return our country to its 1950s, ultraconservative, strongly heterosexist foundation.

Is this about values? Or is this about sex? Perhaps both—but it is definitively about our uneasy relationship with sexual practices that challenge the norm and thus make us uncomfortable. This conflicted relationship with sex then becomes the foundation for a political call to war, which encourages the legislation and enforcement of measures to curb nonheterosexual unions.

And warfare it has become. Hawaii and Vermont are thus far the only states to officially recognize gay marriages, although the implications of this are far-reaching. Opposition to gay marriage is proclaimed adamantly by the mainstream media. "If gay marriage, why not incest?" asks *Time* magazine. "Why not child sexual abuse? Why not polygamy?" A federal court judge is presently deciding whether to overturn a Florida court's decision to award custody of a 12-year-old girl to her father, a convicted murderer, rather than allow her to continue to live with her lesbian mother. When emotions run so high that educated people compare homosexuality to incest and murder and find the latter to be preferable, this signals a war in which there are likely to be few survivors and many wounded.

Gay Families

Gay marriages are here, however, and they are "out" (meaning in your face, not passé). They are challenging our definitions of family in more ways than marriage. Gay adoptions are becoming commonplace. With the development of artificial insemination and the proliferation of sperm banks, lesbian couples have many options for bearing their own children that allow them to avoid the difficult question of involving a biological father in their children's lives.

New children's books with titles like *Janie's Two Mommies* and *I Have a Donor Daddy* have hit the stands, and straight parents of preschoolers are likely to meet gay parents at the PTA.

For some, this is a welcome relief from the oppression, denial, and ostracism that has prevailed until now. In some cases, gay parents may come as couples to their children's school functions without incident (although certainly with some trepidation). But in other cases, there may be tremendous opposition. Churches have taken up the cause with a vengeance. Religious conferences have been splintered by the issue, and long-term church members have found themselves on the outs with others in the congregation if they express gay-positive views. While a number of states have recognized the custodial rights of gay and lesbian partners of biological parents, and many major corporations and universities have extended spousal benefits to same-sex partners, opposition to these changes still runs high.

Other corporations have publicly opposed offering benefits to partners of gay employees, and President Clinton has felt the pressure to make a public statement opposing gay marriage even though in other matters he has been a supporter of homosexual rights. These events occur in the public eye, and thus place the evolution of the traditional family squarely in our view. We cannot avoid noticing that the times are changing. "Families of choice" now offer gays and lesbians, whose "families of lineage" have ostracized them, a community of acceptance and an identity they can embrace.

While gay families are not new, they are no longer hidden—and are hotly debated in the public forum. The debate can sometimes become a bloody battle, bespeaking a cultural climate that continues to promote fear and alienation about sex.

Hope for the Future: Healthy Sexuality for Our Children

Highly publicized instances of the sexual abuse of children have promoted a climate of paranoia, judgment, and accusation. This climate of fear may certainly have saved some children, but victimized some adults in the process. Many parents avoid touching their children for fear someone will decide their actions are inappropriate and the children will be taken by the state. Dear Abby sagely informs us that no 3-year-old child should be sharing the shower with the parent of the opposite sex. Parents are afraid to photograph their infants and small children when they are naked, as a film developer could turn them in to the authorities.

These are not unfounded fears. Cases such as these *have* happened and innocent, loving parents *have* lost their children. How much do we fear our children's sexuality? How much do we fear our own sexuality in relation to our children? The naked, perfect body of my 3-year-old son is perhaps the most delightful sight I can imagine. Dare I say this out loud, much less in print with my name attached?

Finding pleasure in the delicious smell of a child fresh out of the bath, or the intense, four-limbed body hug provided by an enthusiastic and loving small boy now creates fear. The pendulum has swung, and certainly for good reason. The sexual abuse of even one child should be enough to put us all on guard at all times. However, nakedness, bubble baths, and physical closeness do not constitute sexual abuse; rather, they are an integral part of the intimate duties involved in truly "caring" for small children. If we teach our children that their naked bodies and their pleasurable physiological sensations are shameful, we afford them little opportunity to find their own healthy, positive definition of sex as they mature. We risk, as Oxenhandler (1996) notes, throwing the babies out with the bathwater.

How do we respect our own and our children's privacy, offer them graceful acceptance and appreciation of their own bodies, and plant the seeds of intimacy and caring in connection with sex, rather than the seeds of fear, alienation, exploitation, and shame? We must first look at our own choices, our own values, our own daily interactions. We must be willing to offer our children more, to go beyond our fears and help them learn ways to live gently, safely, and passionately on this planet. That willingness represents our chance to go beyond sexual and emotional alienation as we enter this new century.

May the legacy we pass on be one of hope, so that the 21st century may become known as the age of intimacy.

Chapter 30

From Snow White to Esmerelda: A Mother-Daughter Conversation in Three Generations

Anne Hearon Rambo
Shelby Hearon
Rachel Shelby Rambo

Anne's Story

In 1937, when she was 6, my mother, Shelby Hearon, stood in line to see the new Walt Disney movie, *Snow White*. In 1996, I took my 6-year-old daughter, Rachel, to see both the re-release of *Snow White* and the latest animated epic from the Disney studios, *The Hunchback of Notre Dame*.

The movies are not dissimilar. The animation is quite comparable in detail, even though in 1937 the work was done by Depression artists and architects toiling for an hourly pittance, while in 1996 it was largely computer-generated. But the heroes are equally stiff, the animals and gargoyles are identically cute, and the villains similarly villainous. Frollo, the evil judge of Hunchback, even seems to have borrowed the wicked stepmother's flowing black gown.

Only the two heroines, Snow White and Esmerelda, seem radically opposed. Snow White is boyishly slender, undeveloped, with a high-pitched, baby-doll voice. Wholly unable to protect herself, she even endangers her would-be protectors with her lack of survival skills. The birds of the forest chirp at her not to eat that poisoned apple; she eats it anyway. Later, she is revived and borne off in triumph by the first prince to come along. She lies limply passive in his arms, gazing adoringly at him, apparently willing to bond with whoever is willing to take care of her.

Esmerelda, on the other hand, is made of sterner stuff. She appears to have spent numerous hours in the gym pumping iron, assuming that actual cosmetic surgery was not involved. She is depicted gleefully kicking, throwing missiles at, leaping over, and escaping from armed soldiers. As the film progresses, she rescues her male companions at least as often as they attempt to rescue her.

In the film's climactic scene, the villain offers to save her from certain death if she will marry him—essentially the same deal the prince offers Snow White. (Okay, maybe the villain, who is quite possibly a Catholic priest—this is left vague—is not exactly offering legal marriage. On the other hand, who knew precisely what arrangement that prince had in mind?) Esmerelda draws herself up and spits in his face. I found myself quite unable to picture Snow White doing that. The difference between the two heroines made me wonder about what has happened in the past 59 years.

To my daughter, however, the differences were readily explainable. When you are 6, most things that puzzle older and vaguer minds are quite clear to you. "*Obviously*, Mommy," she explains, "Snow White was a kid. Esmeralda was grown up. Because Quasi [the hunchback] doesn't have a mother—remember she gets killed in the beginning—and Esmeralda and Quasi don't get married, Esmeralda is supposed to be Quasi's mother from then on. Probably she adopts him or something. But when you grow up and get to be a mother, you *have* to be brave and strong and smart. Can you imagine Snow White taking care of a baby? She probably doesn't know the difference between a poisoned apple and a healthful one! Also, when you're a mom, you get to have better dresses and better hair, not like Snow White."

A random survey of her 6- to 9-year-old peer group revealed that her belief that Esmeralda is, or soon will be, functionally Quasimodo's mother was universally shared, if not by the scriptwriters (let alone Victor Hugo, who should have thought of that tidy resolution to the dilemma of unrequited love). There was also universal agreement that mothers, by definition, are capable of rescuing self and others. I think something has happened in the past 50 to 60 years to alter our collective view of heroines, women, and mothers.

Perhaps this something is mixed up with the changes in the family over the same time period. We often think of these changes in terms of cycles—Rosie the Riveter in the 1940s, countered by Suzie Homemaker in the 1950s. But the demographic reality is one of steady, incremental change. From 1900 to the present, with each decade women live longer, have fewer children, and accept more paid employment outside the home regardless of the social climate. Each decade has seen a steady increase in life expectancy for women, a decrease, however slight, in family size, and an increase in the percentage of women in the workforce (Glennon, 1996).

The correlation between those first two statistics would not have been lost on my mother's mother, who died last year at the age of 89—this being a 50-year improvement over her own mother's life span.

My grandmother, Evelyn Shelby Roberts Reed, lost her 39-year-old mother while she was still young. As an adult, she made it her cause to see that fewer children were left motherless. She was an early Planned Parenthood activist in both Kentucky and Texas. When I had my first and only child, at the comparatively advanced age of 34, my grandmother stayed up all night for me, lighting candles and worrying. The next morning, when she called the hospital for news, the nurse breezily said, "I bet you want to know *all* the details—how much the baby weighed and everything!" "No," my grandmother said, "I just want to know if she and the baby both lived." The cheery young charge nurse thought this an impossibly macabre question, and delicately suggested to me later that I must come from an "unusual" family. But perhaps what is truly both odd and encouraging is that in one woman's lifetime, and in the cultural leap from rural Kentucky to urban Florida, such a question should have become not a usual one after all.

If we no longer buy our babies' lives with our own, at least not usually, does that mean we love them less? Are the muscular, fierce heroines of today terrifying all the potential husbands and fathers into oblivion? This being an election year, politicians of all persuasions have been calling for a return to traditional family values.

My mother's parents, her father and stepmother, lived a very different lifestyle at the other end of town. One had to be invited to visit. These grandparents drank, unlike my other grandparents. And they danced and summered at their country place. They had friends; they did not often see kin. They looked down on the large sprawling house full of Reeds with all those degrees and protruding teeth. When my daddy returned to Marion, Kentucky, during the war, I was then 10, old enough to observe things I had not before. Why was it that the family with the full city block of land and trees, the big house, all the diplomas, was the "poor relation" and the family in the small pink stucco house on a narrow corner lot, with dark rooms and no hidden closets with old hats and china dolls, was the "rich" branch of the family? What was it that the town, and my parents, subscribed to that I could not see?

It appeared to me that my own parents had defined family in the best possible way. If you were there, you belonged. My mother had more books than the Marion public library, and my friend Patty Jo, who read nearly all of them, was family, especially since her own mother had died giving birth to her and she was raised by elderly, overwhelmed grandparents.

Daddy's friends, geologists, physicists, were always welcome, always stopping by, becoming surrogate parents, and some I still see and treat like parents. *Us* and *Them* were people with and without good sense, good hearts, and good conversation. *Us* and *Them* did not have to do with blood kinship. Now, looking back and looking ahead, I can draw a general conclusion about the inclusive and the exclusive families.

I believe the exclusive family had to do with the primacy of inheritance. My maternal grandmother's family could trace themselves back to the Mayflower (and did, frequently, given the slightest encouragement). This lineage was inherited. So was the silver, the china, the books that had belonged to May Shelby, the great aunt who sent to France for European literature while living on a pig farm in Fredonia, Kentucky. (There was no money, the family story goes, and so May Shelby had no choice but to marry the pig farmer, wealthy and kind even if hopelessly declassé. But she could, and did, read Balzac and pretend the rest of her days.) So were portraits of kin, letters from kin, linens of kin, any evidence that these possessions had come down to you. I believe that the inclusive family was based on common economic and functional goals (the hamburger stand, the bean and corn garden, childrearing, job hunting).

My last uncle, the baby of the family, got help from all the older brothers and sisters to finish up his engineering degree at the height of the Depression. That's what you did for family: saw to it that no one was left behind. I would anticipate that in the next century we'll get back to the concept of inclusive family for defining family. For one thing, even with divorce, name changes, mobility, the ascendancy of communication over property as a goal, the idea of inheritance seems fairly fragile and useless. It belongs only to people with nothing else to worry about, while the need to pool services has become paramount. The whole idea of millions of couples duplicating at the same time the heating of fishsticks, tying of shoes, reading of bedtime stories, and so on, seems a staggering waste.

I think the first thing is to get the forms changed in school so that they no longer ask: NAME OF FATHER, NAME OF MOTHER, NAME OF BROTHER(S), NAME OF SISTER(S). Rather, they will ask: ADULTS TO BE CONTACTED BY SCHOOL. NAMES OF OTHER CHILDREN IN THE SCHOOL. This and other similar shifts in questions will allow children to grow up with a similar shift in the construction of family. Not "Daddy and his new wife," and "Mommy and her new husband," and "my half-brother" and "stepsister," which, much like the South's terms of "second cousin once removed," have a lot to do with inheritance and not much at all to do with a sense of family.

This, needless to say, would solve the "problem" of gay marriages, not by simply allowing gays to get into all the kinship mess of straights but by allowing all adults to live together and make children and gardens and homesteads and art and science and kites and lifelong alliances.

"My family" would then refer to the people who raised you and taught you and loved you. Family would not be those who gave birth to you as a way to hold on to their names and property, but those who elected to take on your care. Family, finally, not those who inherit you but those who select you.

Anne Reminiscing About Herself and Shelby

I remember the woods—when I was small, before I outgrew the circle of my mother's arms. It seems to me in memory that my life was quietly idyllic. There was room to play, the whole neighborhood to wander around in until dark and sometimes after, and what seems like now an incredible amount of free time to dream, to make up stories, to paint, to do whatever I liked. And my mother was always there, in the background, as a constant security figure.

I don't remember my father at all until I was 8. Before then, I know he lived with us. What values *do* we want to bring forward from the past, and where are we going in the future? To explore these questions, I convened my own three-generation panel: my mother, my daughter, and myself. My grandmother was doubtless with us in spirit. In the ensuing conversation, my mother remembers the family she grew up in and the family she raised. I do the same. My daughter comments on us both, and shares her own confident picture of the family she will one day create. My mother is Shelby (born Evelyn Shelty Reed, now Shelby Hearon), and she is 65; I am Anne (born Anne Shelby Hearon, now Anne Hearon Rambo), and I am 40; and my daughter is Rachel (Rachel Shelby Rambo), almost seven years old.

My mother grew up during the Depression in a town of 2,000 people in western Kentucky. My two grandfathers lived at opposite ends of Main Street and did not speak to each other. One was a mining engineer with two degrees; the other owned the mine. Years later, my father, a mining engineer who liked to call himself a geophysicist, returned with my mother and me during World War II to the same town, Marion, Kentucky.

My earliest impression of families, in the 1930s and 1940s, was that they came in two varieties: inclusive, at one end of Main Street, and exclusive, at the other end. My daddy and his six brothers and sisters and their spouses all returned to the old homestead during the Depression, university degrees in hand, to run a hamburger stand where the road from Paducah curved into town. It was called the Green Frog, with the motto, "We hop to serve." They offered a hamburger and a glass of milk for a nickel. Any jobless transients could get leftovers for yard work.

My mother used her college knowledge of nutrition to feed me on dandelion greens and boiled eggs, cheap and healthy. My aunts and uncles claimed various contributions to my upbringing: one claims to have helped raise me but I always remember him as "at the office," a place I confused with the continent of Africa.

My grandmother once pointed this very large continent out to me, on the globe. I thought that was where all the daddies went during the day, returning only at night to sleep and refuel.

When I was 8, the Girl Scouts had a father-daughter banquet, and one of my uncles showed up in place of my father. I remember we played Hangman all evening and discovered we both liked words. From then on he became someone whose attention I sought and valued, but very much as a visitor, an emissary from another world.

In this respect, I was no different from my peers. Male and female alike, we lived in a world of women. Our mommies were women, our teachers were women, the only grown-ups we saw were women. The few exceptions were men such as Mr. Postman and Mr. Doctor. If they were not actually made of cardboard, like the ones on the preschool bulletin board, they might as well have been. The mommies were real and solid and always there, and they hugged you, fed you, and scolded you, whether they were your own or a neighbor child's.

We lived in a neighborhood with many young children, and any doorbell you rang would produce someone's mommy, wiping her hands on her apron, ready to take charge. The daddies would be "at the office." This seemed to me fitting, in the natural order of things.

The house where we lived backed up to still undeveloped land, and my memories of that time are mixed up with the smell of cedar and mountain laurel, and the gamier aroma of the raccoons and possums who came to steal cat food at our back door on summer nights. They were always mommies, too. Only the mothers, gnawed at by the babies growing inside them or squeaking alongside, were brave enough to scavenge at the very door of the humans.

It seemed to me that "family" meant that mother-child bond, especially the mother-daughter bond. I was as at home in the house of my mother's mother as I was in my own house, and as safely rooted in both places as the tiny possum babies, clinging to their mother's fur. Of course, this was how it should be and always had been, small things played in the sun and burrowed snugly up close to their mothers for safety and sleep.

Somewhere in my elementary school years, it began to occur to me that there was a larger, alien outside world, where the men lived. In this world the rules were all different. I liked that world, too. It was mixed up with the sights and smells of downtown, of cars, of "the office," where I now sometimes got to venture, on state occasions.

But it was confusing to me that the rules were all so different. In the raccoon and mountain laurel world of the mothers, it was good to be smart, to ask a lot of questions. Underneath fluorescent lights, meeting your father's law partners, it seemed to be of more importance to be pretty and have nice manners, generally defined as not asking a lot of questions. At home, my mother's word was law—to question her authority would have seemed ludicrous to me. But at the office, my strong, powerful mother turned into someone timorously asking a secretary if this was a good time.

The secretaries themselves were like sentries between the two worlds, guarding the mysterious secrets of the male environs. I hated them on sight; in my dreams, they turned into snarling monsters with high-heeled shoes, keeping me away from my father and his world.

I wanted to go live in my father's world; on the other hand, I wanted to stay at home in my mother's world forever. I wanted to grow up muddy and wild like a baby possum; on the other hand, I longed to wear pearls and gloves and have the wife of the senior partner in my father's law firm marvel at my precociously ladylike behavior. (Instead, as I recall, she manifested some vague difficulty telling me apart from my brother, grubby and inseparable as we were.)

I didn't know what I wanted, but I knew I felt the chasm between the two worlds as a personal grief. I remember tromping through the neighborhood at dusk, vowing with each step that when I grew up, I would figure all this out, and make the two worlds come together, set up a baby possum sanctuary downtown, banish all the secretaries, give all the mommies big shiny cars of their own. (The concept that mommies could employ secretaries themselves would have been far too alien for me to fathom.)

Later on, I saw my mother become visible to the outside world as the writer she is. When I was 12, her first novel was published. To me, she was the same mother I had always known, the same person, scribbling away on the same yellow legal pad; I believe she was also the same person to herself. But in the whole social context, everything began to change with the external validation of her publishers. Five novels later, when I was 19, no one could see her any more as the Junior League president, the wife and mother. She had come too sharply into focus as an individual to fit in that time and place.

When I was 20, my parents divorced. Noticing my mother be seen as a professional brought home to me how invisible she had been before, how constrained she must have been when the world was seeing her as a suburban housewife. I began to worry that she had in some sense sold herself, and who knew at what cost, to give my brother and me our safe, mother-enclosed childhood.

ANNE TODAY

Anne Continues: So at first, when I had my daughter, I was going to do and be everything. I was going to show her how to combine those worlds. By the time she came to me, I had already been working as a family therapist for 12 years. I had a real office and a title and everything. That I could love and mother her I had no doubt. After her breech presentation and a difficult labor, which would unquestionably have killed at least one of us back in rural Kentucky (my grandmother had good intuition), I felt invincible. I felt like I had reached into death and pulled out this slippery, wriggling, new life. (Of course, the big shot of morphine they gave me could have had something to do with my euphoria.) "We will do everything," I promised her, "We will have it all, together." This feeling of invincibility sustained me through her earliest years. When my husband, her father, decided he had not yet found himself and that he could explore better without us, I let him go, not wholly without reproach, but with enough civility that we are frequently introduced as "the world's most civilized divorced couple." I welcomed his visits with her, and their growing bond, but I had no qualms about being the one in the center of her world. I took her to work with me; I took my work home to her. I even brought her into therapy sessions a few times when my other arrangements fell through. ("Stop that," she firmly commanded a squabbling couple when she was 18 months old. "Make nice or go home." Although I had thought she was safely occupied with toys in a corner, I had to admit she was far more effective than I had been with them.)

Somewhere along the line, though, I got tired. I stopped worrying about selling out; I was only too anxious to find a buyer. It occurred to me that a steady diet of No-Doz and Diet Coke was not all that great for me; and that others might find it odd that my child invariably headed for the front door, car keys in hand, when she was hungry. "Us go buy food now, Mommy!" The possibility that there might be food already in our house, perhaps even in the kitchen, would have struck her as remote. Most of all, I worried when she saw a playmate of hers hug me, and admonished him, "Don't touch; no one but me touches my Mommy." It was all too true, that she had never seen me as the recipient of anyone's affection but hers. So I set about finding her a stepfather.

But in a certain sense, it was already too late. I found someone willing to provide her with the nice house in the suburbs, the pet dog, all the things I wanted for her. I felt he could provide me with the respectability and stability I would need to be a better mother, a mother who could take her through the judgmental world of elementary school and beyond. I was willing to make whatever compromises it took; I was ready to buy the pearls and gloves.

But Rachel and he could never adjust to each other. It turned out she actually liked our life before; she thought the suburbs were boring and missed our meals on the run. He demanded of her a respect and obedience she was not prepared to grant. At 6, she said to him coolly, "You do not understand the things that are most important." He slapped her, and I made the choice any mother possum would make. We were gone from there, and back on our own. How will all this work in the future? I think we are living the future now and I don't think anyone yet knows.

Rachel's Story as Told to Anne

Rachel's section of this chapter was dictated to her mother. Initially reluctant to contribute—"I don't want those graduate students saying I'm cute again"—she was eventually lured to our modern equivalent of the communal hearth, the food court at the nearby mall, and shamelessly plied with cinnamon sugar pretzels and lemonade until she agreed to let herself be tape-recorded. What follows is a verbatim transcript of her comments.

(*After a synopsis of Grandmother Shelby's childhood*) That sounds cool. I would like to have a hamburger stand. What is a depression? (*After a synopsis of mother Anne's childhood*) That sounds really weird. Are you sure that is right? Your mother didn't have an office at all? Where did you go when you didn't want to go to school or day camp? Who did your mom play with while you were at school? And how come the daddies had offices if the moms didn't? That doesn't make any sense. Besides, if your mom didn't have an office, how did she make money? Because you have to have a job to make money. Yes, I know you said your daddy gave her money, but daddies don't know what you really need to buy.

Mostly daddies buy you everything you want, unless they just read a book and it said not to and so they don't buy you hardly anything for awhile, but only your mom can tell the difference between, like, a toy that you just want and a toy that you really, really need to have because Shannon has had it for weeks already and everybody has it and you really *need* it. So moms obviously have to have their own money.

I think you must have gotten that part wrong. This is not more of your graduate students, is it? Why would people want to read about what is a family? What are they, babies? Everyone knows what a family is. Okay, if you want me to say, I will say, but everybody knows. A family is when you agree about the rules. Not the little rules, like brush your teeth and don't be fussy, because everybody is fussy sometimes, but the *big* rules, like don't be mean to hunchbacks. All of you agree about what's important. Like, people are most important, second, animals, third, music, last are things. Animals are really almost as important as people, because they are alive, too. And music is sort of alive. But things are way last. So, like, if you break a glass, it is not a big deal in my family. Yes, I know my daddy collects antiques, but I am teaching him about it is not so important if they get a little broken. My family is you [mom], me, my daddy, my two baby cats, my dog, my hamster that we haven't got yet, Grandmama Shelby, Granddaddy Bob that lives in Texas, my friend Ashley, my very best friend Elizabeth, your work friend that lets me play on his computer, your other work friend that has a real snake in her office and she let me name it, George that used to be my babysitter when I was a child and now he's in college, George's mom and stepdad that he is your boss at work, too. . . . This is taking too long to tell about everybody in my family and I need another pretzel.

Uncle Reed is in my family, all the way in my family—you know, Uncle Reed that used to be your brother when you were little. Even though he lives way far away in California, he owns all those restaurants and he took me to eat dim sum in Chinatown and never laughed at me, not once, not even when I dropped my chopsticks. He doesn't have any children or even a wife, so I am his child now, too, because we agree about let's eat interesting things and stay up late and talk. That duck that used to live next door to us, before the bad dog, not my dog, that other dog, ate him, is in my family, too. Not the boys next door that bought him at the pet store because they used to forget to feed him and they left his cage open and so the dog got him, and not that big bad dog, not ever, but that duck. That duck used to sit in my lap and eat crackers with me and we would agree about things. So that duck is in my family still, even though he's in heaven now, except for the part of him that the dog spit out, which I think used to be his beak. I saved that; it will be very cool for show and tell. What? I have to answer more questions? About when I get big, okay.

When I grow up, I will be a vet and fix sick ducks and turtles, or maybe save dangered species. I will live in a *big* house, with stairs, just like where we live now has stairs. I like stairs because then where you live is big enough for everyone to have their own places to read and play. It will be just like where we live now, because that is the best place, except even bigger. And maybe I'll get Disney wallpaper and Disney sheets and by that time probably you could buy whole Disney houses, where the walls make music for you. That would be cool. I will have all my friends living there and I will pick one of them—a boy one, maybe Ryan, *not* Vinnie, you have to pick a boy one and just one at a time that you like the best—to be my husband and make a baby with me.

I will have a girl baby and three or four brothers for her. When I am at my office, she can come, too, or my husband will watch her. It would be okay for him to get a job, too, because she could come Xerox at his office, or if she wanted to stay home, you could watch her, Mom. You will be old then but I will let you watch her. And my house will have cats and dogs and hamsters and horses and ducks and turtles. It will be so fun. I can hardly wait.

But it is still a long time until I get big. You have to be in school forever first, I think. When I grow up, I want to be just like you, Mom. Now buy me another pretzel, I talked a lot already.

Anne Reflects

After I finished transcribing this, I sat for a long time in my office, thinking. I thought of my mother and my daughter, so much alike in their embrace of life. I lack their courage; but in its place, I have a compelling and urgent desire to protect them both from whatever might cloud their bright spirits.

I sat in the twilight and thought about them, and all the people I love and can't always protect. As it grew darker outside, I heard a scraping noise downstairs, then a thud. My office is on my university's east campus and backs up to the edge of a vacant lot, thick with pine trees. I stole downstairs to surprise the intruder; it was a raccoon, coming in from the thicket near the pine trees to scavenge in the dumpster. Her four hungry babies rolled in the garbage as she backed up and prepared to face me down, ready to snarl and bite if need be, but too tired to look forward to the battle. Instead, I coaxed her to my side with bits of a granola bar and finally she laid her little paw in my hand, while snuffling for more crumbs. I took this as a good omen for the future of our families, hers and mine both.

As the woods recede, the dangers increase, and we mothers will have to get braver. But sometimes also, even though we cannot yet see very clearly in the changing light, we surprise ourselves and come close enough to trust in ourselves.

References

Glennon, L. (1996). Celebrating 70 years of the American family. *Parents*, 71(8): 49–113.

Index